Management of Type 2 Diabetes: Current Insights and Future Directions

Management of Type 2 Diabetes: Current Insights and Future Directions

Editors

Andrej Belančić
Sanja Klobučar
Dario Rahelić

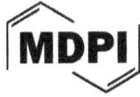

Basel • Beijing • Wuhan • Barcelona • Belgrade • Novi Sad • Cluj • Manchester

Editors

Andrej Belančić
Clinical Hospital Centre Rijeka
Rijeka
Croatia

Sanja Klobučar
Clinical Hospital Centre Rijeka
Rijeka
Croatia

Dario Rahelić
Merkur University Hospital
Zagreb
Croatia

Editorial Office
MDPI
St. Alban-Anlage 66
4052 Basel, Switzerland

This is a reprint of articles from the Special Issue published online in the open access journal *Diabetology* (ISSN 2673-4540) (available at: https://www.mdpi.com/journal/diabetology/special_issues/F84Y056927).

For citation purposes, cite each article independently as indicated on the article page online and as indicated below:

Lastname, A.A.; Lastname, B.B. Article Title. *Journal Name* **Year**, *Volume Number*, Page Range.

ISBN 978-3-7258-0647-8 (Hbk)
ISBN 978-3-7258-0648-5 (PDF)
doi.org/10.3390/books978-3-7258-0648-5

© 2024 by the authors. Articles in this book are Open Access and distributed under the Creative Commons Attribution (CC BY) license. The book as a whole is distributed by MDPI under the terms and conditions of the Creative Commons Attribution-NonCommercial-NoDerivs (CC BY-NC-ND) license.

Contents

Andrej Belančić, Sanja Klobučar and Dario Rahelić
Current Obstacles (With Solutions) in Type 2 Diabetes Management, Alongside Future Directions
Reprinted from: *Diabetology* 2023, 4, 31, doi:10.3390/diabetology4030031 1

Timothy J. Renier, Htun Ja Mai, Zheshi Zheng, Mary Ellen Vajravelu, Emily Hirschfeld, Diane Gilbert-Diamond, et al.
Utilizing the Glucose and Insulin Response Shape of an Oral Glucose Tolerance Test to Predict Dysglycemia in Children with Overweight and Obesity, Ages 8–18 Years
Reprinted from: *Diabetology* 2024, 5, 8, doi:10.3390/diabetology5010008 4

Anwar Althubyani, Clarice Tang, Jency Thomas and Sabrina Gupta
Evaluating the Use of Web-Based Technologies for Self-Management among Arabic-Speaking Immigrants Living with Type 2 Diabetes Mellitus: A Cross-Sectional Study in Saudi Arabia
Reprinted from: *Diabetology* 2024, 5, 7, doi:10.3390/diabetology5010007 18

Simon Lebech Cichosz, Clara Bender and Ole Hejlesen
A Comparative Analysis of Machine Learning Models for the Detection of Undiagnosed Diabetes Patients
Reprinted from: *Diabetology* 2024, 5, 1, doi:10.3390/diabetology5010001 29

Musawenkosi Ndlovu, Phiwayinkosi V. Dludla, Ndivhuwo Muvhulawa, Yonela Ntamo, Asanda Mayeye, Nomahlubi Luphondo, et al.
Global Trends in Risk Factors and Therapeutic Interventions for People with Diabetes and Cardiovascular Disease: Results from the WHO International Clinical Trials Registry Platform
Reprinted from: *Diabetology* 2023, 4, 50, doi:10.3390/diabetology4040050 40

Vilma Kolarić, Valentina Rahelić and Zrinka Šakić
The Quality of Life of Caregivers of People with Type 2 Diabetes Estimated Using the WHOQOL-BREF Questionnaire
Reprinted from: *Diabetology* 2023, 4, 37, doi:10.3390/diabetology4040037 54

Marco Mancuso, Rocco Bulzomì, Marco Mannisi, Francesco Martelli and Claudia Giacomozzi
3D-Printed Insoles for People with Type 2 Diabetes: An Italian, Ambulatory Case Report on the Innovative Care Model
Reprinted from: *Diabetology* 2023, 4, 29, doi:10.3390/diabetology4030029 64

Mariza Brandão Palma, Elisa Paolin, Ismaela Maria Ferreira de Melo, Francisco De Assis Leite Souza, Álvaro Aguiar Coelho Teixeira, Leucio Duarte Vieira, et al.
Biological Evidence of Improved Wound Healing Using Autologous Micrografts in a Diabetic Animal Model
Reprinted from: *Diabetology* 2023, 4, 26, doi:10.3390/diabetology4030026 82

Dominik Strikić, Andro Vujević, Dražen Perica, Dunja Leskovar, Kristina Paponja, Ivan Pećin, et al.
Importance of Dyslipidaemia Treatment in Individuals with Type 2 Diabetes Mellitus—A Narrative Review
Reprinted from: *Diabetology* 2023, 4, 48, doi:10.3390/diabetology4040048 101

Bright Test and Jay H. Shubrook
Prevention of Type 2 Diabetes: The Role of Intermittent Fasting
Reprinted from: *Diabetology* 2023, 4, 44, doi:10.3390/diabetology4040044 116

Filip Mustač, Tin Galijašević, Eva Podolski, Andrej Belančić, Martina Matovinović and Darko Marčinko
Recent Advances in Psychotherapeutic Treatment and Understanding of Alexithymia in Patients with Obesity and Diabetes Mellitus Type 2
Reprinted from: *Diabetology* **2023**, *4*, 41, doi:10.3390/diabetology4040041 . . . . **128**

Nikol Georgieva, Viktor Tenev, Maria Kamusheva and Guenka Petrova
Diabetes Mellitus—Digital Solutions to Improve Medication Adherence: Scoping Review
Reprinted from: *Diabetology* **2023**, *4*, 40, doi:10.3390/diabetology4040040 . . . . **137**

Erik M. Donker, Andrej Belančić, Joost D. Piët, Dinko Vitezić, Jelle Tichelaar and on behalf of the Clinical Pharmacology and Therapeutics Teach the Teacher (CP4T) Program and the Early Career Pharmacologists of the European Association for Clinical Pharmacology and Therapeutics (EACPT)
Educating Medical Students on How to Prescribe Anti-Hyperglycaemic Drugs: A Practical Guide
Reprinted from: *Diabetology* **2023**, *4*, 43, doi:10.3390/diabetology4040043 . . . . **153**

Elvira Meni Maria Gkrinia, Andrea Katrin Faour, Andrej Belančić, Jacques Bazile, Emma Marland and Dinko Vitezić
A Systematic Review of Economic Evaluations of Insulin for the Management of Type 2 Diabetes
Reprinted from: *Diabetology* **2023**, *4*, 38, doi:10.3390/diabetology4040038 . . . . **161**

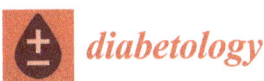

Editorial

Current Obstacles (With Solutions) in Type 2 Diabetes Management, Alongside Future Directions

Andrej Belančić [1,2,*,†], Sanja Klobučar [3,4,†] and Dario Rahelić [5,6,7,†]

1. Department of Clinical Pharmacology, Clinical Hospital Centre Rijeka, Krešimirova 42, 51000 Rijeka, Croatia
2. Department of Basic and Clinical Pharmacology with Toxicology, Faculty of Medicine, University of Rijeka, Braće Branchetta 20, 51000 Rijeka, Croatia
3. Department of Internal Medicine, Division of Endocrinology, Diabetes and Metabolic Diseases, Clinical Hospital Centre Rijeka, Krešimirova 42, 51000 Rijeka, Croatia; sanja.klobucarm@gmail.com
4. Department of Internal Medicine, Faculty of Medicine, University of Rijeka, Braće Branchetta 20, 51000 Rijeka, Croatia
5. Vuk Vrhovac University Clinic for Diabetes, Endocrinology and Metabolic Diseases, Merkur University Hospital, 10000 Zagreb, Croatia; dario.rahelic@gmail.com
6. School of Medicine, Catholic University of Croatia, 10000 Zagreb, Croatia
7. School of Medicine, J.J. Strossmayer University of Osijek, 31000 Osijek, Croatia
* Correspondence: a.belancic93@gmail.com or andrej.belancic@uniri.hr
† These authors contributed equally to this work.

Citation: Belančić, A.; Klobučar, S.; Rahelić, D. Current Obstacles (With Solutions) in Type 2 Diabetes Management, Alongside Future Directions. *Diabetology* 2023, 4, 376–378. https://doi.org/10.3390/diabetology4030031

Received: 28 August 2023
Accepted: 30 August 2023
Published: 5 September 2023

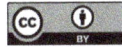

Copyright: © 2023 by the authors. Licensee MDPI, Basel, Switzerland. This article is an open access article distributed under the terms and conditions of the Creative Commons Attribution (CC BY) license (https://creativecommons.org/licenses/by/4.0/).

Dear Reader,

The world is grappling with increasing rates of obesity (a 650 million to 2 billion increase by 2035) and type 2 diabetes–T2D (a 500 million to 1.3 billion increase by 2050), which have therefore been positioned among the highest public health and scientific priorities, demanding a prompt and thorough multidisciplinary approach [1–4]. Large diabetes-associated costs are a problem in low-, middle-, and high-income nations alike, and hence it is urgently (and continuously) necessary to consider and discuss (re)making policies, (re)allocating medical resources, (re)editing clinical guidelines, and thus balancing healthcare expenditures well while simultaneously improving patients' T2D care and quality-of-life determinants [5,6].

The authors of this Editorial will expand, in this manuscript, on their perspectives on current obstacles (with solutions) in T2D management, alongside future directions in the present setting. Bearing in mind the aforementioned epidemiological rates and the interconnection of the two diseases/'friends', it is clear that more force should be put into T2D prevention by optimizing lifestyle modifications and obesity prevention/treatment principles, as well as through timely diagnosis/early detection (before the development of complications/comorbidities) through structured regional/national screening programs. Another issue that should be taken into account is the individualization of therapeutic approaches (bearing in mind the effectiveness, risk of hypoglycemia, potential cardiometabolic and renal benefits, comorbidities, safety profile, and pharmacoeconomics) by delineating subgroups of type 2 diabetes that would benefit the most (e.g., phenotype-approach, precision medicine principles, etc.), as well as considering factors of medication adherence (e.g., education and digital solutions) and timing (e.g., a question on using metformin, GLP-1 RA and/or SGLT-2i in prediabetes) [7–14]. In addition to standard dietary and physical activity and pharmacological interventions, (co)management approaches such as metabolic surgery and gut microbiome modification/fecal transplantation may become more important in the years yet to come, and may even potentially help us as clinicians to achieve T2D remission (as an ultimate goal) in some of our patient candidates [15–17]. Increasing the accessibility of multidisciplinary health care teams in all settings/regions, diagnostics and glucose monitoring (e.g., the availability of CGMs for T2D patients), medications (reimbursement issues), and comprehensive diabetes education programs are definitely on a list of future directions/improvements needed [18–21]. What is more, both clinical- and science-wise, decision support and information systems (patient registers, systems to recall patients to the practice, templates for care plans and guidelines for health professionals) are areas in which thorough work also needs to be carried out [22].

Bearing in mind the aforementioned, the authors (editors) aimed at organizing the present Special Issue, "Management of type 2 diabetes—Current insights and future directions", within the Diabetology journal [23], which we see as an excellent platform to support an overview of current evidence and insights regarding novelties in the diabetology (co)management field (e.g., digital solutions to improve medication adherence, gut microbiome modifications, psychological and quality-of-life aspects, predictors of therapeutic success and therapy individualization principles, and pharmacoeconomic and reimbursement obstacles/solutions, as well as teachings on the pharmacological management of T2D and evidence-based medicine principles, etc.) that we are currently facing or that we will face soon.

As the field of diabetology is full of novelties, with numerous management and therapeutic innovations, we deliberately chose to discuss those that are currently improving or will improve today's management of the diseases mentioned. This is especially important since we all know that diabetology is a growing field with constant developments in innovations, so it is highly important to stay up to date with all the novelties. Thus, we hope that our Special Issue will draw the attention of readers, patients, students, scientists, clinicians, and policymakers, and ultimately result in an overall improvement in diabetes care/management quality.

Author Contributions: Conceptualization: A.B. and S.K.; Writing—Original Draft: A.B.; Preparation: A.B.; Writing—Review and Editing: A.B., S.K. and D.R. All authors have read and agreed to the published version of the manuscript.

Conflicts of Interest: A.B. is the secretary of the Croatian Society of Obesity of the Croatian Medical Association and has no conflicts of interest to declare; S.K. is the vice president of the Croatian Society for Diabetes and Metabolic Disorders of the Croatian Medical Association and the vice president of the Croatian Society for Obesity of the Croatian Medical Association. She serves as an Executive Committee member of the Croatian Endocrine Society. She has served as principal investigator or co-investigator in clinical trials of Eli Lilly, MSD, Novo Nordisk, and Sanofi Aventis. She has received honoraria for speaking or advisory board engagements and consulting fees from Abbott, AstraZeneca, Boehringer Ingelheim, Eli Lilly, Lifescan—Johnson & Johnson, Novartis, Novo Nordisk, MSD, Merck Sharp & Dohme, Mylan, Pliva, and Sanofi Aventis; D.R. is the director of the Vuk Vrhovac University Clinic for Diabetes, Endocrinology, and Metabolic Diseases at Merkur University Hospital, Zagreb, Croatia. He is the president of the Croatian Society for Diabetes and Metabolic Disorders of the Croatian Medical Association. He serves as an Executive Committee member of the Croatian Endocrine Society, Croatian Society for Obesity, and Croatian Society for Endocrine Oncology. He was a board member and secretary of IDF Europe, and the chair of the IDF Young Leaders in Diabetes (YLD) Program. He has served as an Executive Committee member of the Diabetes and Nutrition Study Group of the European Association for the Study of Diabetes (EASD), and currently he serves as an Executive Committee member of the Diabetes and Cardiovascular Disease Study Group of EASD. He has served as a principal investigator or co-investigator in clinical trials for AstraZeneca, Eli Lilly, MSD, Novo Nordisk, Sanofi Aventis, Solvay, and Trophos. He has received honoraria for speaking or advisory board engagements and consulting fees from Abbott, Amgen, AstraZeneca, Bauerfeund, Bayer, Boehringer Ingelheim, Eli Lilly, Lifescan—Johnson & Johnson, Krka, Novartis, Novo Nordisk, Medtronic, Merck, MSD, Mylan, Pfizer, Pliva, Roche, Salvus, Sanofi, and Takeda.

References

1. World Obesity Federation. World Obesity Atlas. 2023. Available online: https://www.worldobesity.org/resources/resource-library/world-obesity-atlas-2023 (accessed on 25 August 2023).
2. Štimac, D.; Klobučar Majanović, S.; Baretić, M.; Bekavc Bešlin, M.; Belančić, A.; Crnčević Orlić, Ž.; Đorđević, V.; Marčinko, D.; Miličić, D.; Mirošević, G.; et al. Hrvatske Smjernice za Liječenja Odraslih Osoba s Debeljinom. *Acta Med. Croat.* **2022**, *76*, 3–18. Available online: https://hrcak.srce.hr/285231 (accessed on 27 August 2023).

3. Ong, K.L.; Stafford, L.K.; McLaughlin, S.A.; Boyko, E.J.; Vollset, S.E.; Smith, A.E.; Dalton, B.E.; Duprey, J.; Cruz, J.A.; Hagins, H.; et al. Global, regional, and national burden of diabetes from 1990 to 2021, with projections of prevalence to 2050: A systematic analysis for the Global Burden of Disease Study 2021. *Lancet* **2023**, *402*, 203–234. [CrossRef] [PubMed]
4. Sun, H.; Saeedi, P.; Karuranga, S.; Pinkepank, M.; Ogurtsova, K.; Duncan, B.B.; Stein, C.; Basit, A.; Chan, J.C.N.; Mbanya, J.C.; et al. IDF Diabetes Atlas: Global, regional and country-level diabetes prevalence estimates for 2021 and projections for 2045. *Diabetes Res. Clin. Pract.* **2022**, *183*, 109119. [CrossRef]
5. Trikkalinou, A.; Papazafiropoulou, A.K.; Melidonis, A. Type 2 diabetes and quality of life. *World J. Diabetes* **2017**, *8*, 120–129. [CrossRef]
6. Bommer, C.; Heesemann, E.; Sagalova, V.; Manne-Goehler, J.; Atun, R.; Bärnighausen, T.; Vollmer, S. The global economic burden of diabetes in adults aged 20-79 years: A cost-of-illness study. *Lancet Diabetes Endocrinol.* **2017**, *5*, 423–430. [CrossRef] [PubMed]
7. Davies, M.J.; Aroda, V.R.; Collins, B.S.; Gabbay, R.A.; Green, J.; Maruthur, N.M.; Rosas, S.E.; Del Prato, S.; Mathieu, C.; Mingrone, G.; et al. Management of Hyperglycemia in Type 2 Diabetes, 2022. A Consensus Report by the American Diabetes Association (ADA) and the European Association for the Study of Diabetes (EASD). *Diabetes Care* **2022**, *45*, 2753–2786. [CrossRef]
8. Evans, M.; Engberg, S.; Faurby, M.; Fernandes, J.D.D.R.; Hudson, P.; Polonsky, W. Adherence to and persistence with antidiabetic medications and associations with clinical and economic outcomes in people with type 2 diabetes mellitus: A systematic literature review. *Diabetes Obes. Metab.* **2022**, *24*, 377–390. [CrossRef]
9. Kardas, P.; Ágh, T.; Dima, A.; Goetzinger, C.; Potočnjak, I.; Wettermark, B.; van Boven, J.F.M. Half a Century of Fragmented Research on Deviations from Advised Therapies: Is This a Good Time to Call for Multidisciplinary Medication Adherence Research Centres of Excellence. *Pharmaceutics* **2023**, *15*, 933. [CrossRef]
10. van Boven, J.F.M.; Fonseca, J.A. Editorial: Digital Tools to Measure and Promote Medication Adherence. *Front. Med. Technol.* **2021**, *3*, 751976. [CrossRef]
11. Yu, O.H.Y.; Shin, J.Y. Treating type 2 diabetes: Moving towards precision medicine. *Lancet Digit. Health* **2022**, *4*, e851–e852. [CrossRef]
12. Dennis, J.M. Precision Medicine in Type 2 Diabetes: Using Individualized Prediction Models to Optimize Selection of Treatment. *Diabetes* **2020**, *69*, 2075–2085. [CrossRef]
13. Chung, W.K.; Erion, K.; Florez, J.C.; Hattersley, A.T.; Hivert, M.F.; Lee, C.G.; McCarthy, M.I.; Nolan, J.J.; Norris, J.M.; Pearson, E.R.; et al. Precision Medicine in Diabetes: A Consensus Report from the American Diabetes Association (ADA) and the European Association for the Study of Diabetes (EASD). *Diabetes Care* **2020**, *43*, 1617–1635. [CrossRef] [PubMed]
14. Pilla, S.J.; Mathioudakis, N.N.; Maruthur, N.M. Trialing precision medicine for type 2 diabetes. *Nat. Med.* **2023**, *29*, 309–310. [CrossRef] [PubMed]
15. Su, L.; Hong, Z.; Zhou, T.; Jian, Y.; Xu, M.; Zhang, X.; Zhu, X.; Wang, J. Health improvements of type 2 diabetic patients through diet and diet plus fecal microbiota transplantation. *Sci. Rep.* **2022**, *12*, 1152. [CrossRef]
16. Hou, K.; Zhang, S.; Wu, Z.; Zhu, D.; Chen, F.; Lei, Z.N.; Liu, W.; Xiao, C.; Chen, Z.S. Reconstruction of intestinal microecology of type 2 diabetes by fecal microbiota transplantation: Why and how. *Bosn. J. Basic Med. Sci.* **2022**, *22*, 315–325. [CrossRef]
17. Zhou, X.; Zeng, C. Diabetes remission of bariatric surgery and nonsurgical treatments in type 2 diabetes patients who failure to meet the criteria for surgery: A systematic review and meta-analysis. *BMC Endocr. Disord.* **2023**, *23*, 46. [CrossRef]
18. Beck, R.W.; Riddlesworth, T.D.; Ruedy, K.; Ahmann, A.; Haller, S.; Kruger, D.; McGill, J.B.; Polonsky, W.; Price, D.; Aronoff, S.; et al. Continuous Glucose Monitoring Versus Usual Care in Patients with Type 2 Diabetes Receiving Multiple Daily Insulin Injections: A Randomized Trial. *Ann. Intern. Med.* **2017**, *167*, 365–374. [CrossRef]
19. Martens, T.; Beck, R.W.; Bailey, R.; Ruedy, K.J.; Calhoun, P.; Peters, A.L.; Pop-Busui, R.; Philis-Tsimikas, A.; Bao, S.; Umpierrez, G.; et al. Effect of Continuous Glucose Monitoring on Glycemic Control in Patients With Type 2 Diabetes Treated With Basal Insulin: A Randomized Clinical Trial. *JAMA* **2021**, *325*, 2262–2272. [CrossRef]
20. Pozniak, A.; Olinger, L.; Shier, V. Physicians' perceptions of reimbursement as a barrier to comprehensive diabetes care. *Am. Health Drug Benefits* **2010**, *3*, 31–40.
21. Fralick, M.; Jenkins, A.J.; Khunti, K.; Mbanya, J.C.; Mohan, V.; Schmidt, M.I. Global accessibility of therapeutics for diabetes mellitus. *Nat. Rev. Endocrinol.* **2022**, *18*, 199–204. [CrossRef]
22. Leonard, C.E.; Flory, J.H.; Likić, R.; Ogunleye, O.O.; Wei, L.; Wong, I. Spotlight commentary: A role for real-world evidence to inform the clinical care of patients with diabetes mellitus. *Br. J. Clin. Pharmacol.* **2021**, *87*, 4549–4551. [CrossRef] [PubMed]
23. Diabetology Journal. Available online: https://www.mdpi.com/journal/diabetology (accessed on 25 August 2023).

Disclaimer/Publisher's Note: The statements, opinions and data contained in all publications are solely those of the individual author(s) and contributor(s) and not of MDPI and/or the editor(s). MDPI and/or the editor(s) disclaim responsibility for any injury to people or property resulting from any ideas, methods, instructions or products referred to in the content.

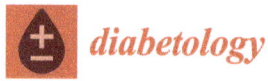

Article

Utilizing the Glucose and Insulin Response Shape of an Oral Glucose Tolerance Test to Predict Dysglycemia in Children with Overweight and Obesity, Ages 8–18 Years

Timothy J. Renier [1], Htun Ja Mai [1], Zheshi Zheng [2], Mary Ellen Vajravelu [3], Emily Hirschfeld [4], Diane Gilbert-Diamond [1,5,6], Joyce M. Lee [4] and Jennifer L. Meijer [1,5,6,7,*]

1. Department of Epidemiology, Geisel School of Medicine at Dartmouth, Hanover, NH 03755, USA; timothy.j.renier.gr@dartmouth.edu (T.J.R.); htun.ja.mai@dartmouth.edu (H.J.M.); diane.gilbert-diamond@dartmouth.edu (D.G.-D.)
2. Department of Biostatistics, School of Public Health, University of Michigan, Ann Arbor, MI 48109, USA; zszheng@umich.edu
3. Division of Pediatric Endocrinology, Diabetes and Metabolism, UPMC—Children's Hospital of Pittsburgh, Pittsburgh, PA 15224, USA; vajravelume@upmc.edu
4. Department of Pediatrics, Division of Pediatric Endocrinology, Susan B. Meister Child Health Evaluation and Research Center, University of Michigan, Ann Arbor, MI 48109, USA; ehirschf@med.umich.edu (E.H.); joyclee@med.umich.edu (J.M.L.)
5. Department of Medicine, Geisel School of Medicine at Dartmouth, Hanover, NH 03755, USA
6. Department of Pediatrics, Geisel School of Medicine at Dartmouth, Hanover, NH 03755, USA
7. Department of Medicine, Dartmouth-Hitchcock Medical Center, Lebanon, NH 03756, USA
* Correspondence: jennifer.l.meijer@dartmouth.edu

Abstract: Common dysglycemia measurements including fasting plasma glucose (FPG), oral glucose tolerance test (OGTT)-derived 2 h plasma glucose, and hemoglobin A1c (HbA1c) have limitations for children. Dynamic OGTT glucose and insulin responses may better reflect underlying physiology. This analysis assessed glucose and insulin curve shapes utilizing classifications—biphasic, monophasic, or monotonically increasing—and functional principal components (FPCs) to predict future dysglycemia. The prospective cohort included 671 participants with no previous diabetes diagnosis (BMI percentile ≥ 85th, 8–18 years old); 193 returned for follow-up (median 14.5 months). Blood was collected every 30 min during the 2 h OGTT. Functional data analysis was performed on curves summarizing glucose and insulin responses. FPCs described variation in curve height (FPC1), time of peak (FPC2), and oscillation (FPC3). At baseline, both glucose and insulin FPC1 were significantly correlated with BMI percentile (Spearman correlation r = 0.22 and 0.48), triglycerides (r = 0.30 and 0.39), and HbA1c (r = 0.25 and 0.17). In longitudinal logistic regression analyses, glucose and insulin FPCs predicted future dysglycemia (AUC = 0.80) better than shape classifications (AUC = 0.69), HbA1c (AUC = 0.72), or FPG (AUC = 0.50). Further research should evaluate the utility of FPCs to predict metabolic diseases.

Keywords: oral glucose tolerance test; insulin; glucose; curve shape; functional data analysis; pediatrics; hemoglobin A1C; longitudinal prediction; prediabetes

Citation: Renier, T.J.; Mai, H.J.; Zheng, Z.; Vajravelu, M.E.; Hirschfeld, E.; Gilbert-Diamond, D.; Lee, J.M.; Meijer, J.L. Utilizing the Glucose and Insulin Response Shape of an Oral Glucose Tolerance Test to Predict Dysglycemia in Children with Overweight and Obesity, Ages 8–18 Years. *Diabetology* **2024**, *5*, 96–109. https://doi.org/10.3390/diabetology5010008

Academic Editors: Andrej Belančić, Sanja Klobučar and Dario Rahelić

Received: 5 December 2023
Revised: 6 February 2024
Accepted: 23 February 2024
Published: 1 March 2024

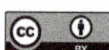

Copyright: © 2024 by the authors. Licensee MDPI, Basel, Switzerland. This article is an open access article distributed under the terms and conditions of the Creative Commons Attribution (CC BY) license (https://creativecommons.org/licenses/by/4.0/).

1. Introduction

The incidence of youth-onset type 2 diabetes (T2D) continues to increase by 4.8% each year, related to a high and increasing prevalence of pediatric obesity [1–3]. In the United States, diabetes care is among the highest health care expenditures, increasing by 26% from 2012 to 2017, further emphasizing the need for early detection of risk and prevention in youth [4]. The American Diabetes Association (ADA) recommends T2D screening using fasting plasma glucose (FPG), hemoglobin A1c (HbA1c), or a 2 h plasma glucose (2hrPG) during an oral glucose tolerance test (OGTT) [5,6]. During an OGTT, individuals consume a 75 g bolus of glucose after an overnight fast. The 2 h plasma glucose (2hrPG) level is indicative of normal glycemia, prediabetes, or T2D, with higher levels suggesting diminished beta cell response and/or decreased insulin sensitivity. However, cut-offs for FPG, HbA1c, and 2hrPG are crude estimates of dysglycemia [7], with uncertain implications for pediatric patients [8]. Recent studies have explored derived variables from insulin and glucose responses in an OGTT, including the sum of insulin across an OGTT [9] and one hour plasma glucose [9,10], which may better predict impaired glucose metabolism than HbA1c. Classifying the temporal response of glucose and insulin to an OGTT may provide a deeper understanding of metabolic risk than a single glucose or HbA1c measurement.

The pattern of glucose response to an OGTT reflects the ability of ß-cells to secrete insulin and the sensitivity of cells to lower glucose levels [11]. A study by Tschritter et al. [12] defined the shape of glucose in response to an OGTT as monophasic (one-peak of glucose), biphasic (second phasic insulin secretion), and incessant increase (continual rise of glucose, henceforth "monotonically increasing") by collecting blood samples at baseline (0 min) and 30, 60, 90, and 120 min post-glucose bolus. In youth with obesity, a monotonically increasing glucose response is associated with the fastest deterioration of ß-cell function [13]. Furthermore, a monophasic glucose response is related to diminished ß-cell function, lower insulin sensitivity, and increased risk of metabolic syndrome in adults [14]. In a sample of adolescents with obesity, a biphasic glucose response was associated with the highest insulin sensitivity and lowest area under an OGTT insulin curve [15]. Another study found that adolescents with obesity who had a monophasic glucose response had lower insulin sensitivity and impaired β-cell function compared to those with a biphasic response, despite similar FPG and 2hrPG in the two groups [16]. Shape classifications are reasonably stable; a study of adults without a history of diabetes found that 59% maintained the same shape over three years, with either newly developing or maintaining a previous monophasic shape being associated with impaired glucose metabolism [17]. However, manually classifying the shape of glucose response to an OGTT is a relatively crude method of summarizing glucose response profiles, failing to account for multiple other ways in which profiles differ, such as the timing of the response peak and overall height [18,19].

Computational methods have been developed to systematically classify a curve shape, creating scores to optimally explain how participants vary in a study population. For instance, Frøslie et al. [20] used functional data analysis (FDA) to generate three functional principal components (FPCs) to classify the glycemic response to an OGTT among pregnant women in the first trimester ($n = 974$). They observed that the FPCs explained over 99% of variation in fitted OGTT curves, with the second FPC more accurately predicting gestational diabetes in the third trimester compared to traditional dysglycemia measures [20]. FDA methods have further been used to classify longitudinal trends of glucose, insulin, and blood pressure throughout pregnancy, identifying phenotypes through FDA that were associated with pregnancy-related outcomes [21]. Furthermore, FDA methods have been explored by Gecili et al. [22] for quantifying data from continuous glucose monitoring (CGM) in children with type 1 diabetes. They derived FPCs using data from CGMs to generate accurate real-time predictions of glycemic excursions. There have been no studies to our knowledge that have used computational FDA methods to classify the OGTT glucose and insulin response curve shape in youth without diabetes. Furthermore, there have been no studies that have compared computational methods with manual shape classifications and ADA classifications of dysglycemia to predict future dysglycemia in this population. The objectives of these analyses in youth with overweight and obesity were to evaluate cross-sectional associations of manual estimates of glucose response shape (monophasic, biphasic, and monotonically increasing) and a quantitative FDA method with markers of metabolic health, and to evaluate the longitudinal associations between these OGTT response characteristics and future dysglycemia.

2. Materials and Methods

2.1. Research Design

Participants in this analysis were a subset of 8–18-year-olds from a prospective cohort study designed to assess the longitudinal performance of tests for dysglycemia in children [23–26]. Participants were recruited through flyers, web postings, mailings, and research assistants at primary care and pediatric specialty clinics in southeast Michigan (2007–2019). Among previously documented exclusion criteria [24], participants were excluded if they had known diabetes or used medications known to affect the metabolism of glucose (oral steroids, metformin, insulin). For this analysis, all participants had overweight or obesity at baseline, defined by $\geq$85th percentile BMI from CDC 2000 growth charts [27]. Written informed consent was obtained from the parent/guardian for all participants. Written assent was obtained from participants $\geq$ 10 years old and verbal assent was obtained from participants < 10 years old. This study was approved by the University of Michigan Institutional Review Board (HUM#00006955).

Participants attended study visits at the Michigan Clinical Research Unit, where a medical history, vital signs, anthropometrics, and laboratory evaluation were performed. Our cohort represents a "convenience sample" with variations in the number of visits completed due to several grant mechanisms supporting different study aims. All participants attended an initial study visit, "Visit 1", as previously documented and henceforth coined "baseline" [24]. All participants arrived at Visit 1 after an overnight fast (12 h). At Visit 1, participants underwent a 2 h OGTT with plasma glucose and insulin measurements; lab testing for HbA1c and lipids; blood pressure (measured twice with a pediatric cuff); measurement of height (twice), weight (twice, wearing a hospital gown), and body mass index (BMI) percentile per CDC growth curves [28]; waist circumference; and provided demographic information. Of 679 total participants with Visit 1 data, we excluded participants with incomplete OGTT glucose and insulin measurements (n = 7) and a missing HbA1c lab (n = 1), for a total cross-sectional analysis sample of N = 671.

Among this sample, a subset of the participants (n = 333) were recruited for longitudinal visits, supported by R01HD074559. This subset of participants completed two baseline OGTTs—Visit 1 (after an overnight fast) and Visit 2 (random fasted or fed state)—and two follow-up fasted OGTTs—Visit 3 and Visit 4—that were <4 weeks apart to assess for reproducibility in OGTT response. More details regarding the cohort structure are represented by Vajravelu et al. [24]. For this analysis, the longitudinal sample consisted of participants who returned for a follow-up OGTT after an overnight fast (n = 218), "Visit 3", as previously described and henceforth coined "follow-up" [24]. Those with <6 months between Visit 1 and Visit 3 were excluded (n = 25), for a total longitudinal analysis sample of N = 193.

2.2. The Oral Glucose Tolerance Test

2.2.1. OGTT Administration and Laboratory Parameters

An oral glucose load of 1.75 g per kg of body weight was administered up to a maximum of 75 g (Glucola, Fisherbrand, Waltham, MA, USA). Serial blood draws were performed at 30 min intervals for two hours and glucose homeostasis assays were conducted by the Michigan Diabetes Research Center (Ann Arbor, MI, USA). A Randox rX Daytona Chemistry Analyzer (Randox Laboratories Limited, Crumlin, UK) measured lipids (total cholesterol with the cholesterol enzymatic end point method, triglycerides with the GPO-PAP method, and HDL and LDL with the two step-direct method) and glucose with the glucose hexokinase method. A double-antibody radioimmunoassay was used to measure insulin. Both glucose and insulin were measured from plasma. Derived summary variables included FPG (0 min glucose), 2hrPG (120 min glucose), and dysglycemia, defined as having FPG > 100 mg/dL or 2hrPG > 140 mg/dL. HbA1c was quantified with a Tosoh G7 HPLC Analyzer (Tosoh Biosciences Inc., San Francisco, CA, USA).

2.2.2. Manual OGTT Shape Classifications

Baseline OGTT profiles were manually classified as "biphasic," "monophasic," or "monotonically increasing" (previously also described as "incessant increase") using criteria previously described in published literature [13,15,29]. A "biphasic" profile was defined by a rise in glucose over time with a subsequent decrease of at least 4.5 mg/dL from the initial peak, and a subsequent second increase of at least 4.5 mg/dL (Figure 1). A "monophasic" profile was defined by a rise in blood glucose that reached a peak with a subsequent decrease of at least 4.5 mg/dL from the maximum and no further increase exceeding 4.5 mg/dL. A "monotonically increasing" profile was defined as increasing blood glucose over time without a drop of more than 4.5 mg/dL from the maximum. An OGTT profile shape was considered "inconclusive" if there was no rise in glucose from baseline by 60 min. Manual shape classifications were only applied to glucose responses, not to insulin.

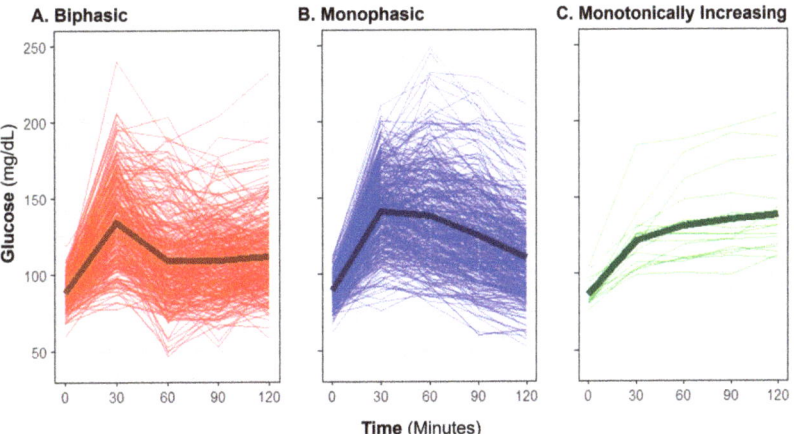

Figure 1. Observed oral glucose tolerance test biphasic, monophasic, and monotonically increasing glucose shape classifications. The plot displays profiles of glucose measurement for individuals (thin lines) and group means (bold lines) with each classification group: (**A**) biphasic, (**B**) monophasic, and (**C**) monotonically increasing.

2.2.3. OGTT Shape Classifications Using Functional Data Analysis (FDA)

The overall FDA procedure was previously described by Frøslie et al. [20]. Each participant's five measurements of glucose and insulin were described by smooth curves in time. Then, FDA was applied to summarize each participant's curve using a prefixed number of three principal component scores. The idea of FDA was to find the combination of basis functions that explain the most variance of the smooth curve and summarize them into the principal components. The implementation is briefly explained below.

The smooth curves were fitted with the *fda* package in R [30], using 7 basis functions and 5 measurements (knots). Thus, the glucose and insulin measurements could be viewed as a function of time, and formulized below:

$$glucose_i(t_j) = \sum_{k=1}^{7} \phi_k^{glucose}(t_j) c_{ik}^{glucose} + e_i^{glucose}(t_j), \; i = 1, \ldots, n; \; j = 1, \ldots, 5$$
$$insulin_i(t_j) = \sum_{k=1}^{7} \phi_k^{insulin}(t_j) c_{ik}^{insulin} + e_i^{insulin}(t_j), \; i = 1, \ldots, n; \; j = 1, \ldots, 5$$

(1)

where $t_1, \ldots, t_5$ were the five measurement time points, $\phi_k^{glucose}(\cdot)$, $\phi_k^{insulin}(\cdot)$ were the k-th basis function for glucose and insulin, $c_{ik}^{glucose}$, $c_{ik}^{insulin}$ were the coefficients to be estimated for k-th basis function of i-th participant, and $e_i^{glucose}(\cdot)$, $e_i^{insulin}(\cdot)$ were the measurement error terms. The above formula could be simplified by using matrix notation:

$$Glucose = \Phi^{glucose}C^{glucose} + E^{glucose}; \quad Insulin = \Phi^{insulin}C^{insulin} + E^{insulin} \qquad (2)$$

where $Glucose$, $Insulin$ were $5 \times n$ matrices of glucose and insulin measurements, $\Phi^{glucose}$, $\Phi^{insulin}$ were 5×7 matrices of basis functions taking value at the measurement time points, $C^{glucose}$, $C^{insulin}$ were $7 \times n$ matrices of coefficients to be estimated, and $E^{glucose}$, $E^{insulin}$ were the measurement error matrices. Following the estimation methods described by Frøslie et al. [20], $C^{glucose}$, $C^{insulin}$ could be estimated with a penalized least squares method:

$$\begin{aligned} C^{glucose} &= \underset{C}{\arg\min}(Glucose - \Phi^{glucose}C)^T(Glucose - \Phi^{glucose}C) + \lambda_1 C^T R_1 C \\ C^{insulin} &= \underset{C}{\arg\min}(Insulin - \Phi^{insulin}C)^T(Insulin - \Phi^{insulin}C) + \lambda_2 C^T R_2 C \end{aligned} \qquad (3)$$

where the penalty term included R_1, R_2 that summarized the curvature of the curves, λ_1, λ_2 were nuisance parameters that control the penalty, and the nuisance parameters were determined by cross-validation [20].

After obtaining the smoothed curve, we used functional principal component analysis to summarize each participant's curve into three scores. We fitted a series of FPC denoted as $\xi_k^{glucose}(\cdot)$, $\xi_k^{insulin}(\cdot)$ of the k-th component, such that they sequentially maximized the variance of the FPC scores $z_{ik}^{glucose} = \int \xi_k^{glucose}(t) glucose_i(t) dt$ and $z_{ik}^{insulin} = \int \xi_k^{insulin}(t) insulin_i(t) dt$ with constraints that $\int \xi_k^{glucose}(t)^2 dt = 1$, $\int \xi_k^{insulin}(t)^2 dt = 1$ and the glucose and insulin FPCs were orthogonal to each other separately. Following the choice made in Frøslie et al. [20], we chose to use the first three principal components for both glucose and insulin, and we found that the first three FPCs successfully explained over 99% of the variance for both glucose and insulin curves. We also standardized all three FPCs (mean = 0, standard deviation (SD) = 1) to enhance interpretability in statistical models.

2.3. Statistical Analysis

2.3.1. Cross-Sectional Analysis

The summary statistics of participant demographics with respect to age, sex, race, and ethnicity were presented for the cross-sectional and longitudinal subsets, separately. Differences in demographics and measures of glucose regulation at baseline among those with and without follow-up were assessed with a Wilcoxon rank sum test (continuous variables) [31] or Fisher's Exact Test (categorical variables) [32].

Classified by the three shaped glucose profiles "biphasic," "monophasic," or "monotonically increasing", participants' OGTT glucose profiles were plotted for the three subgroups. Classified by quartiles of the top three FPC scores, participants' OGTT glucose and insulin mean fitted curves were plotted and compared for the four sub-groups. The proportion of variance explained by the top three FPCs in glucose and insulin curves were calculated and reported. Using Spearman correlation coefficients, we also quantified the association of our classification measurements (manual shape classification and glucose/insulin FPC scores) with glucose and insulin measurements (at time point 0, 30, 60, 90 and 120 min), HbA1c, lipid labs, systolic and diastolic blood pressure, BMI percentile, and waist circumference. A Bonferroni correction was applied to adjust for multiple hypotheses in assessing numerous correlations ($p < 0.0003$, 171 comparisons). Differences in age, sex, race, ethnicity, and metabolic health parameters by manual OGTT shape classifications were assessed with Kruskal–Wallis' Test [31] or Fisher's Exact Test [32]. Linear regression evaluated associations between demographic variables with glucose and insulin FPC scores. To assess if associations between metabolic health parameters and FPCs were independent of demographic factors, we fit linear regression models for each FPC (dependent variable) by metabolic health parameters (independent variable), adjusting for demographic covariates.

2.3.2. Longitudinal Analysis

Differences in FPG, 2hrPG, HbA1c, and BMI percentile between baseline and follow-up visits were assessed with paired Wilcoxon signed rank tests [31]. The difference in the rate of dysglycemia was assessed with McNemar's test [32]. To assess the prediction ability of OGTT summary measures to predict future dysglycemia, a series of logistic regression models was used with dysglycemia at follow-up as the outcome variable and OGTT summary measures at baseline as predictors within the longitudinal subset. Seven different predictors or combinations of predictors were compared: FPG, 2hrPG, HbA1c, shape classifications, glucose FPCs, insulin FPCs, and glucose + insulin FPCs. Predictions for each participant's probability of dysglycemia at follow-up from each model were used to generate receiver–operator curves (ROC), and the area under the ROC (AUC) was used to compare the performance of the predictors using the *pROC* R package [33]. All data analysis was conducted using the R Language for Statistical Computing [34].

3. Results

3.1. Sample Characteristics

Among the total cross-sectional analysis sample (N = 671), median age was 13.5 years (8.13 to 18.0 years), and 362 participants (53.9%) were female (Table 1). The sample was 42.5% non-white. Median BMI was at the 97th percentile, classified as having obesity.

Table 1. Participant Characteristics at Baseline.

	Overall (N = 671) [1]
Study Visits Completed	
Baseline and Follow-Up	193 (28.8%)
Baseline Only	478 (71.2%)
Age (Years)	13.5 [11.5, 15.4]
Sex	
Female	362 (53.9%)
Male	309 (46.1%)
Race	
White	386 (57.5%)
Black or African American	212 (31.6%)
Other/Multiracial	52 (7.8%)
Unknown/Not Reported	21 (3.1%)
Ethnicity	
Non-Hispanic/Latino	632 (94.2%)
Hispanic/Latino	39 (5.8%)
BMI Percentile	97.0 [94.1, 98.8]
OGTT Curve Shape Classification	
Monophasic	367 (54.7%)
Biphasic	282 (42.0%)
Monotonically Increasing	17 (2.5%)
Inconclusive	5 (0.7%)

Abbreviations: BMI, body mass index; OGTT, oral glucose tolerance test; Q1, 1st quartile; Q3, 3rd quartile.
[1] Median [Q1, Q3] or n (%).

3.2. Cross-Sectional Analysis

3.2.1. Glucose Profile Manual Shape Classifications

The manual OGTT shape classifications yielded 42.0% of participants having the lowest risk associated [15,16] classification of "biphasic", with a majority having "monophasic" shape (54.7%), and few with "monotonically increasing" (2.5%). For five participants (0.7%), the shape of the curve was inconclusive due to a lack of rise in glucose within the first hour in the test. The average profile for each shape subgroup is representative of the morphology expected for each (Figure 1); however, individual participant glucose responses varied widely in height and peak time within each classification.

3.2.2. Glucose and Insulin FDA Shape Characteristics

The first three glucose FPCs explained 89.6%, 7.9%, and 2.1% of the variance in the glucose curves, respectively (Figure S1A–C). FPC1 score successfully characterized the height of the glucose curve, meaning participants with higher FPC1 score are more likely to have a higher glucose level throughout the OGTT (Figure 2A), FPC2 and FPC3 scores characterized the shape of the glucose curve, with FPC2 relating to the timing and height of the peak value (Figure 2B) and FPC3 relating to oscillation (Figure 2C). These shape characteristics are further demonstrated by plotting the glucose curves for participants with the highest and lowest decile of each FPC score (Figure S2A–C).

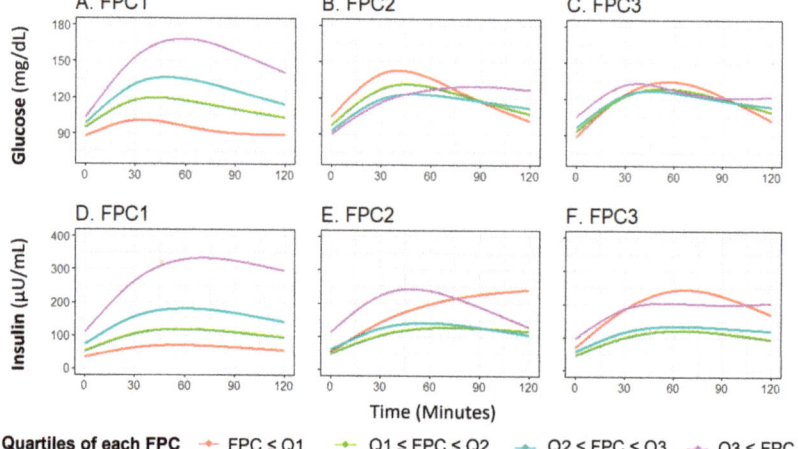

Figure 2. Means of fitted curves of the oral glucose tolerance test curves for glucose and insulin by FPC scores quartile classification. The plot shows average fitted curves of glucose (**A–C**) and insulin (**D–F**) responses, classified by the quartile of each FPC score ((**A,D**): FPC1 score; (**B,E**): FPC2 score, and (**C,F**): FPC3 score). Abbreviations: FPC, functional principal component.

The first three insulin FPCs captured similar variation, with 92.2%, 7.0%, and 0.7% of variation in the insulin curves explained by the first three FPCs, respectively (Figure S1D–F). Similar to the findings with glucose, FPC1 score characterized the overall height of the insulin curve (Figure 2D), FPC2 score characterized the timing of peak (Figure 2E), and FPC3 score related to the oscillation (Figure 2F). The difference of insulin curves between participants with extreme high/low deciles of FPC scores are presented in Figure S2D,E.

3.2.3. Cross-Sectional Associations with Metabolic Health Parameters

Glucose manual profile shapes (coded as dichotomous variables) and FPC scores summarizing glucose and insulin curve shapes (coded as continuous variables) were compared with metabolic health parameters, cross-sectionally (Figure 3). The monophasic shape was significantly associated with higher 60- ($r = 0.42$), and 90- ($r = 0.24$) minute glucose, monotonically increasing shape with higher 120 min glucose ($r = 0.17$), and biphasic with lower 60- ($r = -0.44$) and 90- ($r = -0.27$) minute glucose. The monophasic glucose shape was associated with higher 60- ($r = 0.29$) and 90- ($r = 0.22$) minute insulin, and biphasic with significantly lower 60- ($r = -0.29$) and 90- ($r = -0.24$) minute insulin. The directions of associations of glucose shape classifications with glucose and insulin values support the validity of these classifications to describe the general shape of responses. Although the shape classifications capture the general shape of intra-person response in plasma glucose, these moderate correlations highlight substantial response variability utilizing the manual shape classifications. Other metabolic health parameters were associated with manual shape classification (Figure 3, Table S1): waist circumference (WC) was positively associated with monophasic shape (r = 0.18, median monophasic WC = 93 cm) and negatively with biphasic shape (r = −0.16, median biphasic WC = 88 cm). The shape classifications differed significantly by age and ethnicity, but not by sex or race (Table S1).

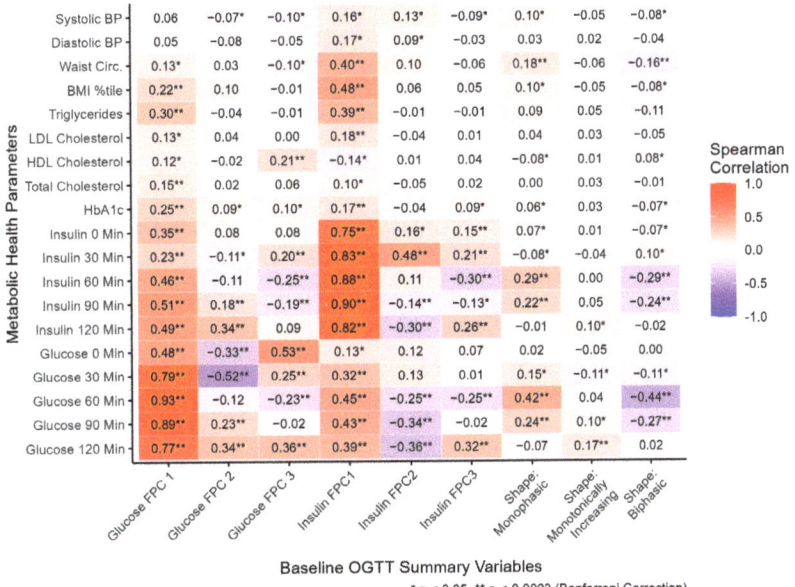

Figure 3. At baseline, the relationship between oral glucose tolerance test shape variables and metabolic health parameters. All FPC scores were standardized as continuous variables. Shape classifications were coded as separate dichotomous variables, with five participants excluded with unclassified shapes. Spearman correlations were utilized to assess associations. Units: systolic/diastolic BP (mmHg), waist circumference (cm), triglycerides/HDL/LDL/total cholesterol (mg/dL), HbA1c (%), insulin (µU/mL), glucose (mg/dL). Abbreviations: BP, blood pressure; BMI, body mass index; LDL, low-density lipoprotein; HDL, high-density lipoprotein; HbA1c, hemoglobin A1c; FPC, functional principal component. Variable-specific missingness existed for BP (n = 21), waist circumference (n = 24), and lipid labs (n = 10).

Glucose FPC1 score was positively correlated with glucose at each time point throughout the OGTT (r = 0.48, 0.79, 0.93, 0.89, and 0.77; Figure 3), consistent with its general explanation of overall curve height. Glucose FPC2 score was negatively correlated with 0- (r = −0.33), and 30- (r = −0.52) minute glucose and positively correlated with 90- (r = 0.23) and 120- (r = 0.34) minute glucose, consistent with a general explanation of time to peak captured by FPC2 score. Glucose FPC3 score was positively correlated with 0- (r = 0.53), 30- (r = 0.25), and 120- (r = 0.36) minute glucose and negatively correlated with 60 min glucose (r = −0.23), consistent with its general explanation of oscillation in each curve. All three insulin FPC scores followed similar patterns of association with insulin at each time as the glucose FPC scores did with glucose at each time, supporting the characteristics qualitatively captured by each FPC. Furthermore, multiple significant associations were found between glucose FPCs and plasma insulin, and between insulin FPCs and plasma glucose, suggesting each type of FPC (glucose or insulin) is strongly related to levels of the other marker.

Glucose FPC1 score was significantly correlated with HbA1c (r = 0.25), total cholesterol (r = 0.15), triglycerides (r = 0.30), and BMI percentile (r = 0.22). Glucose FPC2 score was not significantly correlated with any metabolic health parameters. Glucose FPC3 score was significantly correlated with HDL cholesterol (r = 0.21). Insulin FPC1 score was significantly correlated with HbA1c (r = 0.17), LDL cholesterol (r = 0.18), triglycerides (r = 0.39), BMI percentile (r = 0.48), and waist circumference (r = 0.40). Insulin FPC2 and FPC3 scores were not significantly correlated with any metabolic health parameters after multiple hypothesis correction.

We evaluated associations of age, sex, race, and ethnicity (independent variable) with glucose and insulin FPC scores (dependent variables) in separate linear regression models. Several significant associations were found between these demographic factors and the FPC scores, as reported in Tables S2 (glucose FPC scores) and S3 (insulin FPC scores). Therefore, to evaluate associations between the metabolic health parameters (independent variables) and glucose and insulin FPC scores (dependent variables) independent of demographic factors, we fit linear regression models adjusting for age, sex, race, and ethnicity. As reported in Tables S4 (models for glucose FPC scores) and S5 (models for insulin FPC scores), numerous significant associations were found. Notably, these adjusted regression findings concurred with all significant correlations of metabolic health parameters and glucose and insulin FPC scores reported in Figure 3, suggesting these associations are independent of demographic factors.

3.3. Longitudinal Analysis

A total of 193 participants completed the follow-up assessment at least six months after baseline. Age at baseline, sex, and ethnicity did not differ significantly among participants who also had complete longitudinal data compared with those in the cross-sectional analysis alone, though there were significant differences in race and some baseline metabolic health parameters (Table S6). In the longitudinal subset, median follow-up time was 14.5 months (Table 2). Paired FPG ($p < 0.001$) and HbA1c (HbA1c) changed significantly between baseline and follow-up, though 2hrPG and BMI percentile did not. Though the overall rate of dysglycemia was 7.3% ($n = 14$) at both baseline and follow-up, just four participants with dysglycemia at baseline still had dysglycemia at follow-up (28.6%), meaning the same number of participants ($n = 10$) newly developed dysglycemia as those who no longer had it.

Table 2. Comparison of characteristics of participants between baseline and follow-up from the longitudinal subset ($N = 193$).

Characteristic	At Baseline [1]	At Follow-Up [1]	p-Value [2]
Age (years)	13.3 [11.5, 15.3]	14.7 [12.9, 16.5]	
Δ Age (months)		14.5 [12.6, 17.2]	
Dysglycemia			1.000
No (%)	179 (92.7%)	179 (92.7%)	
Yes (%)	14 (7.3%)	14 (7.3%)	
FPG (mg/dL)	83 [79, 90]	87 [83, 91]	<0.001
2hrPG (mg/dL)	99 [86, 114]	102 [86, 114]	0.438
HbA1c (%) [3]	5.2 [5.0, 5.4]	5.2 [5.0, 5.4]	<0.001
BMI Percentile	96.2 [92.1, 98.6]	96.3 [91.5, 98.8]	0.567

Abbreviations: FPG, fasting plasma glucose; 2hrPG, 2 h plasma glucose; HbA1c, hemoglobin A1c; BMI, body mass index; Q1, 1st quartile; Q3, 3rd quartile. [1] Median [Q1, Q3] or n (%). [2] Paired Wilcoxon signed rank tests (continuous variables) or McNemar's test (dysglycemia). [3] One participant had missing HbA1c at follow-up. Median change in HbA1c was 0.1 [−0.1, 0.2].

Of all measures assessed to predict future dysglycemia, FPG performed the poorest (AUC = 0.50) (Figure 4A). Though the manual shape classifications (AUC = 0.69) (Figure 4B) exceeded the performance of FPG, greater prediction accuracy was achieved by 2hrPG (AUC = 0.78) and HbA1c (AUC = 0.72) (Figure 4A). The combination of glucose and insulin FPCs yielded the greatest prediction accuracy (AUC = 0.80) (Figure 4B), with notable improvements in test sensitivity at higher values of specificity for all FPC approaches when compared to the other approaches.

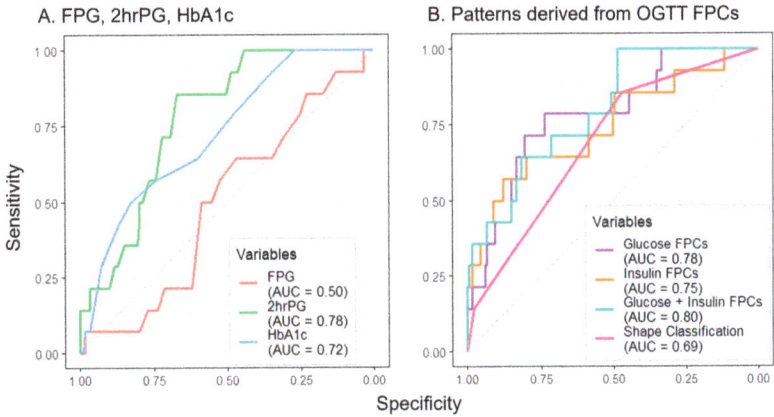

Figure 4. Utilizing baseline oral glucose tolerance test parameters to predict follow-up dysglycemia. Predictors include single laboratory values (**A**) and methods using OGTT response shape information (**B**). Abbreviations: FPG, fasting plasma glucose; 2hrPG, 2 h plasma glucose; HbA1c, hemoglobin A1c; OGTT, oral glucose tolerance test; FPC, functional principal component; AUC, area under the curve.

4. Discussion

To our knowledge, this is the first study that has used FDA for summarizing OGTT glucose and insulin responses to evaluate the association of FPC scores with metabolic health markers and future dysglycemia in a diverse adolescent population. We sought to utilize FDA to characterize the glucose and insulin response to an OGTT because single measures and manual shape classifications may be missing information on the dynamic response to a glucose bolus. Glucose and insulin FPC scores had substantially stronger associations with metabolic health parameters than manual shape classifications, being significantly correlated with waist circumference, BMI percentile, LDL/HDL/total cholesterol, triglycerides, and HbA1c. Though differences in FPC scores by age, sex, and race were noted, these associations were still observed in models adjusting for demographic covariates. In longitudinal logistic regression analyses, glucose and insulin FPC scores predicted future dysglycemia better than manual shape classifications, HbA1c, or FPG.

Multiple characteristics of glucose and insulin curves were captured by the FPCs. Glucose and insulin FPC1 explained variation in overall curve height, FPC2 explained the positioning of the peak, and FPC3 explained oscillations in the curves. These attributes are similar to previous findings from use of this method in OGTTs from the first trimester of pregnancy, supporting this method as consistent across OGTTs for multiple applications [20]. Given this extent of variance explained, the FPC scores numerically captured some variation qualitatively related to the glucose shape classifications. Additional exploratory analysis revealed monophasic shape was positively correlated with FPC1 (r = 0.28) and negatively with FPC2 (r = −0.18) and FPC3 (r = −0.51) scores, indicating a high curve that peaks mid/late with little curvature. The biphasic shape was notably negatively correlated with FPC1 (r = −0.30), and positively with FPC3 (r = 0.50) scores, indicating a curve with a low overall level and high amount of oscillation. Monotonically increasing shape was notably positively associated with FPC2 score (r = 0.27), indicating a late peak.

Previously, manual glucose curve shape classifications have been associated with differences in β-cell function and insulin sensitivity in both children and adults [13,14,16]. Furthermore, measures of insulin in an OGTT may enhance the assessment of impaired glucose metabolism [9]. By using glucose and insulin FPCs, multiple modes of variation in both glucose and insulin are captured across time and may more comprehensively assess disordered glucose regulation and metabolism. To our knowledge, no other method captures this variation in both glucose and insulin. The performance of the FPC scores for predicting future dysglycemia supports their utility. Consistent with concerns about generalizing methods of classifying dysglycemia using single laboratory values to children [7,8], only 28.6% of children with dysglycemia at baseline (defined by a composite of elevated FPG or 2hrPG) still had it at follow-up. When predicting this longitudinal dysglycemia, the glucose and insulin FPC scores outperformed both single laboratory values (FPG, 2hrPG, HbA1c) and the manual shape classifications. Though for the application of gestational diabetes, this is consistent with a previous findings that glucose FPC2 score in the first trimester of pregnancy is a significant predictor of gestational diabetes in the third, while other glucose summary measures were not [20].

The sample was large, racially and ethnically diverse, and had a reasonably long median follow-up time over which to observe longitudinal changes in dysglycemia. These findings are therefore reasonably generalizable to children ages 8–18 with overweight or obesity and without a previous diagnosis of diabetes. Several limitations are important to note. First, the study cohort did not consistently collect physician-assessed tanner staging to determine pubertal status and puberty is associated with a physiologically normal decrease in insulin sensitivity [35]. However, obesity and metabolic disease are known to affect this physiologic change during puberty [35,36], so it is unclear how to best account for puberty in relation to fitting and using FPC scores. This analysis adjusted for age and sex in cross-sectional models to account for puberty-related differences. Additionally, few participants had dysglycemia at follow-up, preventing the split of the cohort into training and validation samples for longitudinal prediction. This low overall rate of dysglycemia at follow-up seems to be related to observed differential follow-up completion by health status, where "healthier" children were more likely to complete follow-up. The longitudinal predictive value of the FPC scores should be further confirmed in other cohorts.

Though the OGTT method used in this study required serial blood draws and would likely be burdensome to use as a clinical predictive screening test for otherwise healthy children, future work should validate and adapt the use of OGTT FPCs for a clinical setting. Further research is needed to translate individual glucose and insulin FPC scores to clinically useful classifications of risk, a potentially valuable tool to include in an electronic medical record. Additionally, previous studies have used similar functional data analysis methods with continuous glucose monitoring (CGM) data in type I diabetes [22]. A CGM-based screening tool could be developed to detect early abnormal glucose regulation for children without known diabetes; such a method would be minimally burdensome to the patient and could incorporate many more data points to better fit precise glucose curves.

5. Conclusions

This analysis suggested that beyond simple plasma glucose values, glucose and insulin curve shape information derived from OGTTs more directly profiles underlying physiology in a way that is meaningfully associated with metabolic health parameters and longitudinally with future dysglycemia in children with overweight or obesity. Glucose and insulin FPC scores from an OGTT present a powerful way to summarize this shape information. FPCs may be clinically useful to predict future dysglycemia among children at elevated risk due to their body weight, allowing for enhanced early intervention.

Supplementary Materials: The following supporting information can be downloaded at: https://www.mdpi.com/article/10.3390/diabetology5010008/s1, Table S1: Metabolic health parameters by shape classification (cross-sectional); Figure S1: Fitted FPC curves for glucose and insulin (% variance explained); Figure S2: Curves from extreme deciles of each FPC; Table S2: Univariate linear regression of standardized glucose FPCs by demographic characteristics (cross-sectional); Table S3: Univariate linear regression of standardized insulin FPCs by demographic characteristics (cross-sectional); Table S4: Adjusted linear regression models of standardized glucose FPCs by metabolic health parameters (cross-sectional); Table S5: Adjusted linear regression models of standardized insulin FPCs by metabolic health parameters (cross-sectional); Table S6: Longitudinal subset participant characteristics at baseline, comparison to cross-sectional sample.

Author Contributions: Conceptualization, T.J.R., H.J.M., J.M.L. and J.L.M.; methodology, T.J.R., H.J.M., Z.Z., E.H., D.G.-D. and J.L.M.; software, T.J.R., H.J.M. and J.L.M.; validation, T.J.R., H.J.M. and J.L.M.; formal analysis, T.J.R., H.J.M., Z.Z. and J.L.M.; investigation, M.E.V., E.H. and J.M.L.; resources, M.E.V., E.H. and J.M.L.; data curation, T.J.R., M.E.V., H.J.M., E.H., D.G.-D., J.M.L. and J.L.M.; writing—original draft preparation, T.J.R.; writing—review and editing, all authors; visualization, T.J.R. and J.L.M.; supervision D.G.-D., J.M.L. and J.L.M.; project administration, M.E.V., E.H., J.M.L. and J.L.M.; funding acquisition, J.M.L. All authors have read and agreed to the published version of the manuscript.

Funding: This research was funded by the National Institute of Child Health & Human Development, grant number R01HD074559 and was supported by services from the National Institute of Diabetes and Digestive and Kidney Diseases, grant numbers P30DK020572 (MDRC), P30DK092926 (MCDTR) and P30DK089503 (MNORC), the National Institutes of Health, grant numbers UL1RR024986, UL1TR000433, and UL1TR002240 (MICHR), and the Elizabeth Weiser Caswell Diabetes Institute at the University of Michigan. T.J.R. was supported by a training fellowship from the National Cancer Institute, T32CA260262.

Institutional Review Board Statement: This study was conducted according to the guidelines of the Declaration of Helsinki and approved by the Institutional Review Board (or Ethics Committee) of The University of Michigan (HUM#00006955 and initial date of approval 26 July 2007).

Informed Consent Statement: Informed consent was obtained from all subjects involved in this study.

Data Availability Statement: The datasets presented in this article are not readily available due to privacy and IRB regulatory restrictions. Requests to access the datasets should be directed to the authors.

Acknowledgments: We thank the staff of the Michigan Clinical Research Unit and Michigan Diabetes Research Center for their contributions to perform the study visits and laboratory measurements.

Conflicts of Interest: The authors declare no conflict of interest. The funders had no role in the design of the study; in the collection, analyses, or interpretation of data; in the writing of the manuscript; or in the decision to publish the results.

References

1. Divers, J.; Mayer-Davis, E.J.; Lawrence, J.M.; Isom, S.; Dabelea, D.; Dolan, L.; Imperatore, G.; Marcovina, S.; Pettitt, D.J.; Pihoker, C.; et al. Trends in Incidence of Type 1 and Type 2 Diabetes Among Youths—Selected Counties and Indian Reservations, United States, 2002–2015. *MMWR Morb. Mortal. Wkly. Rep.* **2020**, *69*, 161–165. [CrossRef]
2. Dabelea, D.; Mayer-Davis, E.J.; Saydah, S.; Imperatore, G.; Linder, B.; Divers, J.; Bell, R.; Badaru, A.; Talton, J.W.; Crume, T.; et al. Prevalence of type 1 and type 2 diabetes among children and adolescents from 2001 to 2009. *JAMA* **2014**, *311*, 1778–1786. [CrossRef] [PubMed]
3. Fryar, C.D.; Carroll, M.D.; Ogden, C.L. *Prevalence of Overweight, Obesity, and Severe Obesity among Children and Adolescents Aged 2–19 Years: United States, 1963–1965 through 2015–2016*; National Center for Health Statistics (U.S.): Hyattsville, MD, USA, 2018.
4. American Diabetes Association. Economic costs of diabetes in the US in 2017. *Diabetes Care* **2018**, *41*, 917–928. [CrossRef] [PubMed]
5. American Diabetes Association. 12. Children and Adolescents: Standards of Medical Care in Diabetes-2018. *Diabetes Care* **2018**, *41*, S126–S136. [CrossRef] [PubMed]
6. ElSayed, N.A.; Aleppo, G.; Aroda, V.R.; Bannuru, R.R.; Brown, F.M.; Bruemmer, D.; Collins, B.S.; Hilliard, M.E.; Isaacs, D.; Johnson, E.L.; et al. 2. Classification and Diagnosis of Diabetes: Standards of Care in Diabetes-2023. *Diabetes Care* **2023**, *46*, S19–S40. [CrossRef]

7. Jagannathan, R.; Neves, J.S.; Dorcely, B.; Chung, S.T.; Tamura, K.; Rhee, M.; Bergman, M. The Oral Glucose Tolerance Test: 100 Years Later. *Diabetes Metab. Syndr. Obes. Targets Ther.* **2020**, *13*, 3787–3805. [CrossRef]
8. Di Bonito, P.; Licenziati, M.R.; Corica, D.; Wasniewska, M.; Di Sessa, A.; Miraglia Del Giudice, E.; Morandi, A.; Maffeis, C.; Faienza, M.F.; Mozzillo, E.; et al. Which Is the Most Appropriate Cut-Off of HbA1c for Prediabetes Screening in Caucasian Youths with Overweight or Obesity? *Int. J. Environ. Res. Public Health* **2023**, *20*, 928. [CrossRef]
9. La Valle, A.; d'Annunzio, G.; Campanello, C.; Tantari, G.; Pistorio, A.; Napoli, F.; Patti, G.; Crocco, M.; Bassi, M.; Minuto, N.; et al. Are glucose and insulin levels at all time points during OGTT a reliable marker of diabetes mellitus risk in pediatric obesity? *J. Endocrinol. Investig.* **2023**, *46*, 1685–1694. [CrossRef]
10. Brar, P.C.; Mehta, S.; Brar, A.; Pierce, K.A.; Albano, A.; Bergman, M. Value of 1-Hour Plasma Glucose During an Oral Glucose Tolerance Test in a Multiethnic Cohort of Obese Children and Adolescents. *Clin. Med. Insights. Endocrinol. Diabetes* **2023**, *16*, 11795514231177206. [CrossRef]
11. Yin, C.; Zhang, H.; Xiao, Y.; Liu, W. Shape of glucose curve can be used as a predictor for screening prediabetes in obese children. *Acta Paediatr.* **2014**, *103*, e199–e205. [CrossRef]
12. Tschritter, O.; Fritsche, A.; Shirkavand, F.; Machicao, F.; Haring, H.; Stumvoll, M. Assessing the shape of the glucose curve during an oral glucose tolerance test. *Diabetes Care* **2003**, *26*, 1026–1033. [CrossRef]
13. Arslanian, S.; El Ghormli, L.; Young Kim, J.; Bacha, F.; Chan, C.; Ismail, H.M.; Levitt Katz, L.E.; Levitsky, L.; Tryggestad, J.B.; White, N.H.; et al. The Shape of the Glucose Response Curve During an Oral Glucose Tolerance Test: Forerunner of Heightened Glycemic Failure Rates and Accelerated Decline in beta-Cell Function in TODAY. *Diabetes Care* **2019**, *42*, 164–172. [CrossRef]
14. de Andrade Mesquita, L.; Pavan Antoniolli, L.; Cittolin-Santos, G.F.; Gerchman, F. Distinct metabolic profile according to the shape of the oral glucose tolerance test curve is related to whole glucose excursion: A cross-sectional study. *BMC Endocr. Disord.* **2018**, *18*, 56. [CrossRef]
15. Nolfe, G.; Spreghini, M.R.; Sforza, R.W.; Morino, G.; Manco, M. Beyond the morphology of the glucose curve following an oral glucose tolerance test in obese youth. *Eur. J. Endocrinol.* **2012**, *166*, 107–114. [CrossRef]
16. Kim, J.Y.; Michaliszyn, S.F.; Nasr, A.; Lee, S.; Tfayli, H.; Hannon, T.; Hughan, K.S.; Bacha, F.; Arslanian, S. The Shape of the Glucose Response Curve During an Oral Glucose Tolerance Test Heralds Biomarkers of Type 2 Diabetes Risk in Obese Youth. *Diabetes Care* **2016**, *39*, 1431–1439. [CrossRef] [PubMed]
17. Manco, M.; Nolfe, G.; Pataky, Z.; Monti, L.; Porcellati, F.; Gabriel, R.; Mitrakou, A.; Mingrone, G. Shape of the OGTT glucose curve and risk of impaired glucose metabolism in the EGIR-RISC cohort. *Metabolism* **2017**, *70*, 42–50. [CrossRef] [PubMed]
18. La Grasta Sabolic, L.; Pozgaj Sepec, M.; Cigrovski Berkovic, M.; Stipancic, G. Time to the Peak, Shape of the Curve and Combination of These Glucose Response Characteristics During Oral Glucose Tolerance Test as Indicators of Early Beta-cell Dysfunction in Obese Adolescents. *J. Clin. Res. Pediatr. Endocrinol.* **2021**, *13*, 160–169. [CrossRef] [PubMed]
19. Cree-Green, M.; Xie, D.; Rahat, H.; Garcia-Reyes, Y.; Bergman, B.C.; Scherzinger, A.; Diniz Behn, C.; Chan, C.L.; Kelsey, M.M.; Pyle, L.; et al. Oral Glucose Tolerance Test Glucose Peak Time Is Most Predictive of Prediabetes and Hepatic Steatosis in Obese Girls. *J. Endocr. Soc.* **2018**, *2*, 547–562. [CrossRef]
20. Frøslie, K.F.; Røislien, J.; Qvigstad, E.; Godang, K.; Bollerslev, J.; Voldner, N.; Henriksen, T.; Veierød, M.B. Shape information from glucose curves: Functional data analysis compared with traditional summary measures. *BMC Med. Res. Methodol.* **2013**, *13*, 6. [CrossRef] [PubMed]
21. Szczesniak, R.D.; Li, D.; Duan, L.L.; Altaye, M.; Miodovnik, M.; Khoury, J.C. Longitudinal Patterns of Glycemic Control and Blood Pressure in Pregnant Women with Type 1 Diabetes Mellitus: Phenotypes from Functional Data Analysis. *Am. J. Perinatol.* **2016**, *33*, 1282–1290. [CrossRef] [PubMed]
22. Gecili, E.; Huang, R.; Khoury, J.C.; King, E.; Altaye, M.; Bowers, K.; Szczesniak, R.D. Functional data analysis and prediction tools for continuous glucose-monitoring studies. *J. Clin. Transl. Sci.* **2020**, *5*, e51. [CrossRef]
23. Lee, J.M.; Gebremariam, A.; Wu, E.; LaRose, J.; Gurney, J.G. Evaluation of nonfasting tests to screen for childhood and adolescent dysglycemia. *Diabetes Care* **2011**, *34*, 2597–2602. [CrossRef] [PubMed]
24. Vajravelu, M.E.; Hirschfeld, E.; Gebremariam, A.; Burant, C.F.; Herman, W.H.; Peterson, K.E.; Meijer, J.L.; Lee, J.M. Prospective Test Performance of Nonfasting Biomarkers to Identify Dysglycemia in Children and Adolescents. *Horm. Res. Paediatr.* **2023**, *96*, 316–324. [CrossRef] [PubMed]
25. LaBarre, J.L.; Hirschfeld, E.; Soni, T.; Kachman, M.; Wigginton, J.; Duren, W.; Fleischman, J.Y.; Karnovsky, A.; Burant, C.F.; Lee, J.M. Comparing the Fasting and Random-Fed Metabolome Response to an Oral Glucose Tolerance Test in Children and Adolescents: Implications of Sex, Obesity, and Insulin Resistance. *Nutrients* **2021**, *13*, 3365. [CrossRef] [PubMed]
26. Gallego-Suarez, C.; Bulan, A.; Hirschfeld, E.; Wachowiak, P.; Abrishami, S.; Griffin, C.; Sturza, J.; Tzau, A.; Hayes, T.; Woolford, S.J.; et al. Enhanced Myeloid Leukocytes in Obese Children and Adolescents at Risk for Metabolic Impairment. *Front. Endocrinol.* **2020**, *11*, 327. [CrossRef] [PubMed]
27. CDC. Defining Childhood Weight Status. Available online: https://www.cdc.gov/obesity/childhood/defining.html (accessed on 3 March 2022).
28. Kuczmarski, R.J.; Ogden, C.L.; Guo, S.S.; Grummer-Strawn, L.M.; Flegal, K.M.; Mei, Z.; Wei, R.; Curtin, L.R.; Roche, A.F.; Johnson, C.L. 2000 CDC Growth Charts for the United States: Methods and development. *Vital Health Stat.* **2002**, *11*, 1–190.

29. Utzschneider, K.M.; Younes, N.; Rasouli, N.; Barzilay, J.I.; Banerji, M.A.; Cohen, R.M.; Gonzalez, E.V.; Ismail-Beigi, F.; Mather, K.J.; Raskin, P.; et al. Shape of the OGTT glucose response curve: Relationship with beta-cell function and differences by sex, race, and BMI in adults with early type 2 diabetes treated with metformin. *BMJ Open Diabetes Res. Care* **2021**, *9*, e002264. [CrossRef] [PubMed]
30. Ramsay, J.; Hooker, G.; Graves, S. Package 'fda'. Available online: https://cran.r-project.org/web/packages/fda/fda.pdf (accessed on 4 September 2023).
31. Hollander, M.; Wolfe, D.A. *Nonparametric Statistical Methods*; John Wiley & Sons: New York, NY, USA, 1973.
32. Agresti, A. *Categorical Data Analysis*; John Wiley & Sons: New York, NY, USA, 1990.
33. Robin, X.; Turck, N.; Hainard, A.; Tiberti, N.; Lisacek, F.; Sanchez, J.C.; Muller, M. pROC: An open-source package for R and S+ to analyze and compare ROC curves. *BMC Bioinform.* **2011**, *12*, 77. [CrossRef] [PubMed]
34. R Core Team. R: A Language and Environment for Statistical Computing. Available online: https://www.R-project.org/ (accessed on 3 March 2022).
35. Kelsey, M.M.; Zeitler, P.S. Insulin Resistance of Puberty. *Curr. Diab. Rep.* **2016**, *16*, 64. [CrossRef]
36. Tobisch, B.; Blatniczky, L.; Barkai, L. Cardiometabolic risk factors and insulin resistance in obese children and adolescents: Relation to puberty. *Pediatr. Obes.* **2015**, *10*, 37–44. [CrossRef]

Disclaimer/Publisher's Note: The statements, opinions and data contained in all publications are solely those of the individual author(s) and contributor(s) and not of MDPI and/or the editor(s). MDPI and/or the editor(s) disclaim responsibility for any injury to people or property resulting from any ideas, methods, instructions or products referred to in the content.

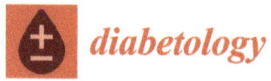

Article

Evaluating the Use of Web-Based Technologies for Self-Management among Arabic-Speaking Immigrants Living with Type 2 Diabetes Mellitus: A Cross-Sectional Study in Saudi Arabia

Anwar Althubyani [1,2,*], Clarice Tang [3,4], Jency Thomas [1] and Sabrina Gupta [5]

[1] Department of Microbiology Anatomy Physiology and Pharmacology (MAPP), School of Agriculture Biomedicine and Environment (SABE), La Trobe University, Melbourne, VIC 3086, Australia; j.thomas@latrobe.edu.au
[2] Department of Public Health, Applied college, University of Tabuk, Tabuk 47713, Saudi Arabia
[3] Institute of Health and Sport, Victoria University, Melbourne, VIC 3011, Australia; clarice.tang@vu.edu.au
[4] School of Health Sciences, Western Sydney University, Campbelltown, NSW 2560, Australia
[5] Department of Public Health, School of Psychology and Public Health, La Trobe University, Melbourne, VIC 3086, Australia; s.gupta@latrobe.edu.au
* Correspondence: aalthubyani@latrobe.edu.au; Tel.: +61-452360155

Abstract: This study aimed to investigate the use of and willingness to adopt web-based technology for self-management of type 2 diabetes among Arabic-speaking immigrants in Saudi Arabia. Conducted in Taif in 2022, it involved participants with type 2 diabetes mellitus, utilizing a study-specific questionnaire to gather data on demographics, disease specifics, and attitudes towards using this technology for diabetes management. Out of the 109 individuals who responded, 91 completed the survey and reported accessing web-based technology and an average usage of two hours per day. The primary use was for social media (90.1%) and information searching (73.6%). The study found a high willingness to use web-based technology for dietary planning (85.7%), physical activity monitoring (94.5%), and communication with healthcare providers (93.41%). Notably, younger participants, those with higher education, and married individuals showed more inclination towards using such technology, as indicated by significant correlations ($p < 0.001$, CI = 0.03–0.38; $p < 0.039$, CI = 1.06–10.26; $p = 0.024$, CI = 1.23–19.74). Over half of the participants (56%) considered web-based technology beneficial for diabetes management, with many finding it time-saving (61.5%). In conclusion, a significant proportion of participants demonstrated a strong preference for integrating web-based technology into their diabetes self-management routines. This preference was particularly evident in key areas such as diet, physical activity, and glucose monitoring. These findings underscore the potential of web-based technologies in supporting effective diabetes management among Arabic-speaking immigrants, highlighting the need for targeted interventions that leverage these digital tools.

Keywords: Arabic-speaking immigrants; type 2 diabetes mellitus; web-based technology; diabetes self-management; Saudi Arabia

Citation: Althubyani, A.; Tang, C.; Thomas, J.; Gupta, S. Evaluating the Use of Web-Based Technologies for Self-Management among Arabic-Speaking Immigrants Living with Type 2 Diabetes Mellitus: A Cross-Sectional Study in Saudi Arabia. *Diabetology* **2024**, *5*, 85–95. https://doi.org/10.3390/diabetology5010007

Academic Editors: Andrej Belančić, Sanja Klobučar and Dario Rahelić

Received: 29 December 2023
Revised: 28 January 2024
Accepted: 26 February 2024
Published: 28 February 2024

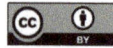

Copyright: © 2024 by the authors. Licensee MDPI, Basel, Switzerland. This article is an open access article distributed under the terms and conditions of the Creative Commons Attribution (CC BY) license (https://creativecommons.org/licenses/by/4.0/).

1. Introduction

Type 2 Diabetes mellitus (T2DM) is a global epidemic [1], affecting 10.5% of adults around the world [2]. Additionally, 374 million individuals have impaired glucose tolerance, putting them at high risk of developing T2DM later in life [3]. The prevalence of T2DM has significantly increased particularly in high-income countries such as the Kingdom of Saudi Arabia (KSA) [4]. KSA is currently within the top 10 countries with the highest reported T2DM diagnosis globally [4].

T2DM poses a significant health challenge, especially for immigrants from low- and middle-income countries who have relocated to high-income nations [5]. This population faces a unique set of risks, with studies indicating that immigrants, particularly those in the first generation, are more susceptible to developing T2DM compared to their host population counterparts [6]. This heightened risk is particularly pronounced among immigrants from the Middle East and North Africa, where a blend of genetic predispositions and environmental factors such as urbanization, mechanization, and shifts in nutrition and lifestyle behaviors contribute to the increased prevalence of T2DM [7].

In Saudi Arabia, managing diabetes for Arabic-speaking immigrants is challenging due to late diagnoses and poor control of blood sugar levels [8,9]. These issues are compounded by difficulties such as adherence to treatment plans, different beliefs, and knowledge about diabetes, money, and healthcare issues [10,11]. Because of the mix of genetic, environmental, and lifestyle factors that make Middle Eastern and North African immigrants more likely to get T2DM, there is a strong need for new, tailored ways to manage T2DM. Web-based technologies (WBT) offer a good solution by providing customized help that meets the specific needs of these communities, which could make diabetes management more effective for this group [12].

In addressing this growing health concern, the integration of assistive WBT into T2DM self-management protocols emerges as a promising solution [13]. These technologies have the potential to significantly augment the diabetes care provided by healthcare professionals, offering crucial educational and motivational support [14]. Particularly when access to primary healthcare is limited or when patients face barriers like time constraints, financial limitations, or geographical isolation, WBT can play a pivotal role in expanding the availability and effectiveness of diabetes education and support [15]. Often, patients may struggle to regularly attend diabetes education classes or consult with diabetes educators due to these barriers [16]. However, through the use of WBT tools, essential education and training can be delivered remotely, enabling patients to learn and implement new practices and routines that are critical for effective diabetes management [15]. Furthermore, it is instrumental in facilitating daily self-management activities for T2DM, including blood glucose monitoring, physical activity, healthy eating, medication adherence, monitoring for potential complications, and developing problem-solving skills [17].

Despite the demonstrated clinical efficacy of WBT in enhancing blood sugar control and weight management for those who are receptive to using them [18–21], there remains a gap in research focusing on patient preferences and attitudes towards these technologies in real-world scenarios [22]. This gap is particularly noteworthy in the context of T2DM management among specific groups such as Arabic-speaking immigrants [23]. Therefore, given the scarcity of research specifically addressing Arabic-speaking immigrants with T2DM in KSA, the study is particularly significant. The study aims to delve into the attitudes and intentions of these individuals towards the adoption of WBT for T2DM self-management. This focus is essential to understand whether these individuals are inclined to incorporate technological strategies into their T2DM management routine. By doing so, the study provides valuable insights into tailoring these technologies to better meet their specific needs and preferences, thereby filling a critical gap in current research.

2. Materials and Methods

2.1. Study Design and Setting

In 2022, this study was carried out in Taif, a city located in western Saudi Arabia known for its diverse population, which includes immigrants from various Arabic-speaking countries. The study employed a convenience sampling method to recruit participants, specifically targeting patients with T2DM who sought care at a prominent tertiary hospital's diabetes clinic. Inclusion criteria encompassed individuals aged 18 and above who self-identified as both living with T2DM and Arabic-speaking immigrants in KSA. The study excluded individuals under the age of 18, those with type 1 diabetes, and those who did not come from Arabic-speaking immigrant backgrounds.

2.2. Questionnaire

In this study, a validated survey instrument originally developed by Dobson et al. [24,25] was adapted to explore the use of WBT for diabetes self-management among Arabic-speaking immigrants in KSA. To ensure accessibility and comfort for all participants, the survey was made available in both Arabic and English, allowing participants to choose the language in which they preferred to respond. Questions related to using apps for diabetes self-management were replaced by use of WBT for managing T2DM. Questions regarding the BMI were removed as the purpose of the study was not to measure the BMI or obesity levels. Additionally, questions from another study by Alzubaidi and colleagues were incorporated to address gaps in Dobson's survey [26]. These questions were related to the measure of self-satisfaction during the previous 7 days regarding diet, blood monitoring and physical activity, education, occupation, marital status, ethnicity, religion, and language spoken at home. These additions enhanced the applicability of the survey to our specific context. Our adoption of this survey was driven by its thoroughness and the validation it received in a similar research setting. This makes it a suitable and reliable tool for our study, allowing us to evaluate the use of WBT for diabetes self-management among Arabic-speaking immigrants in KSA with greater depth and accuracy.

The final questionnaire Survey S1, consisted of 35 questions divided into five sections: demographic information (13 items), disease information (6 items), use of WBT (5 items), intentions for using WBT for T2DM management (10 items), and general explanations (1 item)—this item is deliberately open-ended, allowing participants to share any additional thoughts, experiences, or insights that might not have been captured by the structured items in the previous sections. The demographic section included questions about gender, age, and residence status. The disease information section sought information about the duration of T2DM and other chronic illnesses; these could include, but are not limited to, hypertension, cardiovascular diseases, chronic kidney disease, chronic respiratory diseases, as well as difficulties with diabetes management such as diet, physical activity, communication with healthcare providers, and goal setting. The section on WBT asked about the devices used to access the internet and how they were used. The section of the questionnaire focusing on intentions and attitudes towards using WBT for diabetes management inquired about the types of services participants deemed necessary. It also evaluated their perspectives on employing WBT for self-management. This assessment was conducted using a 5-point Likert scale, where a score of 0 indicated 'highly unlikely' and 5 represented 'extremely likely' to use such technology. Likelihood of intention to use WBT for diabetes management was also ascertained. Prior to initiating data collection, the questionnaire underwent a pilot phase to ensure its readability and ease of understanding. Minor edits were made, such as replacing certain terms, for example, "control" and "management," with more easily understandable Arabic words, before it was administered to the participants.

2.3. Data Collection

Data collection for the study was approved by the Human research ethics committee of La Trobe University (HEC21273). Data collection occurred from February 2022 to August 2022. The researcher (AA) visited the clinic and explained the study objectives and how to complete the questionnaire to patients in the waiting room. Individuals who self-identified as having T2DM, being from an immigrant background, and being interested in participating could access the survey either via a QR code or use of an iPad provided by the researcher at the time of recruitment. Participants were informed that completion of the survey implied consent to the study. A member of the research team (AA) was present to clarify any questions that participants may have had whilst completing the questionnaire.

2.4. Statistical Analyses

Data were analyzed using SPSS version 22.0 [27]. Demographic information, the use of or intention to use WBT and difficulties with self-management questions were descriptively analyzed. The study utilized the median to represent the central point of Likert scale responses and the interquartile range (IQR) to indicate the data's variability. This approach was chosen as it provides a clear and succinct representation of ordinal data, highlighting the main trends while considering potential outliers. Intention score was determined through a single item, "I intend to use WBT for assisting in my diabetes management in the future", with answer options ranging from 0 (not at all) to 5 (very much). To examine the relationship between demographic characteristics like age, gender, educational level, marital status, employment, disease duration, and the intention to use WBT, regression analysis was employed, setting the threshold for statistical significance at $p < 0.05$.

3. Results

Out of the 221 individuals contacted, a total of 109 responded to the survey, with 91 completing it fully, yielding a response rate of 83.49%. Table 1 presents the demographic information of 91 participants. Of the 91 participants, the majority (54%) were female, with ages ranging from 25 to over 65 years. Only 2 participants were aged over 65, while the largest age group consisted of 44 participants in the 45–54-year age bracket. Most of the participants were married (71%) and were employed full-time (71%). As many as 39% of the participants had a bachelor's degree as the highest level of education. Nearly half of the participants were temporary residents (49%), while 31% were permanent residents of KSA. The largest group of immigrants came from Egypt (36%), followed by Yemen (27%). Approximately 41% of the participants had been living with T2DM for more than 5 years. 40% of the participants also had a family history of diabetes.

Table 1. Participants' demographic and disease details.

Demographic Details (N = 91)	n (%)
Gender	
Female	50 (55)
Male	41 (45)
Age Range	
25–34	4 (4)
35–44	33 (36)
45–54	44 (48)
55–64	8 (8)
65 or over	2 (2)
Marital status	
Married	65 (71)
Widowed	12 (13)
Single	8 (8)
Divorced	6 (6)
Employment	
Retired	6 (6)
Full-time employment	65 (71)
Part-time employment	6 (6)
Unemployed	14 (15)
Education level	
Elementary school	1 (1)
Middle school	8 (8)
High school	22 (24)
Diploma	23 (25)
University undergraduate degree	36 (39)
Postgraduate (Master's or PhD)	1 (1)

Table 1. Cont.

Demographic Details (N = 91)	n (%)
Current residential status	
Citizen	17 (18)
Permanent resident	29 (31)
Temporary resident	45 (49)
Ethnicity	
Egyptian	33 (36)
Yemenis	25 (27)
Syrians	16 (17)
Jordanians	5 (5)
Palestinians	6 (6)
Sudanese	4 (4)
Lebanese	1 (1)
Duration of the disease	
1 to 3 years	15 (16)
3 to 5 years	36 (39)
5 years and longer	38 (41)
Unknown/not applicable	2 (2)
Family history	
Yes	37 (40)
No	54 (59)
Other chronic diseases	
Yes	24 (26)
No	24 (26)
Do not know	43 (47)

Table 2 displays the general findings of the participants' use of WBT and their intention to use it to manage T2DM. Ninety of the ninety-one (94%) participants had access to a smart device. As many as 43% of participants had more than one device. Overall, participants spent about 2–3 h per day accessing WBT content, with 41 (45%) spending 2–3 h per day on the internet, while 35 (38%) spent more than 3 h. The participants primarily used their mobile phones for social media n = 82 (90%), watching movies or TV n = 74 (81%), searching for information n = 67 (73%), and reading news or books n = 67 (73%). Moreover, most participants reported they would use WBT for diet planning 78 (85%), physical activity planning 86 (94%), monitoring blood glucose 77 (48%), communicating with healthcare providers 85 (93%), and connecting with other diabetic patients 82 (90%).

Table 2. Use and intention to use web-based technology for diabetes control.

Variables	n (%)
Current technology use	
Having a mobile phone	
Yes	90 (94)
No	1 (5)
Having a computer	
Yes	38 (24)
No	53 (75)
Having a tablet	
Yes	29 (18)
No	62 (81)

Table 2. *Cont.*

Variables	n (%)
Intention to use web-based technology for diabetes control	
Dietary planning	
Yes	78 (85)
No	7 (7)
Don't know	6 (6)
Planning physical activity	
Yes	86 (94)
No	3 (3)
Don't know	2 (2)
Text messaging monitoring and/or reminders	
Yes	63 (69)
No	10 (10)
Don't know	18 (19)
Image messaging monitoring and/or reminders	
Yes	67 (73)
No	11 (12)
Don't know	13 (14)
Glucose reading and tracking option	
Yes	77 (84)
No	7 (7)
Don't know	7 (7)
Contacting healthcare providers	
Yes	85 (93)
No	4 (4)
Don't know	2 (2)
Contacting other patients with diabetes	
Yes	82 (90)
No	5 (5)
Don't know	4 (4)
Average daily use of web-based technology	
from 1–2 h	15 (16)
From 2–3 h	41 (45)
More than 3 h	35 (38)

In addition, Figure 1 illustrates that participants held positive perceptions of WBT for self-management across various descriptors. In this section of the survey, participants were asked about their perceptions and attitudes towards using WBT for diabetes self-management, where a score of 0 indicates 'Strongly Disagree' and 5 signifies 'Strongly agree'. Across a spectrum of descriptors such as 'Good Idea', 'Enjoyable', 'Comforting', 'Exciting', and 'Interesting', participants consistently assigned a median score of 4, indicative of their overall positive perception of WBT in these domains. It is noteworthy that 'Time-saving' garnered the highest rating with a median score of 5, underscoring the participants' strong preference for the efficiency and convenience offered by WBT in managing their T2DM. The IQRs, typically ranging from 3 to 5, signify a degree of agreement among participants, although some variability exists, especially in their assessments of the enjoyability, excitement, and interest associated with WBT usage.

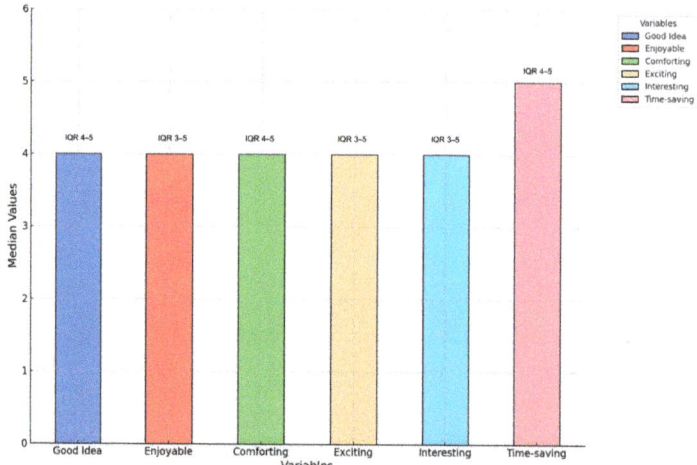

Figure 1. Perceptions of Arabic-Speaking Immigrants on Using Web-Based Technology for Diabetes Self-Management.

The study investigated the relationships between demographic factors and the use of WBT for diabetes self-management, uncovering significant correlations (Table 3). Utilizing binary regression analysis, a negative correlation was observed between age and the willingness to use WBT tools for diabetes care, indicating that older participants were generally less inclined to use these methods (OR = 0.101, $p < 0.001$, 95% CI = 0.027–0.381). Conversely, a positive correlation was found between higher educational attainment and the adoption of WBT tools, suggesting that individuals with more education were more likely to employ this technology for supporting their diabetes management (OR = 3.30, $p < 0.039$, 95% CI = 1.063–10.261). Furthermore, the analysis showed that married people were more likely to use WBT for diabetes self-management (OR = 4.92, $p < 0.024$, 95% CI = 1.230–19.740).

Table 3. Multiple regression analysis of factors influencing intention to use web-based technology for diabetes self-management.

Model	B	SE	Exp(B)	p Value	95% C.I. for Exp(B)	
					Lower	Upper
Age	−2.294	0.678	0.101	<0.001 *	0.027	0.381
Gender	0.206	0.554	1.228	0.710	0.415	3.636
Education level	1.195	0.578	3.303	0.039 *	1.063	10.261
Marital status	1.595	0.708	4.928	0.024 *	1.230	19.740
Employment status	0.710	0.650	2.035	0.274	0.569	7.270
Disease duration	−3.086	1.714	0.046	0.072	0.002	1.314

*: Correlation is significant at the 0.05 level.

4. Discussion

According to the data collected in this study, a significant majority (94%) of the Arabic-speaking immigrants living with T2DM in KSA reported having access to the Internet through devices such as mobile phones, computers, and tablets. This aligns with the general population trends according to the Communications, Space, and Technology Commission, who suggest 98.6% of the general population in KSA have access to or use WBT [28]. This result suggests that access to technology is not an issue regardless of migration status, making it possible for more people to be able to access telemedicine and telehealth via smart devices. Several studies have reported similar findings, revealing that a majority of participants, often from lower socioeconomic backgrounds and diverse cultural and linguistic backgrounds, own mobile phones that are equipped with advanced internet capabilities and a range of app features [29–31]. This result is significant for immigrant groups, who typically encounter difficulties in accessing conventional healthcare services in their new countries due to a lack of familiarity with the local healthcare systems [32]. The ability to access health services via smart devices can significantly mitigate these challenges, providing a more inclusive and accessible healthcare environment for these populations [33]. Moreover, the high level of technology access among immigrants also suggests the potential for a broader adoption of telemedicine and telehealth services [33]. This can lead to improved healthcare outcomes, as telehealth not only offers convenience but also ensures continuity of care, particularly for chronic conditions such as diabetes, where regular monitoring and consultations are crucial [34].

While access to technology did not seem to differ greatly between immigrants and the general population in KSA, the study did find that time spent on the internet by an immigrant (average of 2 h/day) was far shorter than the general population in KSA (average of 7 h/day) [28]. This difference may be because of different online habits among the participants or might be a reflection of the general population, which includes more younger people. This trend is substantiated by reports showing that younger individuals exhibit a higher preference for online activities and spend more time engaged in them compared to older age groups [35,36].

The results from the study found that the majority of participants had the intention to use WBT, particularly for planning their diet, monitoring blood glucose levels, and organizing physical activities. More importantly, they perceived WBT favorably, with many citing that the use of such technology facilitated time-saving and improved enjoyment and engagement with self-management of T2DM. These findings were of no surprise as they are consistent with research conducted in Canada, the United States, and The Netherlands [37–39], where the majority of participants expressed positive attitudes towards the use of technology. While the intention to use WBT was generally positive, this study did not evaluate if participants had previously utilized WBT for diabetes self-management. It is highly plausible that despite best intentions to use WBT, immigrants in KSA may still choose not to engage with the use of such technology for their diabetes management. As shown in the study by Boyle and colleagues, people living with diabetes did not utilize WBT when asked to do so. Reasons for this may have related to their lack of awareness of its existence or potential benefits, lack of recommendation from healthcare providers, lack of confidence in using such technology, and feeling fatigued after its use [40]. Future research should focus on assessing the actual utilization of WBT for diabetes self-management among respondents who expressed intentions to use it, to determine the extent to which these technologies are effectively employed in managing T2DM.

The study, in line with the findings of Dobson et al. [24], revealed significant positive correlations between specific demographic factors such as age, level of education, marital status, and the use of WBT for diabetes self-management. It was observed that younger patients exhibited a heightened interest and a stronger intention to utilize WBT in the future. Moreover, individuals with higher educational levels demonstrated a more favorable attitude towards the use of WBT, corroborating the findings of Song et al. [41] and Jafari et al. [42], which suggest that higher education is linked with increased confidence and better judgment in employing mHealth technologies. In addition, married participants demonstrated a greater interest in utilizing WBT for diabetes management. This finding suggests a potential direction for future research to investigate how health professionals can utilize this knowledge to identify individuals best suited for receiving mHealth technologies and support. Further studies could delve into how individuals' existing knowledge and support systems can be harnessed to optimize the effective use of digital tools in managing chronic conditions such as diabetes.

To the best of our knowledge, our study is the first to investigate the attitudes and intentions of Arabic-speaking immigrants with T2DM in KSA regarding the use of WBT for diabetes self-management. It should be noted that our study was conducted with a sample of 91 patients using convenience sampling, which could be considered a limitation. While the study survey was based on validated questionnaires, the survey was not tested for its face validity to ensure that all questions were presented in a culturally appropriate manner for Arabic-speaking immigrants. However, the lead researcher from this study is an insider to the culture in KSA and did adapt the questionnaire to best suit the cultural needs of the participants.

5. Conclusions

Among Arabic-speaking immigrants residing in KSA and living with T2DM, WBT is commonly used for social interactions and information-seeking purposes. Overall, access to technology does not appear to be a limiting factor, and the majority of participants were positive towards utilizing such technology as a tool for managing their diabetes. Most of these individuals expressed a willingness to integrate WBT into their diabetes care, specifically for diet planning, blood glucose monitoring, and communication with healthcare professionals. Future research needs to evaluate if Arabic-speaking immigrants indeed will utilize WBT when asked to manage T2DM. If utilization of WBT differed from the intention to use WBT, further studies should focus on exploring barriers to utilization of WBT for T2DM management.

Supplementary Materials: The following supporting information can be downloaded at: https://www.mdpi.com/article/10.3390/diabetology5010007/s1, Survey S1: the survey instruments.

Author Contributions: Conceptualization, S.G., C.T. and J.T.; methodology, A.A.; formal analysis, A.A.; data collection, A.A.; writing—original draft preparation, A.A.; writing—review and editing, S.G., C.T. and J.T.; funding acquisition, no formal funding; however, A.A. is a PhD student who received full scholarship from University of Tabuk (KSA). All authors have read and agreed to the published version of the manuscript.

Funding: This research received no external funding.

Institutional Review Board Statement: The study was conducted in accordance with the Declaration of Helsinki and approved by the Ethics Committee of La Trobe university (Ethics Application Number (HEC21273).

Informed Consent Statement: Implied informed consent was obtained by completing the survey.

Data Availability Statement: The data presented in this study are available on request from the corresponding author (due to ethical restrictions).

Acknowledgments: The authors wish to extend their sincere gratitude to Al Ameen Hospital, Taif City, Saudi Arabia, for their invaluable support in facilitating the data collection process for this study. The hospital's cooperation was instrumental in providing a conducive environment for gathering essential research data, thereby significantly contributing to the success of this project. Special thanks are also due to Ninorta Morad for her crucial role in translating the survey from English to Arabic. Her meticulous efforts in ensuring the accuracy and cultural relevance of the translation. Her contribution has been a key factor in the smooth execution and overall success of this study. Also, the authors would like to extend special appreciation to Xia Li for her valuable assistance in handling the statistical aspects of this project. Lastly, the authors acknowledge the assistance of AI platforms such as Grammarly and ChatGPT in rephrasing sentences. This support proved particularly valuable as the authors' first language is not English, helping to enhance the clarity and effectiveness of communication.

Conflicts of Interest: The authors declare no conflict of interest.

References

1. Fan, W. Epidemiology in Type 2 Diabetes mellitus and cardiovascular disease. *Cardiovasc. Endocrinol.* **2017**, *6*, 8–16. [CrossRef]
2. International Diabetes Federation. *IDF Diabetes Atlas*, 9th ed.; International Diabetes Federation: Brussels, Belgium, 2021. Available online: http://www.diabetesatlas.org (accessed on 16 November 2023).
3. Al Dawish, M.; Robert, A. Type 2 Diabetes mellitus in Saudi Arabia. In *Handbook of Healthcare in the Arab World*; Springer: Berlin/Heidelberg, Germany, 2019; pp. 1–18.
4. Wani, K.; Alfawaz, H.; Alnaami, A.M.; Sabico, S.; Khattak, M.N.K.; Al-Attas, O.S.; Alokail, M.S.; Alharbi, M.; Chrousos, G.P.; Kumar, S.; et al. Effects of a 12-Month Intensive Lifestyle Monitoring Program in Predominantly Overweight/Obese Arab Adults with Prediabetes. *Nutrients* **2020**, *12*, 464. [CrossRef]
5. Renzaho, A.M. *Globalisation, Migration and Health: Challenges and Opportunities*; Imperial College Press: London, UK, 2016.
6. Reus-Pons, M.; Mulder, C.H.; Kibele, E.U.B.; Janssen, F. Differences in the health transition patterns of migrants and non-migrants aged 50 and older in southern and western Europe (2004–2015). *BMC Med.* **2018**, *16*, 57. [CrossRef]
7. El-Kebbi, I.M.; Bidikian, N.H.; Hneiny, L.; Nasrallah, M.P. Epidemiology of type 2 diabetes in the Middle East and North Africa: Challenges and call for action. *World J. Diabetes* **2021**, *12*, 1401–1425. [CrossRef]
8. Robert, A.; Al Dawish, A.; Braham, B.; Musallam, A.; Al Hayek, A.; Al Kahtany, H. Type 2 Diabetes Mellitus in Saudi Arabia: Major Challenges and Possible Solutions. *Curr. Diabetes Rev.* **2016**, *13*, 59–64. [CrossRef]
9. Alaqeel, A. Pediatric diabetes in Saudi Arabia: Challenges and potential solutions. A review article. *Int. J. Pediatr. Adolesc. Med.* **2019**, *6*, 125–130. [CrossRef]
10. Alzubaidi, H.; Oliveira, H.; Samorinha, C.; Mc Namara, K.; Shaw, J.E. Acculturation and glycaemic control in Arab immigrants with type 2 diabetes in Australia. *Diabetologia* **2024**. ahead of print. [CrossRef] [PubMed]
11. Almutairi, M. Quality of Diabetes Management in Saudi Arabia: A Review of Existing Barriers. *Arch. Iran. Med.* **2015**, *18*, 816–821. [PubMed]
12. Zaho, J.; Freeman, B.; Li, M. Can mobile phone apps influence people's health behavior change? An evidence review. *J. Med. Internet Res.* **2016**, *18*, e287. [CrossRef] [PubMed]
13. Novianto, F.; Putri, M.Y.; Fajrin, F.N.; Fadhilah, M.; Khairunnisa, R. The Effectiveness of Health Management-Assisted Technology on Glycated Hemoglobin Levels in Patients with Type 2 Diabetes Mellitus: Meta-Analysis. 2021. Available online: https://scite.ai/reports/10.26911/thejhpm.2021.06.02.01 (accessed on 24 November 2023).
14. Hunt, C.W. Technology and diabetes self-management: An integrative review. *World J. Diabetes* **2015**, *6*, 225–233. [CrossRef] [PubMed]
15. Glasgow, R.E.; Kurz, D.; King, D.; Dickman, J.M.; Faber, A.J.; Halterman, E.; Woolley, T.; Toobert, D.J.; Strycker, L.A.; Estabrooks, P.A. Twelve-month outcomes of an Internet-based diabetes self-management support program. *Patient Educ. Couns.* **2012**, *87*, 81–92. [CrossRef]
16. Song, M.; Choe, M.A.; Kim, K.S.; Yi, M.S.; Lee, I.; Kim, J.; Lee, M.; Cho, Y.M.; Shim, Y.S. An evaluation of Web-based education as an alternative to group lectures for diabetes self-management. *Nurs. Health Sci.* **2009**, *11*, 277–284. [CrossRef]
17. Bond, G.E. Lessons learned from the implementation of a Web-based nursing intervention. *Comput. Inform. Nurs.* **2006**, *24*, 66–74. [CrossRef]
18. Bandura, A. Health promotion by social cognitive means. *Health Educ. Behav. Off. Publ. Soc. Public Health Educ.* **2004**, *31*, 143–164. [CrossRef] [PubMed]
19. Lorig, K.; Ritter, P.L.; Laurent, D.D.; Plant, K.; Green, M.; Jernigan, V.B.; Case, S. Online diabetes self-management program: A randomized study. *Diabetes Care* **2010**, *33*, 1275–1281. [CrossRef] [PubMed]
20. Norton, S.; Matthews, F.E.; Brayne, C. A commentary on studies presenting projections of the future prevalence of dementia. *BMC Public Health* **2013**, *13*, 1. [CrossRef] [PubMed]
21. Sarkar, U.; Karter, A.J.; Liu, J.Y.; Adler, N.E.; Nguyen, R.; Lopez, A.; Schillinger, D. The literacy divide: Health literacy and the use of an internet-based patient portal in an integrated health system-results from the diabetes study of northern California (DISTANCE). *J. Health Commun.* **2010**, *15* (Suppl. S2), 183–196. [CrossRef] [PubMed]
22. Alaiad, A.; Zhou, L. Patients' Adoption of WSN-Based Smart Home Healthcare Systems: An Integrated Model of Facilitators and Barriers. *IEEE Trans. Prof. Commun.* **2017**, *60*, 4–23. [CrossRef]
23. Lyles, C.R.; Ratanawongsa, N.; Bolen, S.D.; Samal, L. mHealth and Health Information Technology Tools for Diverse Patients with Diabetes. *J. Diabetes Res.* **2017**, *2017*, 1704917. [CrossRef]
24. Dobson, K.G.; Hall, P. A pilot study examining patient attitudes and intentions to adopt assistive technologies into type 2 diabetes self-management. *J. Diabetes Sci. Technol.* **2014**, *9*, 309–315. [CrossRef] [PubMed]
25. Rangraz Jeddi, F.; Nabovati, E.; Hamidi, R. Mobile phone usage in patients with type II diabetes and their intention to use it for self-management: A cross-sectional study in Iran. *BMC Med. Inf. Decis. Mak.* **2020**, *20*, 24. [CrossRef]
26. Alzubaidi, H.; Mc Namara, K.; Versace, V.L. Predictors of effective therapeutic relationships between pharmacists and patients with type 2 diabetes: Comparison between Arabic-speaking and Caucasian English-speaking patients. *Res. Soc. Adm. Pharm.* **2018**, *14*, 1064–1071. [CrossRef] [PubMed]
27. IBM Corp. *IBM SPSS Statistics for Windows*, Version 27.0; IBM Corp: Armonk, NY, USA, 2020.

28. Communications, Space & Technology Commission. Internet System and Its Usage in the Kingdom of Saudi Arabia. Saudi Internet Report. 2022. Available online: https://www.cst.gov.sa/en/mediacenter/pressreleases/Pages/2023030802.aspx (accessed on 8 March 2023).
29. Fox, S.; Duggan, M. *Tracking for Health*; Pew Internet & American Life Project: Washington, DC, USA, 2013.
30. Tirado, M. Role of mobile health in the care of culturally and linguistically diverse US populations. *Perspect. Health Inf. Manag.* **2011**, *8*, 1e. [PubMed]
31. Heath-Brown, N. *Pew Research Center. The Statesman's Yearbook 2016: The Politics, Cultures and Economies of the World*; Palgrave Macmillan: London, UK, 2015; p. 80.
32. Sarría-Santamera, A.; Hijas-Gómez, A.I.; Carmona, R.; Gimeno-Feliú, L.A. A systematic review of the use of health services by immigrants and native populations. *Public Health Rev.* **2016**, *37*, 28. [CrossRef] [PubMed]
33. Anderson-Lewis, C.; Darville, G.; Mercado, R.E.; Howell, S.; Di Maggio, S. mHealth Technology Use and Implications in Historically Underserved and Minority Populations in the United States: Systematic Literature Review. *JMIR Mhealth Uhealth* **2018**, *6*, e128. [CrossRef] [PubMed]
34. Lyles, C.R.; Tieu, L.; Sarkar, U.; Kiyoi, S.; Sadasivaiah, S.; Hoskote, M.; Ratanawongsa, N.; Schillinger, D. A Randomized Trial to Train Vulnerable Primary Care Patients to Use a Patient Portal. *J. Am. Board Fam. Med. JABFM* **2019**, *32*, 248–258. [CrossRef] [PubMed]
35. Australian Government. The digital lives of younger Australians–ACMA. Communications and media in Australia. 2021. Available online: https://www.acma.gov.au/sites/default/files/2021-05/The%20digital%20lives%20of%20younger%20Australians.pdf (accessed on 20 December 2023).
36. Bailey, D.; Wells, A.; Desai, T.; Sullivan, K.; Kass, L. Physical activity and sitting time changes in response to the COVID-19 lockdown in England. *PLoS ONE* **2022**, *17*, e0271482. [CrossRef]
37. Conway, N.; Campbell, I.; Forbes, P.; Cunningham, S.; Wake, D. mHealth applications for diabetes: User preference and implications for app development. *Health Inform. J.* **2016**, *22*, 1111–1120. [CrossRef]
38. Jenkins, C.; Burkett, N.-S.; Ovbiagele, B.; Mueller, M.; Patel, S.; Brunner-Jackson, B.; Saulson, R.; Treiber, F. Stroke patients and their attitudes toward mHealth monitoring to support blood pressure control and medication adherence. *Mhealth* **2016**, *2*, 24. [CrossRef]
39. Hofstede, J.; de Bie, J.; Van Wijngaarden, B.; Heijmans, M. Knowledge, use and attitude toward eHealth among patients with chronic lung diseases. *Int. J. Med. Inform.* **2014**, *83*, 967–974. [CrossRef]
40. Boyle, L.; Grainger, R.; Hall, R.M.; Krebs, J.D. Use of and beliefs about mobile phone apps for diabetes self-management: Surveys of people in a hospital diabetes clinic and diabetes health professionals in New Zealand. *JMIR Mhealth Uhealth* **2017**, *5*, e85. [CrossRef] [PubMed]
41. Song, H.; Cramer, E.M.; McRoy, S.; May, A. Information needs, seeking behaviors, and support among low-income expectant women. *Women Health* **2013**, *53*, 824–842. [CrossRef] [PubMed]
42. Jafari, J.J.; Moonaghi, H.K.; Ahmady, S.; Zary, N.; Masiello, I. Investigating readiness to use internet and mobile services of diabetic patients of a middle-income country. *PeerJ PrePrints* **2015**, *3*, e1111v2. [CrossRef]

Disclaimer/Publisher's Note: The statements, opinions and data contained in all publications are solely those of the individual author(s) and contributor(s) and not of MDPI and/or the editor(s). MDPI and/or the editor(s) disclaim responsibility for any injury to people or property resulting from any ideas, methods, instructions or products referred to in the content.

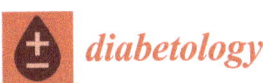

Article

A Comparative Analysis of Machine Learning Models for the Detection of Undiagnosed Diabetes Patients

Simon Lebech Cichosz *, Clara Bender and Ole Hejlesen

Department of Health Science and Technology, Aalborg University, 9000 Aalborg, Denmark
* Correspondence: simcich@hst.aau.dk; Tel.: +45-9940-2020; Fax: +45-9815-4008

Abstract: Introduction: Early detection of type 2 diabetes is essential for preventing long-term complications. However, screening the entire population for diabetes is not cost-effective, so identifying individuals at high risk for this disease is crucial. The aim of this study was to compare the performance of five diverse machine learning (ML) models in classifying undiagnosed diabetes using large heterogeneous datasets. Methods: We used machine learning data from several years of the National Health and Nutrition Examination Survey (NHANES) from 2005 to 2018 to identify people with undiagnosed diabetes. The dataset included 45,431 participants, and biochemical confirmation of glucose control (HbA1c) were used to identify undiagnosed diabetes. The predictors were based on simple and clinically obtainable variables, which could be feasible for prescreening for diabetes. We included five ML models for comparison: random forest, AdaBoost, RUSBoost, LogitBoost, and a neural network. Results: The prevalence of undiagnosed diabetes was 4%. For the classification of undiagnosed diabetes, the area under the ROC curve (AUC) values were between 0.776 and 0.806. The positive predictive values (PPVs) were between 0.083 and 0.091, the negative predictive values (NPVs) were between 0.984 and 0.99, and the sensitivities were between 0.742 and 0.871. Conclusion: We have demonstrated that several types of classification models can accurately classify undiagnosed diabetes from simple and clinically obtainable variables. These results suggest that the use of machine learning for prescreening for undiagnosed diabetes could be a useful tool in clinical practice.

Keywords: undiagnosed diabetes; diabetes mellitus; machine learning; prescreening; clinically obtainable variables; NHANES

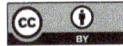

1. Introduction

The prevalence of type 2 diabetes is on the rise, leading to increased occurrences of illness and mortality and escalated healthcare expenditures. The incidence of type 2 diabetes varies across regions such as the UK, the U.S., China, and the United Arab Emirates, encompassing a range of 7% to 34% of the respective population [1,2]. Of individuals in the United States, 9.7% have received a formal diagnosis of diabetes, while an additional 4.3% are living with diabetes but remain undiagnosed. Notably, approximately 30% of those who eventually receive a diabetes diagnosis exhibit associated complications [3].

The timely identification of type 2 diabetes holds significance due to its potential to significantly mitigate long-term complications through rigorous diabetes management. Nevertheless, conducting diabetes screening across the entire population lacks cost-effectiveness, thus emphasizing the need to prioritize the recognition of individuals with a heightened susceptibility to the condition [4,5]. Numerous investigations regarding diabetes screening have been conducted within the previous ten years. Risk prediction or stratification models can serve the purpose of identifying individuals at an elevated risk level for diabetes, allowing for subsequent targeted testing. Typically, these models incorporate a blend of variables, encompassing weight, lifestyle, familial background, and clinical measurements, and are formulated through the utilization of multivariable statistical techniques [6–8].

Nevertheless, numerous of these models are not extensively employed within clinical practice, primarily owing to their foundation on data gathered for alternate objectives. This circumstance can decrease the relevance of these findings when applied to a broader population [9]. Additionally, attempts are often made to create models that are easy to use in clinical practice. This is often accomplished by condensing continuous variables into distinct categories or opting for predictors in a subjective manner. However, such approaches can result in excessive simplification and a consequent decrease in the models' overall efficacy [10,11].

Analyzing data on diabetes can be difficult because medical data often exhibit non-linear, nonnormal, correlated, and complex characteristics [12]. Machine learning (ML) methods have the potential to structure and utilize these complex patterns to classify diseases. It has previously been reported that ML could be utilized in diabetes for different purposes [13–19].

Others have reported ML approaches for the detection of diabetes and prediabetes [20–25]. However, it is still unclear which ML methods are best at capturing the complexity of the data to aid in selecting people at high risk of undiagnosed diabetes.

The objective of this study was to compare the performance of five diverse ML models for classifying undiagnosed diabetes using a large heterogeneous dataset.

2. Methods

2.1. Data Source

To identify individuals with undiagnosed diabetes using machine learning, we used data from multiple years of the National Health and Nutrition Examination Survey (NHANES) from 2005 to 2018 [26], which included HbA1c (glycated hemoglobin) data. HbA1c is recommended for the diagnosis of diabetes in most patient groups by the American Diabetes Association [27]. The NHANES study was executed by the National Center for Health Statistics, a division of the Centers for Disease Control and Prevention. This research employs intricate sampling techniques to determine the demographic composition of the U.S. populace. This inclusivity extends to the overrepresentation of subpopulations, such as elderly individuals and various racial and ethnic minorities. Over the period spanning 2005 to 2018, a comprehensive total of 70,190 participants were enrolled in the NHANES.

The present investigation involved individuals aged >20 years, excluding pregnant individuals and those with a documented diabetes diagnosis. A participant's diabetes diagnosis was ascertained by their affirmative response to the survey. Have you ever been informed by a medical professional that you have diabetes?

Using these data, we developed and compared ML models for diabetes prescreening in patients with undiagnosed diabetes.

2.2. End Points

Our objective was to compare five machine learning models for the detection of undiagnosed diabetes (prevalence) in the NHANES cohort.

We included two binary end points for classification:

The primary endpoint (ap1) for the classification of undiagnosed diabetes was defined as an HbA1c $\geq$ 6.5% (48 mmol/mol) without a previous diagnosis of diabetes.

The secondary endpoint (ap2) was for the classification of undiagnosed diabetes (defined by an HbA1c $\geq$ 6.5% (48 mmol/mol) without a previous diagnosis of diabetes) or known diabetes.

2.3. Variables and Selection

We included simple variables commonly associated with the risk of diabetes that could be used in a practical prescreening procedure. The variables included age, sex, ethnicity, weight, height, waist circumference, sleep duration, BMI, blood pressure (BP), physical activity, smoking, alcohol use, education, and the ratio of family income to poverty. Variable selection were performed according to an automatic approach using the training data, 3-fold cross-validation, and receiver operating characteristic (ROC) area under the curve (AUC) improvements as criteria for the inclusion of variables. Missing data among variables used for classification and prediction are common both in studies and during clinical usage. However, the chosen ML methods implemented in this study can incorporate missing values into the modeling approach without the need for imputation or case deletion [28].

2.4. Model Development

We included five ML models for comparison: random forest, AdaBoost, RUSBoost, LogitBoost, and a neural network. These specific models were compared because previous studies have shown high performance with ensemble and neural network models in general disease classification [29,30]. The rationale behind selecting these models is rooted in the collective strengths they bring to the task of disease classification, which aims to provide a comprehensive comparison across diverse approaches. By including models with different underlying mechanisms (boosting, bagging, or neural networks), we aim to identify the most suitable model for our specific dataset and research objectives.

The models were trained/developed using a sample of 80% (training data) of the individuals in each group and tested on the remaining 20% (test data). This process was conducted in such a manner that 20% of the data were saved for testing the final models; hence, the test data were not used to optimize the models further. The training data were used to select variables through forward selection and to optimize and train the models; cross-validation was used to minimize overfitting of the models. Due to a class imbalance in the dataset, the optimization was conducted with an evaluation criterion based on the precision-recall curve area under the curve (PR-AUC):

A schematic of the procedure is illustrated in Figure 1.

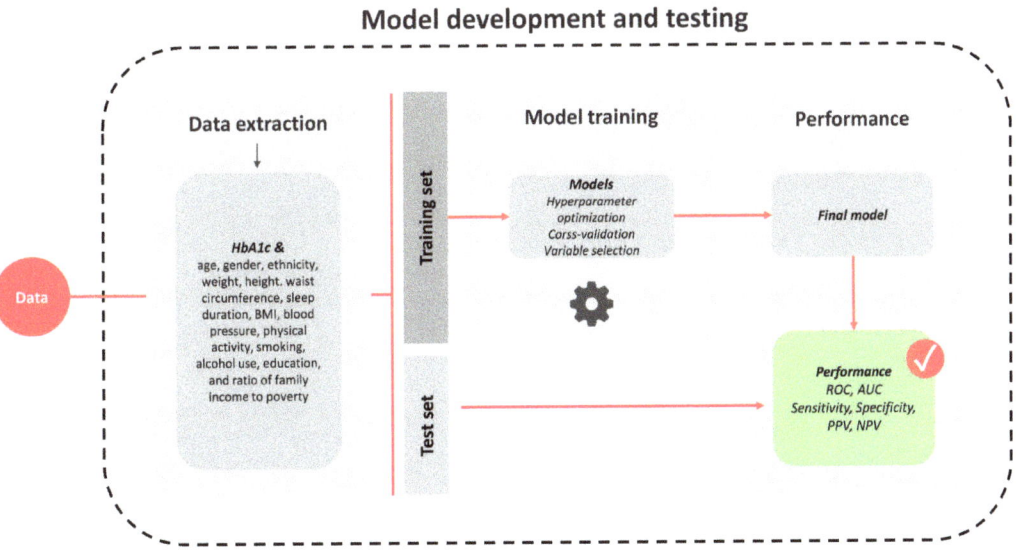

Figure 1. Illustrates model development and performance testing.

All the models were developed and implemented using MATLAB R2021b (MathWorks, Natick, MA, USA).

2.4.1. Random Forest Model

The random forest algorithm is a machine learning method [31] that uses a group of decision trees to make predictions. During the training process, many decision trees are constructed, and the output of the random forest is determined by the majority vote of the trees. Each tree in the forest are based on a random sample of data. The final prediction is made by combining the predictions of all the individual trees. As the number of trees in the forest increases, the accuracy of the predictions tends to improve. Hyperparameter estimation was performed using a grid search strategy. We optimized the number of trees, depth of trees, and minimum number of samples to perform splitting.

2.4.2. AdaBoost

Adaptive boosting (AdaBoost) [32] is an ensemble learning algorithm that is used to improve the accuracy of a weak learner (such as a decision tree). This process involves iteratively training the weak learner and adjusting the weights of the training data at each iteration so that the misclassified examples are given higher weights. The final model is a combination of all the weak learners, with each weak learner contributing a weight to the final prediction. One of the main benefits of AdaBoost is that it is simple to implement and relatively resistant to overfitting problems, making it a good choice for situations where the training data are limited. Hyperparameter estimation was performed using a grid search strategy. We optimized the number of weak learners and the learning rate.

2.4.3. RUSBoost

Random undersampling boosting (RUSBoost) [33] is a variant of the AdaBoost algorithm that are designed to handle imbalanced datasets. The imbalanced datasets are datasets in which one class (the minority class; in our case, individuals with undiagnosed diabetes) has significantly fewer examples than the other class (the majority class; in our cases, individuals without undiagnosed diabetes). In such cases of imbalance, AdaBoost can be prone to bias toward the majority class, leading to poor performance for the minority class. RUSBoost addresses this issue by randomly undersampling the majority class at each iteration. By undersampling the majority class, RUSBoost ensures that each weak learner are trained on a balanced dataset. Hyperparameter estimation was performed using a grid search strategy. We optimized the number of weak learners and the learning rate.

2.4.4. LogitBoost

LogitBoost [34] is a popular boosting modification that can be applied to binary classification problems. From a statistical standpoint, LogitBoost can be seen as an additive tree regression by minimizing the logistic loss. One of the benefits of LogitBoost is that it is relatively easy to implement, and it can often achieve good performance with relatively little hyperparameter tuning. It is also resistant to overfitting, which makes it a good fit for use on noisy or high-dimensional data. Hyperparameter estimation was performed using a grid search strategy. We optimized the number of weak learners and the learning rate.

2.4.5. Neural Network

A neural network is a machine learning model inspired by the structure and function of the human brain. It is composed of layers of interconnected nodes, or neurons, that process and transmit information. We implemented a feedforward neural network with the following architecture: an input layer, three fully connected hidden layers [3, 2, 4 neurons], a softmax layer, and a classification layer. In the training process, 30% of the training dataset were used as the validation dataset to minimize overfitting of the model. Hyperparameter estimation was performed using a grid search strategy. We optimized the number of neurons in the hidden layers.

2.5. Model Assessment

Test datasets were used to assess the performance of the five models. Receiver operating characteristic (ROC) curves and receiver operating characteristic (ROC) curves were used to compare the performance of the models for classifying undiagnosed diabetes (ap1) from that of undiagnosed diabetes and known diabetes (ap2). Ninety-five percent confidence intervals (CIs) for the receiver operating characteristic (ROC) curve were estimated using bootstrap replicates (n = 1000). Furthermore, a specific threshold (based on the maximized Youden index) was used to compare the sensitivity, specificity, positive predictive value (PPV), and negative predictive value (NPV) to better understand the capabilities of the models for usage in clinical practice during a prescreening procedure.

3. Results

A total of 45,431 participants were included in the analysis, and 36,162 participants were excluded from the analysis due to missing HbA1c measurements, age criteria, or pregnancy. Among the included participants, 1297 had undiagnosed diabetes (the prevalence of undiagnosed diabetes was 3.2%), 4772 had known diabetes, and 9556 had prediabetes. The characteristics of the included participants are presented in Table 1.

Table 1. The baseline characteristics of people with prediabetes, undiagnosed diabetes, or diabetes. Significance ($p < 0.05$) is indicated between undiagnosed diabetes and no diabetes (N), prediabetes (P), and diabetes (D).

	No Diabetes	Prediabetes	Undiagnosed Diabetes	Diabetes	Significance $p < 0.05$
n	29,806	9556	1297	4772	
Age, years	36 (19.3)	54.2 (18.4)	57.7 (15)	61.9 (13.9)	NPD
Male, %	48.1	50	52.5	50.5	N
BMI, kg/m^2	26.8 (6.5)	30.1 (7.2)	33.1 (7.8)	32.4 (7.7)	NPD
Height, cm	166.9 (10.1)	166.1 (10.2)	166.1 (9.9)	165.6 (10.7)	N
Weight, kg	75.1 (20.6)	83.5 (22.5)	91.8 (24.2)	89.5 (24.5)	NPD
Systolic BP, mmHg	117.3 (16.5)	127.5 (19)	134.1 (20.9)	131.6 (20.5)	NPD
Diastolic BP, mmHg	67 (13.5)	70.4 (14.4)	72.3 (15.3)	67.7 (14.6)	NPD
Smoking, %	12.6	16.5	17.3	11.7	ND
Physically active, %	36.1	18.7	10.7	8.5	NPD
Drinking alcohol, days/yrs	12.6 (53.2)	10.9 (51.9)	9 (53.8)	10 (54)	N
Family income to poverty ratio	2.5 (1.6)	2.4 (1.6)	2.2 (1.5)	2.3 (1.5)	NP
Sleep, h	7.2 (3.1)	7 (1.6)	7 (3.1)	7.4 (4.8)	ND
Hispanic-Mexican American, %	18.3	15.3	21.6	17.2	NPD
Hispanic-Other Hispanic, %	9.4	9.9	10.4	9.9	
Non-Hispanic White, %	41.9	35.5	27.4	34.3	NPD
Non-Hispanic Black, %	19	28.2	28.5	27.6	N

Table 2 shows the ROC AUCs for the classifiers along with a selected cutoff, which included sensitivity, specificity, positive predictive value (PPV), and negative predictive value (NPV). Figure 2 shows the ROC curves (left) and the precision-recall curves (right) for the five classifiers.

Table 2. The ROC AUC (95% confidence interval) for the classifiers, along with a selected cutoff based on the maximized Youden index, which includes sensitivity, specificity, positive predictive value (PPV), and negative predictive value (NPV).

	ROC AUC	Sensitivity	Specificity	PPV	NPV
Undiagnosed diabetes					
RF	0.786 (0.765; 0.810)	0.855	0.603	0.083	0.99
AdaBoost	0.776 (0.750; 0.797)	0.742	0.674	0.087	0.984
RUSBoost	0.792 (0.767; 0.812)	0.824	0.657	0.091	0.989
LogitBoost	0.799 (0.775; 0.823)	0.871	0.615	0.086	0.991
Neural network	0.806 (0.782; 0.827)	0.848	0.628	0.087	0.99
Diabetes + Undiagnosed diabetes					
RF	0.800 (0.788; 0.815)	0.814	0.637	0.290	0.949
AdaBoost	0.787 (0.775; 0.799)	0.819	0.628	0.287	0.95
RUSBoost	0.796 (0.782; 0.809)	0.818	0.631	0.288	0.95
LogitBoost	0.802 (0.789; 0.814)	0.816	0.645	0.295	0.95
Neural network	0.800 (0.787; 0.810)	0.821	0.64	0.294	0.952

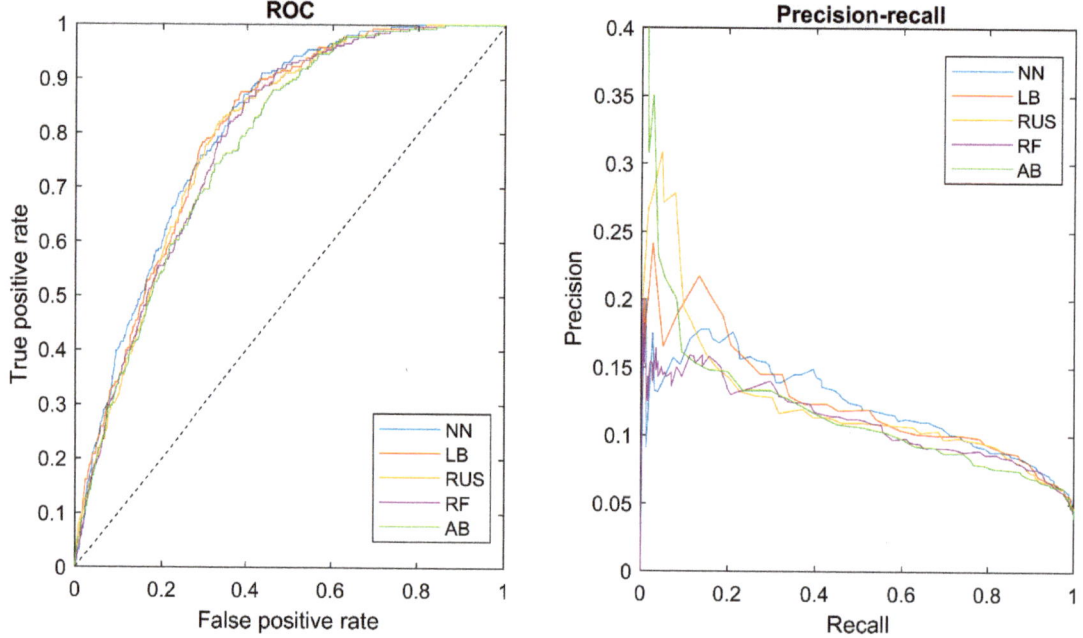

Figure 2. The left figure shows the receiver operating characteristic (ROC) curves for the classifiers: neural network (NN), LogitBoost (LB), RUSBoost (RUS), random forest (RF), and AdaBoost (AB) classifiers. The right figure shows the precision-recall for the classifiers: neural network (NN), LogitBoost (LB), RUSBoost (RUS), random forest (RF), and AdaBoost (AB).

Primary endpoint (ap1): For the classification of undiagnosed diabetes (no diabetes or prediabetes vs. undiagnosed diabetes), the area under the ROC curve (AUC) was between 0.776 and 0.806. The PPV was between 0.083 and 0.091, the NPV was between 0.984 and 0.99, and the sensitivity was between 0.742 and 0.871. Figure 3 shows the selected predictors for each model using forward selection and cross-validation. Age and ethnicity (non-Hispanic white) were selected for all models, and the economic ratio was selected for four out of five models.

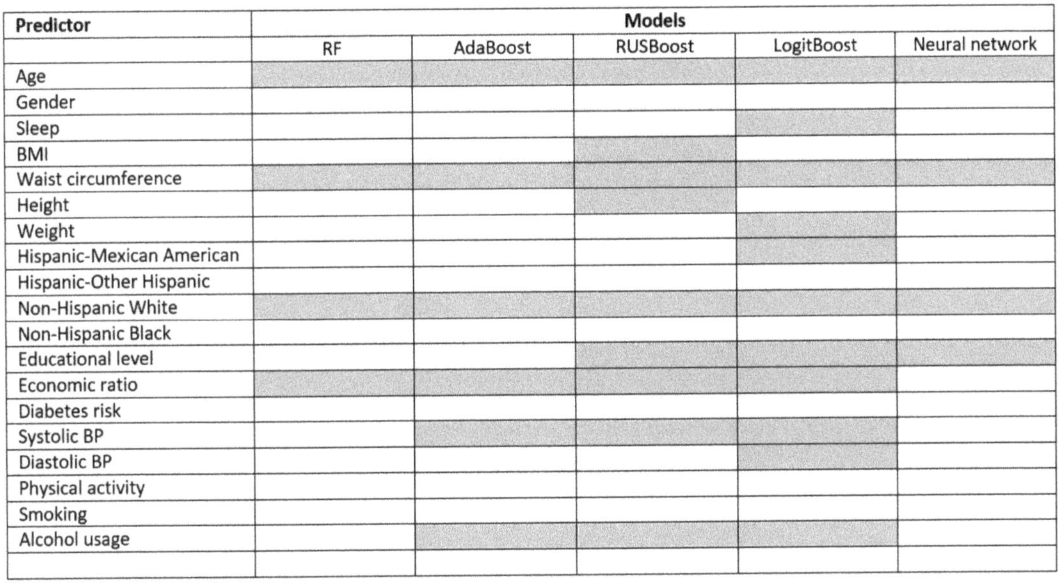

Predictor	Models				
	RF	AdaBoost	RUSBoost	LogitBoost	Neural network
Age	■	■	■	■	■
Gender				■	
Sleep				■	
BMI			■		
Waist circumference			■		
Height			■		
Weight				■	
Hispanic-Mexican American					
Hispanic-Other Hispanic					
Non-Hispanic White	■	■	■	■	■
Non-Hispanic Black					
Educational level			■		■
Economic ratio	■		■	■	■
Diabetes risk					
Systolic BP					
Diastolic BP					
Physical activity					
Smoking					
Alcohol usage			■		■

Figure 3. The selected predictors/features for the model(s). Gray indicates that the selected predictor was selected in the forward feature selection using 3-fold cross-validation.

Secondary endpoint (ap2): For the classification of undiagnosed diabetes + known diabetes (no diabetes or prediabetes vs. undiagnosed diabetes or known diabetes), the receiver operating characteristic (ROC) curves were between 0.787 and 0.802. The PPV was between 0.287 and 295; the NPV was between 0.949 and 952; and the sensitivity was between 0.787 and 802.

4. Discussion

This study aimed to compare the performance of an ML model in classifying undiagnosed diabetes from known diabetes using a large heterogeneous dataset utilizing simple and obtainable clinical information. For the classification of undiagnosed diabetes, the comparison did not reveal large differences in model performance among the five models. All the included models performed well and could be utilized in a clinical prescreening program to identify people for subsequent diabetes testing. The PPV was approximately 8–9%, which is low but is expected for this type of prescreening. Other risk score studies have reported PPVs between 4 and 8% [6,35]. This means that for each of the 1000 people we screened, if a sensitivity of 80% was selected, ~392 people would be eligible for subsequent testing, and out of those people, ~32 would have undiagnosed diabetes. Furthermore, ~8 people will not be diagnosed with diabetes. A substantial portion of the people selected for subsequent testing who did not have undiagnosed diabetes (false positives) were diagnosed with prediabetes. Identifying people with prediabetes could lead to health-promoting initiatives for the group to slow or stop the progression from prediabetes to diabetes.

The exact cutoff for such a prescreening procedure also needs to be considered in a cost-benefit analysis, which is beyond the scope of this paper.

For the classification of undiagnosed diabetes + known diabetes, similar trends were observed—the choice of model did not significantly change the performance. However, the PPV was much greater than that of undiagnosed diabetes alone. This is also expected, as the prevalence of prediabetes at the population level is much greater.

The predictors included in this study can be categorized into three groups: demographic, clinical, and lifestyle predictors. These predictors were used to develop machine learning models to prescreen undiagnosed diabetes patients.

Demographic predictors have been shown to be associated with diabetes incidence [36]. In our study, age and ethnicity were included as predictors in all the proposed models. Clinical variables have been consistently associated with diabetes risk. For example, higher BMI and waist circumference have been shown to be strongly associated with diabetes risk, with individuals with a BMI of 30 or higher being at a greater risk of developing diabetes. Waist circumference and systolic blood pressure were also included as predictors in most of the models. BMI was only selected for one of the compared models; however, studies have shown that waist circumference may be a more specific predictor of dangerous overweight [37]. Lifestyle predictors have also been shown to be associated with diabetes risk [36]. For example, physical activity has been shown to lower diabetes risk, while smoking and alcohol usage have been shown to increase diabetes risk [38]. In our study, alcohol usage and indirect measures of lifestyle, such as education level and economic status, were included as predictors. Surprisingly, physical activity and smoking were not included as predictors. The explanation could be that it might be difficult to capture the discriminative information in these predictors using a questionnaire-based approach or that the information is captured indirectly by other predictors.

4.1. Comparison to Other Related Work

Over the past few decades, several machine learning approaches and classic statistical predictive models have been published on the topic of screening for undiagnosed diabetes. Baan et al. [35] developed three predictive models (logistics regression) based on a sample of participants from the Rotterdam Study (n = 1016) aged 55 to 75 years who were not known to have diabetes. The authors reported ROC AUCs of up to 0.74. Bang et al. [36] developed a simple scoring system (based on logistic regression) based on the Korea National Health and Nutrition Examination Survey (KNHANES) and compared it with previous scoring systems. Bang et al. reported ROC AUCs of up to 0.73. Moreover, Cichosz et al. [23] suggested an extended predictive feature search strategy to model a logistic regression for the prediction of undiagnosed diabetes. They reported an ROC AUC of 0.78.

Yu et al. [24] used a support vector machine (SVM) approach to identify undiagnosed and known diabetes in the 1999–2004 sample of the NHANES with successful performance (AUC = 0.83). However, Yu et al. did not predict undiagnosed diabetes separately, which makes comparison difficult.

4.2. Strengths and Limitations

An important advantage of this research lies in our utilization of a substantial and diverse dataset from the NHANES. This dataset are distinctive because it comprises nationally representative survey data that have been weighted, accurately reflecting the composition of the entire U.S. populace. As a result, the findings are likely to have a reasonable degree of applicability to the broader U.S. population when used in a screening process. Nevertheless, the application of these models in different global regions necessitates careful consideration, and it is imperative to validate their effectiveness in these populations before embracing them on a larger scale.

The approach introduced in this research were rooted in data-driven analysis. We carefully chose variables and refined our models to achieve optimal performance. Although the chosen variables were all characterized as readily available or easily obtainable clinical data, certain pieces of information hold greater clinical practicality, particularly in the context of conducting large-scale population screenings. Should these models be considered for practical clinical use, it becomes important to assess the significance of each variable, with an emphasis on selecting those that offer the most effortlessly attainable information.

A limitation of this study is the definition of undiagnosed diabetes, as it was based on a single lab value of HbA1c above 6.5%. The American Diabetes Association (ADA) recommends that at least two HbA1c levels be measured to fully establish a diabetes diagnosis. Furthermore, known diabetes diagnoses rely on participant self-reports, which are subject to misclassification bias.

Additionally, we explored five distinct, robust machine learning algorithms known for their effective predictive capabilities in healthcare settings for comparative analysis. Numerous alternative methods and implementations, including support vector machines, XGBoost, and K-nearest neighbor methods, are also available. We believe that further exploration and comparison of additional methods could be pertinent, particularly when dealing with more intricate datasets containing extensive additional and complex information for the identification of undiagnosed diabetes.

4.3. Future Directions

In a recent study, Katsimpris et al. [39] demonstrated the potential of leveraging nutritional data for predicting type 2 diabetes mellitus through a logistic regression approach. An avenue for future exploration in the development of a classification model for identifying individuals with undiagnosed diabetes involves integrating dietary information with other pertinent factors. This strategic combination of variables aims to enhance the predictive capabilities of the model, potentially yielding more accurate and comprehensive insights into the identification of undiagnosed diabetes patients.

5. Conclusions

We have demonstrated that several types of classification models can accurately classify undiagnosed diabetes from simple and clinically obtainable variables. Small differences in performance were observed among the compared models, but no one model outperformed the others in terms of classifying undiagnosed diabetes or prediabetes. These results suggest that the use of machine learning for prescreening for undiagnosed diabetes could be a useful tool in clinical practice.

Author Contributions: S.L.C. analyzed the data. S.L.C. and C.B. wrote the main manuscript text and prepared the figures. O.H. assisted in coordinating the various stages of the project and provided critical feedback on the analysis and manuscript. All the authors reviewed this manuscript. All authors have read and agreed to the published version of the manuscript.

Funding: This research received no external funding.

Institutional Review Board Statement: The presented study is a reanalysis of existing, publicly available, and anonymized data NHANES. The presented study in this paper did not need any approval form institutional and/or licensing committee, cf. Danish law on "Bekendtgørelse af lov om videnskabsetisk behandling af sundhedsvidenskabelige forskningsprojekter og sundhedsdatavidenskabelige forskningsprojekter" (Komitéloven, kap. 4, § 14, stk. 3).

Informed Consent Statement: The data were collected with informed consent from participants, and the data were deidentified to protect the privacy of the participants. The NHANES protocol was approved by the NCHS Ethics Review Board (ERB).

Data Availability Statement: All the data are publicly available at: https://www.cdc.gov/nchs/nhanes/index.htm. Accessed on 1 January 2023.

Conflicts of Interest: The authors declare no conflicts of interest.

Abbreviations

National Health and Nutrition Examination Survey (NHANES); positive predictive values (PPVs); negative predictive values (NPVs); machine learning (ML); receiver operating characteristic

(ROC); area under the curve (AUC); Korea National Health and Nutrition Examination Survey (KNHANES)

References

1. Shah, A.; Afzal, M. Prevalence of diabetes and hypertension and association with various risk factors among different Muslim populations of Manipur, India. *J. Diabetes Metab. Disord.* **2013**, *12*, 52. [CrossRef] [PubMed]
2. Noble, D.; Mathur, R.; Dent, T.; Meads, C.; Greenhalgh, T. Risk models and scores for type 2 diabetes: Systematic review. *BMJ* **2011**, *343*, 1243. [CrossRef] [PubMed]
3. Mendola, N.D.; Chen, T.-C.; Gu, Q.; Eberhardt, M.S.; Saydah, S. Prevalence of Total, Diagnosed, and Undiagnosed Diabetes Among Adults: United States, 2013–2016. Key findings Data from the National Health and Nutrition Examination Survey (NHANES). *NCHS Data Brief* **2013**, *319*, 1–8.
4. Gillies, C.L.; Lambert, P.C.; Abrams, K.R.; Sutton, A.J.; Cooper, N.J.; Hsu, R.T.; Davies, M.J.; Khunti, K. Different strategies for screening and prevention of type 2 diabetes in adults: Cost effectiveness analysis. *BMJ* **2008**, *336*, 1180–1184. [CrossRef]
5. Simmons, R.K.; Echouffo-Tcheugui, J.B.; Griffin, S.J. Screening for type 2 diabetes: An update of the evidence. *Diabetes Obes Metab.* **2010**, *12*, 838–844. [CrossRef]
6. Lee, Y.H.; Bang, H.; Kim, H.C.; Kim, H.M.; Park, S.W.; Kim, D.J. A simple screening score for diabetes for the Korean population: Development, validation, and comparison with other scores. *Diabetes Care* **2012**, *35*, 1723–1730. [CrossRef] [PubMed]
7. Liu, M.; Pan, C.; Jin, M. A Chinese diabetes risk score for screening of undiagnosed diabetes and abnormal glucose tolerance. *Diabetes Technol. Ther.* **2011**, *13*, 501–507. [CrossRef]
8. Collins, G.S.; Mallett, S.; Omar, O.; Yu, L.-M. Developing risk prediction models for type 2 diabetes: A systematic review of methodology and reporting. *BMC Med.* **2011**, *9*, 103. [CrossRef]
9. Firdous, S.; Wagai, G.; Sharma, K. A survey on diabetes risk prediction using machine learning approaches. *J. Fam. Med. Prim. Care* **2022**, *11*, 6929.
10. Sun, G.W.; Shook, T.L.; Kay, G.L. Inappropriate use of bivariable analysis to screen risk factors for use in multivariable analysis. *J. Clin. Epidemiol.* **1996**, *49*, 907–916. [CrossRef]
11. Royston, P.; Altman, D.G.; Sauerbrei, W. Dichotomizing continuous predictors in multiple regression: A bad idea. *Stat. Med.* **2006**, *25*, 127–141. [CrossRef]
12. Maniruzzaman, M.; Kumar, N.; Menhazul Abedin, M.; Islam, S.; Suri, H.S.; El-Baz, A.S.; Suri, J.S. Comparative approaches for classification of diabetes mellitus data: Machine learning paradigm. *Comput. Methods Programs Biomed.* **2017**, *152*, 23–34. [CrossRef]
13. Cichosz, S.L.; Xylander, A.A.P. A Conditional Generative Adversarial Network for Synthesis of Continuous Glucose Monitoring Signals. *J. Diabetes Sci. Technol.* **2021**, *16*, 1220–1223. [CrossRef] [PubMed]
14. Cichosz, S.L.; Jensen, M.H.; Hejlesen, O. Short-term prediction of future continuous glucose monitoring readings in type 1 diabetes: Development and validation of a neural network regression model. *Int. J. Med. Inform.* **2021**, *151*, 104472. [CrossRef] [PubMed]
15. Cichosz, S.L.; Johansen, M.D.; Hejlesen, O. Toward Big Data Analytics: Review of Predictive Models in Management of Diabetes and Its Complications. *J. Diabetes Sci. Technol.* **2016**, *10*, 27–34. [CrossRef] [PubMed]
16. Cichosz, S.L.; Frystyk, J.; Tarnow, L.; Fleischer, J. Combining Information of Autonomic Modulation and CGM Measurements Enables Prediction and Improves Detection of Spontaneous Hypoglycemic Events. *J. Diabetes Sci. Technol.* **2014**, *9*, 132–137. [CrossRef]
17. Cichosz, S.L.; Kronborg, T.; Jensen, M.H.; Hejlesen, O. Penalty weighted glucose prediction models could lead to better clinically usage. *Comput. Biol. Med.* **2021**, *138*, 104865. [CrossRef]
18. Cichosz, S.L.; Rasmussen, N.H.; Vestergaard, P.; Hejlesen, O. Precise Prediction of Total Body Lean and Fat Mass from Anthropometric and Demographic Data: Development and Validation of Neural Network Models. *J. Diabetes Sci. Technol.* **2020**, *15*, 1337–1343. [CrossRef]
19. Huang, J.; Yeung, A.M.; Armstrong, D.G.; Battarbee, A.N.; Cuadros, J.; Espinoza, J.C.; Kleinberg, S.; Mathioudakis, N.; Swerdlow, M.A.; Klonoff, D.C. Artificial Intelligence for Predicting and Diagnosing Complications of Diabetes. *J. Diabetes Sci. Technol.* **2023**, *17*, 224–238. [CrossRef]
20. Joshi, R.D.; Dhakal, C.K. Predicting Type 2 Diabetes Using Logistic Regression and Machine Learning Approaches. *Int. J. Environ. Res. Public Health* **2021**, *18*, 7346. [CrossRef]
21. Chen, W.; Chen, S.; Zhang, H.; Wu, T. A hybrid prediction model for type 2 diabetes using K-means and decision tree. In Proceedings of the IEEE International Conference on Software Engineering and Service Sciences, ICSESS, Beijing, China, 24–26 November 2017; pp. 386–390.
22. Sisodia, D.; Sisodia, D.S. Prediction of Diabetes using Classification Algorithms. *Procedia Comput. Sci.* **2018**, *132*, 1578–1585. [CrossRef]
23. Cichosz, S.L.; Johansen, M.D.; Ejskjaer, N.; Hansen, T.K.; Hejlesen, O.K. Improved diabetes screening using an extended predictive feature search. *Diabetes Technol. Ther.* **2014**, *16*, 166–171. [CrossRef]

24. Yu, W.; Liu, T.; Valdez, R.; Gwinn, M.; Khoury, M.J. Application of support vector machine modeling for prediction of common diseases: The case of diabetes and prediabetes. *BMC Med. Inform. Decis. Mak.* **2010**, *10*, 16. [CrossRef]
25. Maniruzzaman, M.; Rahman, M.J.; Ahammed, B.; Abedin, M. Classification and prediction of diabetes disease using machine learning paradigm. *Health Inf. Sci. Syst.* **2020**, *8*, 1–14. [CrossRef]
26. Centers for Disease Control and Prevention (CDC); National Center for Health Statistics (NCHS). National Health and Nutrition Examination Survey Data. Hyattsville MUSD of H and HSC for DC and P. *National Health and Nutrition Examination Survey (NHANES) 2005–2018*. Available online: https://www.cdc.gov/nchs/nhanes/index.htm (accessed on 19 November 2023).
27. Association, A.D. Standards of Medical Care in Diabetes—2022 Abridged for Primary Care Providers. *Clin. Diabetes* **2022**, *40*, 10–38. [CrossRef]
28. García-Laencina, P.J.; Sancho-Gómez, J.L.; Figueiras-Vidal, A.R. Pattern classification with missing data: A review. *Neural Comput. Appl.* **2010**, *19*, 263–282. [CrossRef]
29. Park, D.J.; Park, M.W.; Lee, H.; Kim, Y.-J.; Kim, Y.; Park, Y.H. Development of machine learning model for diagnostic disease prediction based on laboratory tests. *Sci. Rep.* **2021**, *11*, 7567. [CrossRef]
30. Uddin, S.; Khan, A.; Hossain, M.E.; Moni, M.A. Comparing different supervised machine learning algorithms for disease prediction. *BMC Med Inform. Decis. Mak.* **2019**, *19*, 281. [CrossRef]
31. Breiman, L. Random forests. *Mach. Learn.* **2001**, *45*, 5–32. [CrossRef]
32. Freund, Y.; Schapire, R.E. A Decision-Theoretic Generalization of On-Line Learning and an Application to Boosting. *J. Comput. Syst. Sci.* **1997**, *55*, 119–139. [CrossRef]
33. Seiffert, C.; Khoshgoftaar, T.M.; van Hulse, J.; Napolitano, A. RUSBoost: A hybrid approach to alleviating class imbalance. *IEEE Trans. Syst. Man Cybern. Part A Syst. Hum.* **2010**, *40*, 185–197. [CrossRef]
34. Friedman, J.; Hastie, T.; Tibshirani, R. Additive logistic regression: A statistical view of boosting (with discussion and a rejoinder by the authors). *Ann. Statist.* **2000**, *28*, 337–407. [CrossRef]
35. Baan, C.A.; Ruige, J.B.; Stolk, R.P.; Witteman, J.C.; Dekker, J.M.; Heine, R.J.; Feskens, E.J. Performance of a predictive model to identify undiagnosed diabetes in a health care setting. *Diabetes Care* **1999**, *22*, 213–219. [CrossRef]
36. Fletcher, B.; Gulanick, M.; Lamendola, C. Risk factors for type 2 diabetes mellitus. *J. Cardiovasc. Nurs.* **2002**, *16*, 486. [CrossRef]
37. Yang, H.; Xin, Z.; Feng, J.P.; Yang, J.-K. Waist-to-height ratio is better than body mass index and waist circumference as a screening criterion for metabolic syndrome in Han Chinese adults. *Medicine* **2017**, *96*, e8192. [CrossRef]
38. Diabetes Prevention Program Research Group. Reduction in the incidence of type 2 diabetes with lifestyle intervention or metformin. *N. Engl. J. Med.* **2002**, *346*, 393–403. [CrossRef]
39. Katsimpris, A.; Brahim, A.; Rathmann, W.; Peters, A.; Strauch, K.; Flaquer, A. Prediction of type 2 diabetes mellitus based on nutrition data. *J. Nutr. Sci.* **2021**, *10*, 1139. [CrossRef] [PubMed]

Disclaimer/Publisher's Note: The statements, opinions and data contained in all publications are solely those of the individual author(s) and contributor(s) and not of MDPI and/or the editor(s). MDPI and/or the editor(s) disclaim responsibility for any injury to people or property resulting from any ideas, methods, instructions or products referred to in the content.

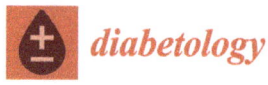

Article

Global Trends in Risk Factors and Therapeutic Interventions for People with Diabetes and Cardiovascular Disease: Results from the WHO International Clinical Trials Registry Platform

Musawenkosi Ndlovu [1], Phiwayinkosi V. Dludla [1,2], Ndivhuwo Muvhulawa [1,3], Yonela Ntamo [1], Asanda Mayeye [1], Nomahlubi Luphondo [1], Nokulunga Hlengwa [2], Albertus K. Basson [2], Sihle E. Mabhida [4], Sidney Hanser [5], Sithandiwe E. Mazibuko-Mbeje [3], Bongani B. Nkambule [6] and Duduzile Ndwandwe [1,*]

[1] Cochrane South Africa, South African Medical Research Council, Tygerberg 7505, South Africa; musawenkosi.ndlovu@mrc.ac.za (M.N.); pdludla@mrc.ac.za (P.V.D.); ndivhuwo.muvhulawa@mrc.ac.za (N.M.); yonela.ntamo@mrc.ac.za (Y.N.); asanda.mayeye@mrc.ac.za (A.M.); nomahlubi.luphondo@mrc.ac.za (N.L.)
[2] Department of Biochemistry and Microbiology, University of Zululand, KwaDlangezwa 3886, South Africa; hlengwan@unizulu.ac.za (N.H.); bassona@unizulu.ac.za (A.K.B.)
[3] Department of Biochemistry, North-West University, Mafikeng Campus, Mmabatho 2735, South Africa; sithandiwe.mazibukombeje@nwu.ac.za
[4] Non-Communicable Diseases Research Unit, South African Medical Research Council, Tygerberg 7505, South Africa; sihle.mabhida@mrc.ac.za
[5] Department of Physiology and Environmental Health, University of Limpopo, Sovenga 0727, South Africa; sidney.hanser@ul.ac.za
[6] School of Laboratory Medicine and Medical Sciences, University of KwaZulu-Natal, Durban 4000, South Africa; nkambuleb@ukzn.ac.za
* Correspondence: duduzile.ndwandwe@mrc.ac.za; Tel.: +27-21-938-0222

Citation: Ndlovu, M.; Dludla, P.V.; Muvhulawa, N.; Ntamo, Y.; Mayeye, A.; Luphondo, N.; Hlengwa, N.; Basson, A.K.; Mabhida, S.E.; Hanser, S.; et al. Global Trends in Risk Factors and Therapeutic Interventions for People with Diabetes and Cardiovascular Disease: Results from the WHO International Clinical Trials Registry Platform. *Diabetology* **2023**, *4*, 560–573. https://doi.org/10.3390/diabetology4040050

Academic Editors: Andrej Belančić, Sanja Klobučar and Dario Rahelić

Received: 20 October 2023
Revised: 17 November 2023
Accepted: 6 December 2023
Published: 8 December 2023

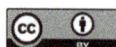

Copyright: © 2023 by the authors. Licensee MDPI, Basel, Switzerland. This article is an open access article distributed under the terms and conditions of the Creative Commons Attribution (CC BY) license (https://creativecommons.org/licenses/by/4.0/).

Abstract: This study presents a comprehensive analysis of 898 clinical trials conducted between 1999 and 2023, focusing on the interplay of metabolic syndrome, cardiovascular diseases (CVDs), and type 2 diabetes mellitus (T2D). This study draws upon data sourced from the International Clinical Trials Registry Platform (ICTRP) until August 2023. The trials were predominantly interventional (67%) or observational (33%). A geographical distribution reveals that while the United States registered approximately 18% of the trials, other regions like Australia, the United Kingdom, and multicounty trials made substantial contributions. Most studies (84%) included both male and female participants, with adults aged 18 to 65 years predominantly represented. The trials aimed at treatment (21%) and prevention (21%), emphasizing the dual focus on addressing existing CVD risk and preventing its development. Notably, CVDs (29%), T2D (8%), and the coexistence of both (21%) constituted the primary conditions of interest. Key interventions encompassed lifestyle and behavioral modifications, dietary supplementation, and drug therapies, with metformin and statins leading in pharmacological treatments. Interestingly, additional interventions such as glucagon-like peptide-1 agonists and dipeptidyl peptidase IV inhibitors are gaining recognition for their potential in managing metabolic syndrome-related conditions. Moreover, the report highlights a growing focus on inflammation, body mass index, blood pressure, body weight, and major adverse cardiovascular events as primary outcomes. Overall, the study highlights the importance of ICTRP as the source of data for clinical trials targeting metabolic syndrome, CVDs, and T2D and the growing recognition of diverse intervention strategies to address this critical global health concern.

Keywords: heart disease; metabolic complications; clinical trials; demographic characteristics; treatment modalities; global health

1. Introduction

The World Health Organization (WHO) has progressively highlighted the significance of cardiovascular diseases (CVDs) in driving the global burden of disease, with evidence suggesting this condition claimed about 17.9 million lives in 2021 [1]. Briefly, CVD incorporates a group of complex disorders affecting the heart and blood vessels, with atherosclerosis recognized as a major contributing factor [2]. These conditions encompass a range of complications, including stroke, coronary artery disease, heart failure, arrhythmias, and cerebrovascular disease, among others [3]. Predominantly studied in the elderly through the Framingham Heart Study [4,5], research on CVD now spans multiple generations of participants [6,7]. Within this context, metabolic complications have significantly contributed to the development and progression of cardiovascular complications [8]. Certainly, increasing evidence indicates that most patients with diabetes are likely to succumb to CVD-related abnormalities when compared to nondiabetic counterparts [9,10].

Epidemiological data unequivocally establish diabetes as an independent risk factor for the development of CVDs [11,12]. As a result, research exploring the relationship between CVD and diabetes, particularly type 2 diabetes (T2D), has garnered significant interest among researchers [13,14]. T2D is characterized by persistent hyperglycemia and a state of insulin resistance that is followed by subsequent damage or dysfunction of pancreatic β-cells [15]. While T2D was historically associated with older adults [16], it is now known that many diverse factors are associated with the development and progression of this condition even in children and adolescents [17,18]. Indeed, research continues to highlight the importance of clarifying factors that contribute to the development of CVD risk in people with diabetes mellitus [19–21]. This includes understanding the influence of factors such as genetic predisposition, lifestyle choices, socioeconomic status, and comorbidities. In fact, risk prediction models are increasingly explored to give insight into the effectiveness of personalized interventions, targeted lifestyle modifications, medication regimens, or novel therapies and how they could contribute to improving CVD outcomes in patients with diabetes [19–21]. Such approaches remain instrumental to a more patient-centered approach to managing CVD risk in individuals with diabetes, potentially leading to more effective prevention and treatment strategies [22,23].

Physical activity and lifestyle modification, when applied consistently, currently remain the most effective interventions to alleviate metabolic complications, including reducing CVD [24–27]. However, only a few people adhere consistently to such strict interventions. Metformin has remained the leading therapeutic intervention for people with T2D [28–30]. This biguanide drug is effective at controlling blood glucose levels, while it is increasingly being investigated for its cardioprotective properties in people with diabetes [28–30]. Alternatively, statins are recommended for people with dyslipidemia [31], with some research indicating cardioprotective effects of these drugs [32]. However, emerging research has reported limitations with statins, especially the limitations associated with their long-term use in reducing the intracellular levels of coenzyme Q_{10} [33], a fat-soluble quinone with a structure similar to that of vitamin K and which is vital to the human body. Beyond the therapeutic effects of metformin and statins [28–30,32], increasing research has progressively evaluated the antidiabetic and cardioprotective effects of various nutrients, especially commonly used foods such as vegetables, fruits, herbal teas, and others [34–36]. Nonetheless, understanding global trends in disease distribution, especially across global regions, has become important before any recommendations can be accepted. For example, adult patients with diabetes are acknowledged to have two–four times higher risk of developing CVD compared to individuals without this condition, and the risk increases with poor glycemic control [37]. Others highlight the significance of understanding trends in the epidemiology of CVD and cardiovascular risk management in T2D for a more individualized patient-centered approach to manage these conditions [38]. Beyond reducing fasting plasma glucose levels, decreasing blood pressure, as well as triglycerides, and low-density lipoprotein cholesterol remains instrumental to lower CVD risk in individuals with diabetes [39].

The International Clinical Trials Registry Platform (ICTRP) plays a pivotal role in advancing our understanding of metabolic diseases by serving as a centralized repository for clinical trial data. Metabolic diseases, including T2D and CVD, present significant global health challenges. The ICTRP provides a valuable resource for researchers, healthcare practitioners, and policymakers, facilitating the registration and dissemination of data from clinical trials focused on metabolic diseases. Through the comprehensive analysis of data from diverse clinical trials, the ICTRP enables the identification of trends, patterns, and emerging insights in the field of metabolic diseases. Such data are instrumental in informing evidence-based practices, guiding the development of targeted interventions, and ultimately improving the management and prevention of CVD-related complications in patients with diabetes. This study also highlights the importance of the ICTRP as the source of data for clinical trials targeting metabolic syndrome, CVDs, and T2D, including the growing recognition of diverse intervention strategies to address this critical global health concern.

2. Methodology

2.1. Source and Data Description

The ICTRP registry (https://www.who.int/clinical-trials-registry-platform, accessed on 3 September 2023) was accessed for a comprehensive analysis of data on clinical trials reporting on the global trends in CVD risk in people with diabetes [40]. This registry contains clinical data from registries across the globe and has become an important tool to monitor disease surveillance or to evaluate the effects on health outcomes [41,42]. An advanced search function of the ICTRP was used to identify relevant clinical trials, registered on 2 August 2023. This study is a cross-sectional analysis of registered clinical trials for people with diabetes at risk of CVD. We conducted searches in the ICTRP, which is a repository hosted by the WHO that contains regularly updated clinical trial data from primary clinical trial registries of the WHO network. Importantly, a growing number of reports have used this registry to analyze and inform on clinical data that remain significant for public health [43–46].

2.2. An Approach for Data Analysis and Management

Two researchers (M.N. and N.M.) independently accessed the WHO ICTRP portal to download relevant data on 2 August 2023. The downloaded Excel spreadsheet was checked by other researchers (P.V.D. and D.N.) before data extractions were performed, especially accuracy in collection of information concerning trial registry source, date of registration, retrospective flag, gender, trial phases, and intervention model. Other relevant information that was collected was based on intervention model prominently used, disease condition, and primary outcomes measured, corresponding to CVD risk in people with diabetes. This information allowed for a comprehensive analysis of global trends in CVD risk for people with T2D within an Excel spreadsheet.

3. Results

3.1. Study Inclusion

Briefly, a total of 935 records (registered from 1999 to 2023) of clinical studies were retrieved from the WHO ICTRP registry. After eligibility assessment, including duplicate removal and exclusion of trials that did not focus on CVD and diabetes, 116 studies were excluded (Figure 1). As a result, a total number of 898 studies were suitable for the analysis, predominantly interventional (n = 602), and observational (n = 295) studies (Figure 1).

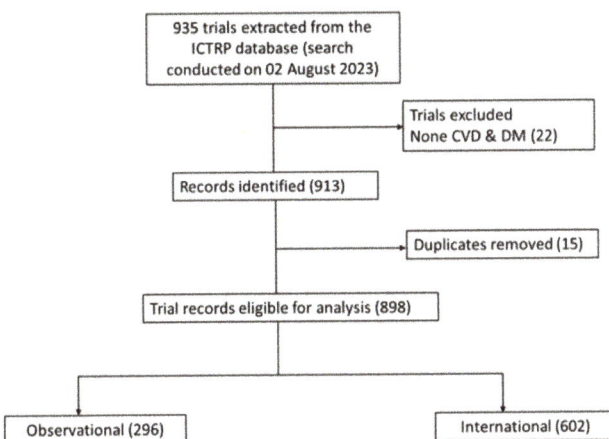

Figure 1. Flow chart repressing clinical trial selection. Briefly, after eligibility assessment, including duplicate removal and exclusion of trials that did not focus on cardiovascular disease (CVD) and diabetes mellitus (DM), 898 studies were suitable for the analysis, predominantly including interventional (n = 602), and observational (n = 296).

3.2. Data Distribution Based on Country of Origin, Clinical Trial Registry Sources, and Year of Publication

When exploring the regions of registered trials, it was observed that about 18% of trials were registered in the United States, while other regions like Australia, the United Kingdom, and multiple countries trials recorded 10%, 7%, and 9%, respectively (Figure 2A,B). Single-country recruitment centers registered 91% in comparison to multicountry multicenter (9%) trials. The ClinicalTrials.gov registry registered the most trials (56%), followed by ANZCTR (12%), ISRCTN (9%), JPRN (6%), EU-CTR (4%), and CTRI (3%) (Figure 2C). Other registries registered ≤1% of trials related to diabetes and CVDs between 1999 and 2023 (Figure 2C). The highest number of trials recorded per year during the reporting period was 7% in 2016. Even though there was no consistency, in the registration of clinical trials on participants with diabetes and CVD, there was a significant increment from 1999 to 2022, with a probability to rise even in 2023 (Figure 3).

A

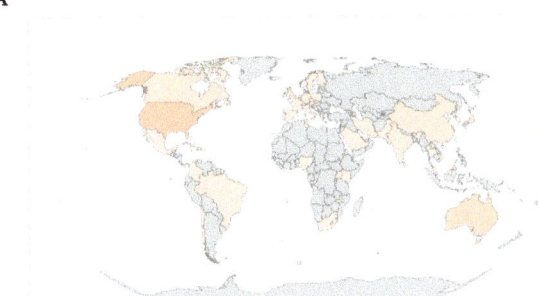

Figure 2. *Cont.*

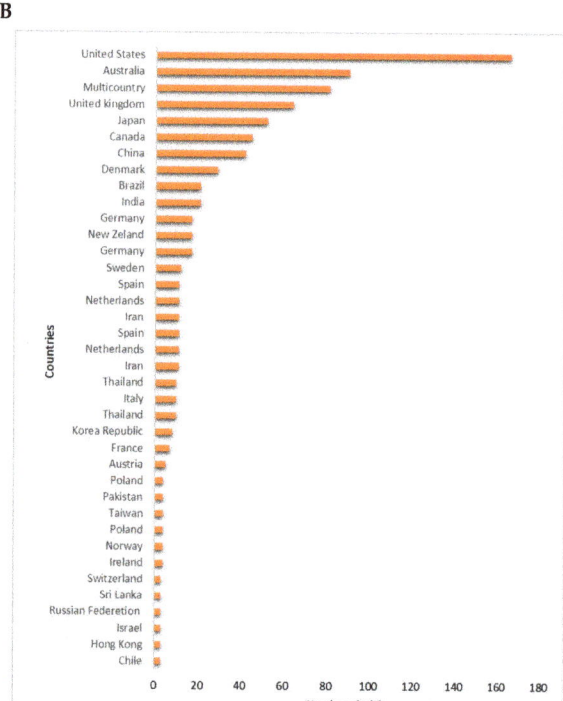

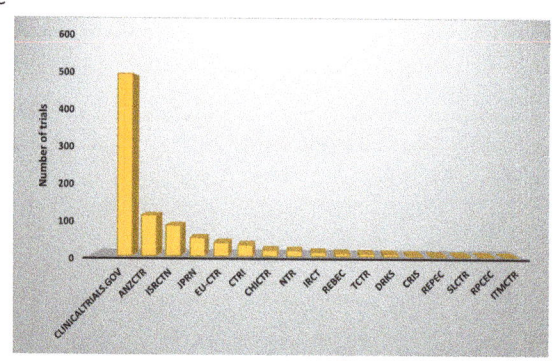

Figure 2. Global distribution of registered trials per country. (**A**) depicts a global map color-coded with strong-shaded regions describing a high number of trials registered in that specific region. (**B**) demonstrates the distribution of trials per country. Briefly, the United States registered the most clinical trials, while other regions like Australia, the United Kingdom, and multiple countries trials recorded 10%, 7%, and 9%, respectively. (**C**) gives an overview of the distribution of trials across different clinical trial registries. Briefly, some of the listed registries included Australian New Zealand Clinical Trials Registry (ANZCTR), International Standard Randomized Controlled Trial Number (ISRCTN), Japan Primary Registries Network (JPRN), Iranian Registry of Clinical Trials (IRCT), Peruvian Clinical Trials Registry (REPEC), Sri Lanka Clinical Trials Registry (SLCTR), Cuban Public Registry of Clinical Trials (RPCEC), International Traditional Medicine Clinical Trial Registry (ITMCTR), Clinical Research Information Service of the Republic of Korea (CRiS), Thai Clinical Trials Registry (TCTR), Chinese Clinical Trial Register (ChiCTR), and the Clinical Trials Registry India (CTRI).

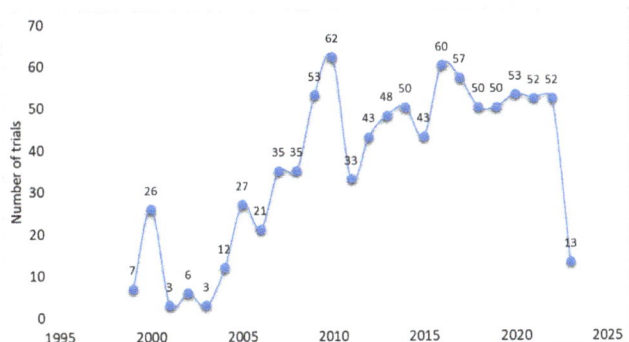

Figure 3. Distribution of registered trials per year from 1999 to 2023. These data show that a steady increase in trial registration is observed between 1999 and 2022.

3.3. Data Distribution Based on Gender of Participants

Most trials (84%) included both females and males in their studies (Figure 4A). When exploring age differences of those registered, it was observed that most trials recruited adults between 18 and 65 years of age for both minimum and maximum age inclusion (Figure 4B).

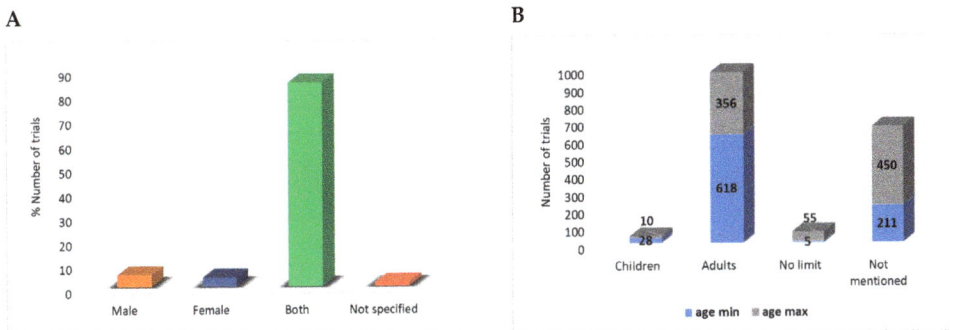

Figure 4. Overview of gender distribution within the included clinical trials. Most trials, 700 (84%), included both females and males in their studies (**A**). When exploring age differences of those registered, it is observed that most trials recruited adults (18 to 65 years) for both minimum and maximum age inclusion (**B**).

3.4. Data Distribution Based on Intervention Model and Disease Type

Mostly, recorded trials focused on different groups of participants receiving different interventions, predominantly of parallel assignment (Figure 5A). Forty-two trials employed cross-over intervention, twenty-eight single group assignments, seventeen factorial, and five sequential. We further explored the primary purpose of individual trials, and we observed that the treatment (21%) and prevention (21%) primary purposes show almost equal percentage numbers of clinical trials (Figure 5A). Other primary purposes of the trials include observation (7%), health service (3%), supportive care (2%), basic science (4%), and diagnostic (1%).

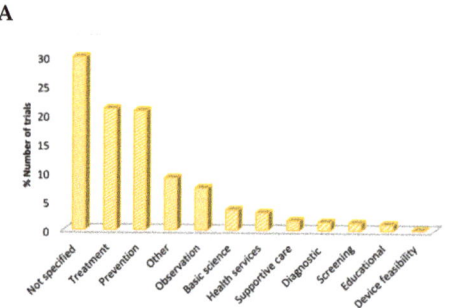
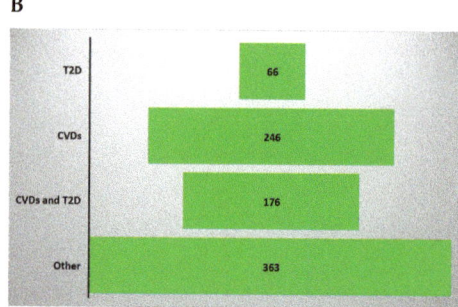

Figure 5. (**A**) lists registered trials distributed according to the primary purpose of the study. Except for those that were not specified, most included clinical trials were focused on treatment and prevention. (**B**) Disease conditions of participants in registered trials included type 2 diabetes (T2D), cardiovascular diseases (CVDs), both conditions (diabetes and CVDs), and others, which were mostly a cluster of metabolic anomalies, such as dyslipidemia, obesity, nonalcoholic fatty liver disease, and hypercholesterolemia.

3.5. Data on Disease Classification and Interventions Being Used in People with Diabetes and CVD

The most common conditions investigated in the trials were CVDs (29%) and T2D (8%) (Figure 5B). Other trials included participants with both T2D and CVDs (21%). Other conditions included a cluster of metabolic complications, characterizing metabolic syndrome (43%) (Figure 5B). Correspondingly, it was obvious that measurements of blood lipid profiles, like cholesterol, low-density lipoprotein, high-density lipoproteins, as well as glucose and insulin or glycated hemoglobin levels, were predominant in these trials reflecting primary outcomes in people with diabetes or those at CVD risk (Table 1). Notably, inflammation, body mass index, blood pressure, body weight, and major adverse cardiovascular events were also evaluated and were also increasingly evaluated as primary outcomes in people with diabetes at risk of CVD (Table 1).

Table 1. Selective reporting for primary outcomes per condition.

Primary Outcome	Number of Trials			
	T2D	CVDs	Both CVDs and T2D	Other
Blood glucose	7	8	10	18
Blood lipids	7	3	6	5
Blood cholesterol	2	13	4	66
LDL	4	6	3	21
HDL		5		7
Insulin	5	2	8	23
HbA1c	9	2	13	18
Inflammation	3	3	6	5
BMI	2	11	4	5
Blood pressure		11	8	64
Body weight	2	3	3	12
MACE		10	12	
Other	2	5	8	20

BMI = body mass index, CVD = cardiovascular disease, HbA1c = glycated hemoglobin, LDL = low-density lipoprotein, HDL = high-density lipoprotein, MACE = major adverse cardiovascular event, T2D: type 2 diabetes.

3.6. Data on Disease Classification and Interventions Being Used in People with Diabetes at Risk of CVDs

We further evaluated a variety of interventions that are being tested in trials being conducted. In Table 2, the interventions being currently explored are distributed according to the health conditions, including T2D, CVDs, both CVDs and T2D, and other conditions. Notably, lifestyle and behavioral modifications as well as dietary supplementation are the interventions implemented in trials across different disease conditions. Drug intervention for both CVDs and T2D included the use of statins, metformin, and pioglitazone (Table 2). Most interestingly, some trials evaluated drug combinations and drug plus physical activity interventions. For intervention against T2D, metformin, dapagliflozin, and empagliflozin were among the drug interventions implemented. Similarly, lifestyle, physical exercise, and behavioral changes were also encouraged. Against cardiovascular diseases, statin (atorvastatin, simvastatin, rosuvastatin, pravastatin) therapy was among the drug interventions implemented. Drug combination therapy, such as ezetimibe plus statins, was investigated by other trials.

Table 2. Selective reporting for intervention per health condition.

Intervention	Number of Studies
Other	
Behavioral	40
Lifestyle modifications	54
Placebo	47
Dietary supplement	17
Statin	13
Metformin	9
Empagliflozin	3
Pioglitazone	7
Type 2 diabetes	
Behavioral	4
Dietary supplement	3
Empagliflozin	2
Metformin	2
Dapagliflozin	3
Ertugliflozin	2
Exercise	5
Placebo	18
Cardiovascular diseases	
Behavioral	33
Dietary supplement	8
Statins	14
Other	102
Both cardiovascular diseases and type 2 diabetes	
Behavioral	34
Dietary supplement	23
Pioglitazone	3
Empagliflozin	7
Statins	3
Other drugs	30

4. Discussion

The comprehensive analysis of clinical trial data on global trends in risk factors associated with diabetes and CVD provides valuable insights into the state of research in this critical area of public health concern. One of the notable aspects of the study is the diversity in trial registration and recruitment patterns. The analysis of the ICTRP data revealed that while the United States accounted for approximately 18% of registered trials, other regions like Australia, the United Kingdom, and multicountry trials also made substantial contributions. This geographic distribution highlights the global relevance and collaborative nature of research addressing CVD risk in individuals with diabetes. This also corroborates information from other studies, showing that ClinicalTrials.gov is the predominant source for clinical trial data, informing on many disease conditions [43,47]. This also aligns with increasing trends in data on the prevalence of metabolic disease in developed nations, including the United States [48]. However, the limited clinical data available underscore the need for research to be conducted in developing nations, like those within the sub-Saharan Africa region where there is an increasing surge in metabolic diseases [49].

The study identified a consistent increase in the registration of clinical trials from 1999 to 2022, with indications of continued growth in 2023. Consistent with growing reports [9,50], this trend reflects the growing recognition of the significance of CVD risk in individuals with diabetes and the urgent need for research in this field. This is in agreement with a growing number of studies [12,51,52] while also pointing to the need to contain diabetes-related abnormalities in order to minimize long-term CVD complications [9] This also does not exclude a gap in prospective and active research, which could provide more timely and actionable insights into CVD risk management in this population. A commendable aspect of the analyzed trials is the inclusion of both genders, with 84% of trials incorporating both males and females. This balanced representation is crucial for generating results that are applicable to a broader population. Furthermore, the trials predominantly recruited adults aged between 18 and 65 years, which is relevant given that diabetes and CVD risk often develop in adulthood [53]. However, it is essential to continue assessing the impact of interventions on pediatric and elderly populations, as these age groups also face significant health challenges related to diabetes and CVD [54].

In examining the primary purposes of the trials, the study found that treatment and prevention were the most common objectives, each accounting for 21% of the trials. This balance suggests that researchers are not only focused on managing existing CVD risk but also on preventing its development in individuals with diabetes. These findings highlight the comprehensive approach to managing this dual health burden. More so, the analysis revealed that trials predominantly investigated CVDs (29%) and T2D (8%), with a substantial proportion focusing on both conditions (21%). Currently, there is conflicting evidence in terms of CVD burden in developing nations. For example, some research has suggested that incidence, prevalence, and mortality rates remain high in low- and middle-income countries [55], while others have seen a decline in trends for CVD incidence and mortality rates and stable survival rates in patients with CVD [56]. Policymakers have predominantly highlighted the importance of focusing on the management of ischemic heart disease, stroke, and congestive heart failure, which contribute most to the burden of CVD globally [22,57]. Other CVD-related conditions, like diabetic cardiomyopathy, are also a concern [58], primarily due to the increasing prevalence of diabetes [17]. Anyway, there is an urgent need to channel resources toward implementing cost-effective policies and interventions to reduce premature mortalities due to noncommunicable diseases.

Additionally, a significant number of trials examined a cluster of metabolic complications characterizing metabolic syndrome (43%). This reflects the strong link between diabetes and CVD risk within a broader metabolic context. As expected, primary outcomes measured in these trials often included blood lipid profiles, glucose levels, and insulin or glycated hemoglobin levels. These biomarkers are central to understanding CVD risk in individuals with diabetes, as elevated levels are associated with increased risk. For example, while management of blood glucose is essential for people with diabetes [59], ongoing research has strongly reported on the importance of assessing blood lipid profiles, especially low-density lipoprotein cholesterol to predict CVD risk in individuals with T2D [60,61]. The interventions being explored in the trials encompassed a wide range of approaches, including lifestyle and behavioral modifications, dietary supplementation, and drug interventions. Although physical activity and lifestyle medications are widely favored to improve the metabolic state [24–27], the use of statins, metformin, and pioglitazone in drug interventions underscores the importance of both glycemic control and lipid management in mitigating CVD risk [62,63]. In fact, metformin is being increasingly investigated for its potential benefits in alleviating CVD-related complications, beyond its well-known properties to improve glycemic levels in patients with T2D [28–30]. A previously published systematic review and meta-analysis involving nine clinical trials with 12,026 participants presented results supporting the potential benefits of pioglitazone in reducing major adverse cardiovascular events in people with insulin resistance, pre-diabetes, and diabetes mellitus [64]. However, these results further indicated that pioglitazone may potentially increase the risk of heart failure, edema, and weight gain. This also highlights the emerging use of nutraceuticals and dietary supplements as alternative or combination therapy to manage metabolic disease, including reducing CVD risk in people with diabetes [65,66]. Nutraceuticals and dietary supplements may encompass food sources rich in antioxidants and anti-inflammatory properties that are necessary to diffuse the harmful effects of oxidative stress and inflammation to reduce CVD risk. Both oxidative stress and inflammation remain the predominant pathological features implicated in the progression of many metabolic diseases; this extends to their link with damage to the cardiovascular system [15,67,68]. Beyond the management of blood glucose levels within a diabetic state, many dietary interventions, such as turmeric, herbal teas, cinnamon, mango, blueberries, red wine, chocolate, fish, and extra virgin olive oil, are increasingly being studied for their potential benefits in alleviating CVD risk [34–36]. In fact, the growth in clinical trials on the potential benefits of these interventions may be more pronounced when used in combination with currently used therapeutic interventions, like metformin or even statins [69–71]. However, as demonstrated by limited data within our reporting, clinical evidence demonstrating the potential benefits of nutraceuticals and dietary interventions against metabolic diseases remains scarce.

Strengths of the report include its comprehensive analysis of clinical trial data, which offers valuable insights into the global trends in risk factors associated with diabetes and CVD. The study's notable strength lies in the diversity of trial registration and recruitment patterns, with contributions from regions worldwide, highlighting the global relevance and collaborative nature of research addressing CVD risk in individuals with diabetes. The increasing trend in the registration of clinical trials underscores the growing recognition of the significance of CVD risk in this population, emphasizing the urgent need for more research. The balanced representation of both genders and the focus on adults aged between 18 and 65 years in the analyzed trials ensures the applicability of the results to a broader population.

However, the report also has limitations, particularly the lack of clinical data from developing nations, where there is a rising surge in metabolic diseases [72,73]. This geographic gap in research highlights the need for more studies in these regions. Additionally, while the report addresses a broad spectrum of metabolic complications characterizing metabolic syndrome, it may benefit from further exploration of interventions on pediatric and elderly populations, as these age groups also face significant health challenges related to diabetes and CVD [74]. Furthermore, the focus on specific biomarkers, such as blood lipid profiles and glucose levels, might not encompass the full range of relevant indicators for understanding CVD risk. In fact, determination of cholesterol efflux capacity is also another important indicator for those potentially at increased risk of CVD. Nonetheless, the report's emphasis on the comprehensive approach to managing both existing CVD risk and its prevention in individuals with diabetes is commendable, offering a valuable perspective on this dual health burden.

5. Conclusions

The analysis of clinical trial data from the ICTRP provides a comprehensive overview of research trends in CVD risk among individuals with diabetes. The findings reflect a global effort to understand and address this critical health issue. The study's insights into trial registration, participant inclusion, trial phases, intervention models, primary purposes, disease classification, and interventions serve as a valuable resource for guiding future research and public health strategies aimed at reducing CVD risk in this vulnerable population. Limitations associated with statistical analysis or analysis of only one clinical trial registry, well beyond research on interventions informing on the status of CVD risk in the pediatric population, are well acknowledged and should be addressed in future studies.

Author Contributions: Conceptualization and data analysis, M.N., N.M., P.V.D. and D.N.; writing—original draft preparation, review, and editing, M.N., N.M., P.V.D., Y.N., A.M., N.L., N.H., A.K.B., S.E.M., S.H., S.E.M.-M., B.B.N. and D.N. All authors have read and agreed to the published version of the manuscript.

Funding: The South African Medical Research Council supports this work on project code: 43500. The content hereof is the sole responsibility of the authors and do not necessarily represent the official views of the funders.

Institutional Review Board Statement: Not applicable.

Informed Consent Statement: Not applicable.

Data Availability Statement: All data generated or analyzed during this study are included in this published article.

Conflicts of Interest: The authors declare no conflict of interest.

Abbreviations

ANZCTR, Australian New Zealand Clinical Trials Registry; ChiCTR, Chinese Clinical Trial Registry; CTRI, Clinical Trials Registry India; CVD, cardiovascular disease; DRKS, German Clinical Trials Register; EU-CTR, EU Clinical Trials Register; GMT, geometric mean titers; ICTRP, International Clinical Trials Registry Platform; IRCT, Iranian Registry of Clinical Trials; ISRCTN, International Standard Randomised Controlled Trial Number; ITMCTR, International Traditional Medicine Clinical Trial Registry; JPRN, Japan Primary Registries Network; Dutch Trial Registry; MMSE, Mini Mental State Examination; NaT, neutralizing antibody titers; PACTR, Pan African Clinical Trials Registry; PSQI, Pittsburgh Sleep Quality Index; ReBec, Brazilian Clinical Trials Registry; REPEC, Peruvian Clinical Trials Registry; RPCEC, Cuban Public Registry of Clinical Trials; SLCTR, Sri Lanka Clinical Trials Registry; T2D, type 2 diabetes; TCTR, Thai Clinical Trials Registry; WHO, World Health Organization.

References

1. World Health Organization. The Leading Causes of Death Globally. Available online: https://www.who.int/news-room/fact-sheets/detail/the-top-10-causes-of-death (accessed on 3 October 2023).
2. Wong, N.D.; Budoff, M.J.; Ferdinand, K.; Graham, I.M.; Michos, E.D.; Reddy, T.; Shapiro, M.D.; Toth, P.P. Atherosclerotic cardiovascular disease risk assessment: An American Society for Preventive Cardiology clinical practice statement. *Am. J. Prev. Cardiol.* **2022**, *10*, 100335. [CrossRef] [PubMed]
3. Kereliuk, S.M.; Dolinsky, V.W. Recent Experimental Studies of Maternal Obesity, Diabetes during Pregnancy and the Developmental Origins of Cardiovascular Disease. *Int. J. Mol. Sci.* **2022**, *23*, 4467. [CrossRef] [PubMed]
4. Andersson, C.; Johnson, A.D.; Benjamin, E.J.; Levy, D.; Vasan, R.S. 70-year legacy of the Framingham Heart Study. *Nat. Rev. Cardiol.* **2019**, *16*, 687–698. [CrossRef] [PubMed]
5. Mahmood, S.S.; Levy, D.; Vasan, R.S.; Wang, T.J. The Framingham Heart Study and the epidemiology of cardiovascular disease: A historical perspective. *Lancet* **2014**, *383*, 999–1008. [CrossRef] [PubMed]
6. Glovaci, D.; Fan, W.; Wong, N.D. Epidemiology of Diabetes Mellitus and Cardiovascular Disease. *Curr. Cardiol. Rep.* **2019**, *21*, 21. [CrossRef] [PubMed]
7. Damaskos, C.; Garmpis, N.; Kollia, P.; Mitsiopoulos, G.; Barlampa, D.; Drosos, A.; Patsouras, A.; Gravvanis, N.; Antoniou, V.; Litos, A.; et al. Assessing Cardiovascular Risk in Patients with Diabetes: An Update. *Curr. Cardiol. Rev.* **2020**, *16*, 266–274. [CrossRef] [PubMed]
8. Alshehri, A.M. Metabolic syndrome and cardiovascular risk. *J. Fam. Community Med.* **2010**, *17*, 73–78. [CrossRef] [PubMed]
9. Leon, B.M.; Maddox, T.M. Diabetes and cardiovascular disease: Epidemiology, biological mechanisms, treatment recommendations and future research. *World J. Diabetes* **2015**, *6*, 1246–1258. [CrossRef]

10. Fan, W. Epidemiology in diabetes mellitus and cardiovascular disease. *Cardiovasc. Endocrinol.* **2017**, *6*, 8–16. [CrossRef]
11. Kannel, W.B.; McGee, D.L. Diabetes and cardiovascular disease. The Framingham study. *JAMA* **1979**, *241*, 2035–2038. [CrossRef]
12. Martín-Timón, I.; Sevillano-Collantes, C.; Segura-Galindo, A.; Del Cañizo-Gómez, F.J. Type 2 diabetes and cardiovascular disease: Have all risk factors the same strength? *World J. Diabetes* **2014**, *5*, 444–470. [CrossRef] [PubMed]
13. Wu, Y.; Ding, Y.; Tanaka, Y.; Zhang, W. Risk factors contributing to type 2 diabetes and recent advances in the treatment and prevention. *Int. J. Med. Sci.* **2014**, *11*, 1185–1200. [CrossRef] [PubMed]
14. Ntzani, E.E.; Kavvoura, F.K. Genetic risk factors for type 2 diabetes: Insights from the emerging genomic evidence. *Curr. Vasc. Pharmacol.* **2012**, *10*, 147–155. [CrossRef] [PubMed]
15. Dludla, P.V.; Mabhida, S.E.; Ziqubu, K.; Nkambule, B.B.; Mazibuko-Mbeje, S.E.; Hanser, S.; Basson, A.K.; Pheiffer, C.; Kengne, A.P. Pancreatic β-cell dysfunction in type 2 diabetes: Implications of inflammation and oxidative stress. *World J. Diabetes* **2023**, *14*, 130–146. [CrossRef]
16. Bradley, D.; Hsueh, W. Type 2 Diabetes in the Elderly: Challenges in a Unique Patient Population. *J. Geriatr. Med. Gerontol.* **2016**, *2*, 14. [CrossRef] [PubMed]
17. International Diabetes Federation. 10th Diabetes Atlas. Available online: https://diabetesatlas.org/ (accessed on 5 October 2023).
18. Ma, C.X.; Ma, X.N.; Guan, C.H.; Li, Y.D.; Mauricio, D.; Fu, S.B. Cardiovascular disease in type 2 diabetes mellitus: Progress toward personalized management. *Cardiovasc. Diabetol.* **2022**, *21*, 74. [CrossRef]
19. Kee, O.T.; Harun, H.; Mustapha, N.; Abdul Murad, N.A.; Chin, S.F.; Jaafar, R.; Abdullah, N. Cardiovascular complications in a diabetes prediction model using machine learning: A systematic review. *Cardiovasc. Diabetol.* **2023**, *22*, 13. [CrossRef]
20. Galbete, A.; Tamayo, I.; Librero, J.; Enguita-Germán, M.; Cambra, K.; Ibáñez-Beroiz, B. Cardiovascular risk in patients with type 2 diabetes: A systematic review of prediction models. *Diabetes Res. Clin. Pract.* **2022**, *184*, 109089. [CrossRef]
21. Liang, J.; Li, Q.; Fu, Z.; Liu, X.; Shen, P.; Sun, Y.; Zhang, J.; Lu, P.; Lin, H.; Tang, X.; et al. Validation and comparison of cardiovascular risk prediction equations in Chinese patients with Type 2 diabetes. *Eur. J. Prev. Cardiol.* **2023**, *30*, 1293–1303. [CrossRef]
22. Roth, G.A.; Mensah, G.A.; Johnson, C.O.; Addolorato, G.; Ammirati, E.; Baddour, L.M.; Barengo, N.C.; Beaton, A.Z.; Benjamin, E.J.; Benziger, C.P.; et al. Global Burden of Cardiovascular Diseases and Risk Factors, 1990–2019: Update From the GBD 2019 Study. *J. Am. Coll. Cardiol.* **2020**, *76*, 2982–3021. [CrossRef]
23. Saeedi, P.; Petersohn, I.; Salpea, P.; Malanda, B.; Karuranga, S.; Unwin, N.; Colagiuri, S.; Guariguata, L.; Motala, A.A.; Ogurtsova, K.; et al. Global and regional diabetes prevalence estimates for 2019 and projections for 2030 and 2045: Results from the International Diabetes Federation Diabetes Atlas, 9(th) edition. *Diabetes Res. Clin. Pract.* **2019**, *157*, 107843. [CrossRef] [PubMed]
24. Myers, J.; Kokkinos, P.; Nyelin, E. Physical Activity, Cardiorespiratory Fitness, and the Metabolic Syndrome. *Nutrients* **2019**, *11*, 1652. [CrossRef] [PubMed]
25. Mthembu, S.X.H.; Mazibuko-Mbeje, S.E.; Ziqubu, K.; Nyawo, T.A.; Obonye, N.; Nyambuya, T.M.; Nkambule, B.B.; Silvestri, S.; Tiano, L.; Muller, C.J.F.; et al. Impact of physical exercise and caloric restriction in patients with type 2 diabetes: Skeletal muscle insulin resistance and mitochondrial dysfunction as ideal therapeutic targets. *Life Sci.* **2022**, *297*, 120467. [CrossRef] [PubMed]
26. Nyawo, T.A.; Pheiffer, C.; Mazibuko-Mbeje, S.E.; Mthembu, S.X.H.; Nyambuya, T.M.; Nkambule, B.B.; Sadie-Van Gijsen, H.; Strijdom, H.; Tiano, L.; Dludla, P.V. Physical Exercise Potentially Targets Epicardial Adipose Tissue to Reduce Cardiovascular Disease Risk in Patients with Metabolic Diseases: Oxidative Stress and Inflammation Emerge as Major Therapeutic Targets. *Antioxidants* **2021**, *10*, 1758. [CrossRef] [PubMed]
27. Jakobsen, I.; Solomon, T.P.; Karstoft, K. The Acute Effects of Interval-Type Exercise on Glycemic Control in Type 2 Diabetes Subjects: Importance of Interval Length. A Controlled, Counterbalanced, Crossover Study. *PLoS ONE* **2016**, *11*, e0163562. [CrossRef] [PubMed]
28. Chen, C.; Yuan, S.; Zhao, X.; Qiao, M.; Li, S.; He, N.; Huang, L.; Lyu, J. Metformin Protects Cardiovascular Health in People With Diabetes. *Front. Cardiovasc. Med.* **2022**, *9*, 949101. [CrossRef] [PubMed]
29. Dludla, P.V.; Nyambuya, T.M.; Johnson, R.; Silvestri, S.; Orlando, P.; Mazibuko-Mbeje, S.E.; Gabuza, K.B.; Mxinwa, V.; Mokgalaboni, K.; Tiano, L.; et al. Metformin and heart failure-related outcomes in patients with or without diabetes: A systematic review of randomized controlled trials. *Heart Fail. Rev.* **2021**, *26*, 1437–1445. [CrossRef] [PubMed]
30. Han, Y.; Xie, H.; Liu, Y.; Gao, P.; Yang, X.; Shen, Z. Effect of metformin on all-cause and cardiovascular mortality in patients with coronary artery diseases: A systematic review and an updated meta-analysis. *Cardiovasc. Diabetol.* **2019**, *18*, 96. [CrossRef]
31. Clark, L.T. Treating dyslipidemia with statins: The risk-benefit profile. *Am. Heart J.* **2003**, *145*, 387–396. [CrossRef]
32. Zhou, Q.; Liao, J.K. Statins and cardiovascular diseases: From cholesterol lowering to pleiotropy. *Curr. Pharm. Des.* **2009**, *15*, 467–478. [CrossRef]
33. Mthembu, S.X.H.; Orlando, P.; Silvestri, S.; Ziqubu, K.; Mazibuko-Mbeje, S.E.; Mabhida, S.E.; Nyambuya, T.M.; Nkambule, B.B.; Muller, C.J.F.; Basson, A.K.; et al. Impact of dyslipidemia in the development of cardiovascular complications: Delineating the potential therapeutic role of coenzyme Q(10). *Biochimie* **2023**, *204*, 33–40. [CrossRef] [PubMed]
34. Russell, C.; Keshavamurthy, S.; Saha, S. Nutraceuticals in the Management of Cardiovascular Risk Factors: Where is the Evidence? *Cardiovasc. Hematol. Disord. Drug Targets* **2021**, *21*, 150–161. [CrossRef] [PubMed]
35. Sosnowska, B.; Penson, P.; Banach, M. The role of nutraceuticals in the prevention of cardiovascular disease. *Cardiovasc. Diagn. Ther.* **2017**, *7*, S21–S31. [CrossRef]

36. Carrizzo, A.; Izzo, C.; Forte, M.; Sommella, E.; Di Pietro, P.; Venturini, E.; Ciccarelli, M.; Galasso, G.; Rubattu, S.; Campiglia, P.; et al. A Novel Promising Frontier for Human Health: The Beneficial Effects of Nutraceuticals in Cardiovascular Diseases. *Int. J. Mol. Sci.* **2020**, *21*, 8706. [CrossRef]
37. Dal Canto, E.; Ceriello, A.; Rydén, L.; Ferrini, M.; Hansen, T.B.; Schnell, O.; Standl, E.; Beulens, J.W. Diabetes as a cardiovascular risk factor: An overview of global trends of macro and micro vascular complications. *Eur. J. Prev. Cardiol.* **2019**, *26*, 25–32. [CrossRef] [PubMed]
38. Yun, J.S.; Ko, S.H. Current trends in epidemiology of cardiovascular disease and cardiovascular risk management in type 2 diabetes. *Metabolism* **2021**, *123*, 154838. [CrossRef]
39. Malekzadeh, H.; Lotfaliany, M.; Ostovar, A.; Hadaegh, F.; Azizi, F.; Yoosefi, M.; Farzadfar, F.; Khalili, D. Trends in cardiovascular risk factors in diabetic patients in comparison to general population in Iran: Findings from National Surveys 2007–2016. *Sci. Rep.* **2020**, *10*, 11724. [CrossRef] [PubMed]
40. Ghersi, D.; Pang, T. En route to international clinical trial transparency. *Lancet* **2008**, *372*, 1531–1532. [CrossRef]
41. World Health Organization. *International Standards for Clinical Trial Registries: The Registration of all Interventional Trials is a Scientific, Ethical and Moral Responsibility*, version 3.0 ed.; World Health Organization: Geneva, Switzerland, 2018; Available online: https://iris.who.int/bitstream/handle/10665/274994/9789241514743-eng.pdf?sequence=1 (accessed on 20 September 2023).
42. Ndwandwe, D.E.; Runeyi, S.; Pienaar, E.; Mathebula, L.; Hohlfeld, A.; Wiysonge, C.S. Practices and trends in clinical trial registration in the Pan African Clinical Trials Registry (PACTR): A descriptive analysis of registration data. *BMJ Open* **2022**, *12*, e057474. [CrossRef]
43. Mathebula, L.; Malinga, T.; Mokgoro, M.; Ndwandwe, D.; Wiysonge, C.S.; Gray, G. Cholera vaccine clinical trials: A cross-sectional analysis of clinical trials registries. *Hum. Vaccines Immunother.* **2023**, *19*, 2261168. [CrossRef]
44. He, Y.; Yang, J.; Lv, Y.; Chen, J.; Yin, F.; Huang, J.; Zheng, Q. A Review of Ginseng Clinical Trials Registered in the WHO International Clinical Trials Registry Platform. *BioMed Res. Int.* **2018**, *2018*, 1843142. [CrossRef] [PubMed]
45. Feizabadi, M.; Fahimnia, F.; Mosavi Jarrahi, A.; Naghshineh, N.; Tofighi, S. Iranian clinical trials: An analysis of registered trials in International Clinical Trial Registry Platform (ICTRP). *J. Evid. Based Med.* **2017**, *10*, 91–96. [CrossRef] [PubMed]
46. Merson, L.; Ndwandwe, D.; Malinga, T.; Paparella, G.; Oneil, K.; Karam, G.; Terry, R.F. Promotion of data sharing needs more than an emergency: An analysis of trends across clinical trials registered on the International Clinical Trials Registry Platform. *Wellcome Open Res.* **2022**, *7*, 101. [CrossRef] [PubMed]
47. Mayo-Wilson, E.; Heyward, J.; Keyes, A.; Reynolds, J.; White, S.; Atri, N.; Alexander, G.C.; Omar, A.; Ford, D.E.; Atri, N.; et al. Clinical trial registration and reporting: A survey of academic organizations in the United States. *BMC Med.* **2018**, *16*, 60. [CrossRef] [PubMed]
48. Saklayen, M.G. The Global Epidemic of the Metabolic Syndrome. *Curr. Hypertens. Rep.* **2018**, *20*, 12. [CrossRef] [PubMed]
49. Okafor, C.I. The metabolic syndrome in Africa: Current trends. *Indian J. Endocrinol. Metab.* **2012**, *16*, 56–66. [CrossRef] [PubMed]
50. Grundy, S.M.; Benjamin, I.J.; Burke, G.L.; Chait, A.; Eckel, R.H.; Howard, B.V.; Mitch, W.; Smith, S.C., Jr.; Sowers, J.R. Diabetes and cardiovascular disease: A statement for healthcare professionals from the American Heart Association. *Circulation* **1999**, *100*, 1134–1146. [CrossRef]
51. Einarson, T.R.; Acs, A.; Ludwig, C.; Panton, U.H. Prevalence of cardiovascular disease in type 2 diabetes: A systematic literature review of scientific evidence from across the world in 2007–2017. *Cardiovasc. Diabetol.* **2018**, *17*, 83. [CrossRef]
52. De Rosa, S.; Arcidiacono, B.; Chiefari, E.; Brunetti, A.; Indolfi, C.; Foti, D.P. Type 2 Diabetes Mellitus and Cardiovascular Disease: Genetic and Epigenetic Links. *Front. Endocrinol.* **2018**, *9*, 2. [CrossRef]
53. Joseph, J.J.; Deedwania, P.; Acharya, T.; Aguilar, D.; Bhatt, D.L.; Chyun, D.A.; Di Palo, K.E.; Golden, S.H.; Sperling, L.S. Comprehensive Management of Cardiovascular Risk Factors for Adults With Type 2 Diabetes: A Scientific Statement From the American Heart Association. *Circulation* **2022**, *145*, e722–e759. [CrossRef]
54. Jaul, E.; Barron, J. Age-Related Diseases and Clinical and Public Health Implications for the 85 Years Old and Over Population. *Front. Public Health* **2017**, *5*, 335. [CrossRef] [PubMed]
55. Gaziano, T.A.; Bitton, A.; Anand, S.; Abrahams-Gessel, S.; Murphy, A. Growing epidemic of coronary heart disease in low- and middle-income countries. *Curr. Probl. Cardiol.* **2010**, *35*, 72–115. [CrossRef] [PubMed]
56. Amini, M.; Zayeri, F.; Salehi, M. Trend analysis of cardiovascular disease mortality, incidence, and mortality-to-incidence ratio: Results from global burden of disease study 2017. *BMC Public Health* **2021**, *21*, 401. [CrossRef]
57. Gaziano, T.A. Cardiovascular disease in the developing world and its cost-effective management. *Circulation* **2005**, *112*, 3547–3553. [CrossRef] [PubMed]
58. Wang, S.; Tian, C.; Gao, Z.; Zhang, B.; Zhao, L. Research status and trends of the diabetic cardiomyopathy in the past 10 years (2012–2021): A bibliometric analysis. *Front. Cardiovasc. Med.* **2022**, *9*, 1018841. [CrossRef] [PubMed]
59. Weinstock, R.S.; Aleppo, G.; Bailey, T.S.; Bergenstal, R.M.; Fisher, W.A.; Greenwood, D.A.; Young, L.A. *The Role of Blood Glucose Monitoring in Diabetes Management*; American Diabetes Association Clinical Compendia: Arlington, VA, USA, 2020. [CrossRef]
60. Wang, Y.; Lammi-Keefe, C.J.; Hou, L.; Hu, G. Impact of low-density lipoprotein cholesterol on cardiovascular outcomes in people with type 2 diabetes: A meta-analysis of prospective cohort studies. *Diabetes Res. Clin. Pract.* **2013**, *102*, 65–75. [CrossRef] [PubMed]
61. Khil, J.; Kim, S.M.; Chang, J.; Choi, S.; Lee, G.; Son, J.S.; Park, S.M.; Keum, N. Changes in total cholesterol level and cardiovascular disease risk among type 2 diabetes patients. *Sci. Rep.* **2023**, *13*, 8342. [CrossRef] [PubMed]

62. van Stee, M.F.; de Graaf, A.A.; Groen, A.K. Actions of metformin and statins on lipid and glucose metabolism and possible benefit of combination therapy. *Cardiovasc. Diabetol.* **2018**, *17*, 94. [CrossRef]
63. Gandhi, G.Y.; Mooradian, A.D. Management of Hyperglycemia in Older Adults with Type 2 Diabetes. *Drugs Aging* **2022**, *39*, 39–58. [CrossRef]
64. Liao, H.W.; Saver, J.L.; Wu, Y.L.; Chen, T.H.; Lee, M.; Ovbiagele, B. Pioglitazone and cardiovascular outcomes in patients with insulin resistance, pre-diabetes and type 2 diabetes: A systematic review and meta-analysis. *BMJ Open* **2017**, *7*, e013927. [CrossRef]
65. Le, Y.; Wang, B.; Xue, M. Nutraceuticals use and type 2 diabetes mellitus. *Curr. Opin. Pharmacol.* **2022**, *62*, 168–176. [CrossRef]
66. Derosa, G.; Limas, C.P.; Macías, P.C.; Estrella, A.; Maffioli, P. Dietary and nutraceutical approach to type 2 diabetes. *Arch. Med. Sci.* **2014**, *10*, 336–344. [CrossRef] [PubMed]
67. Hussain, T.; Tan, B.; Yin, Y.; Blachier, F.; Tossou, M.C.; Rahu, N. Oxidative Stress and Inflammation: What Polyphenols Can Do for Us? *Oxid. Med. Cell Longev.* **2016**, *2016*, 7432797. [CrossRef] [PubMed]
68. Dludla, P.V.; Nkambule, B.B.; Jack, B.; Mkandla, Z.; Mutize, T.; Silvestri, S.; Orlando, P.; Tiano, L.; Louw, J.; Mazibuko-Mbeje, S.E. Inflammation and Oxidative Stress in an Obese State and the Protective Effects of Gallic Acid. *Nutrients* **2018**, *11*, 23. [CrossRef] [PubMed]
69. Ragheb, S.R.; El Wakeel, L.M.; Nasr, M.S.; Sabri, N.A. Impact of Rutin and Vitamin C combination on oxidative stress and glycemic control in patients with type 2 diabetes. *Clin. Nutr. ESPEN* **2020**, *35*, 128–135. [CrossRef] [PubMed]
70. Miller, B.F.; Thyfault, J.P. Exercise-Pharmacology Interactions: Metformin, Statins, and Healthspan. *Physiology* **2020**, *35*, 338–347. [CrossRef] [PubMed]
71. Cicero, A.F.; Colletti, A. Statins and nutraceuticals/functional food: Could they be combined? In *Combination Therapy in Dyslipidemia*; Adis: Cham, Switzerland, 2015; pp. 127–142. [CrossRef]
72. Bowo-Ngandji, A.; Kenmoe, S.; Ebogo-Belobo, J.T.; Kenfack-Momo, R.; Takuissu, G.R.; Kengne-Ndé, C.; Mbaga, D.S.; Tchatchouang, S.; Kenfack-Zanguim, J.; Lontuo Fogang, R.; et al. Prevalence of the metabolic syndrome in African populations: A systematic review and meta-analysis. *PLoS ONE* **2023**, *18*, e0289155. [CrossRef] [PubMed]
73. Burnett, R.J.; Larson, H.J.; Moloi, M.H.; Tshatsinde, E.A.; Meheus, A.; Paterson, P.; François, G. Addressing public questioning and concerns about vaccination in South Africa: A guide for healthcare workers. *Vaccine* **2012**, *30* (Suppl. S3), C72–C78. [CrossRef]
74. Sahoo, K.; Sahoo, B.; Choudhury, A.K.; Sofi, N.Y.; Kumar, R.; Bhadoria, A.S. Childhood obesity: Causes and consequences. *J. Fam. Med. Prim. Care* **2015**, *4*, 187–192. [CrossRef]

Disclaimer/Publisher's Note: The statements, opinions and data contained in all publications are solely those of the individual author(s) and contributor(s) and not of MDPI and/or the editor(s). MDPI and/or the editor(s) disclaim responsibility for any injury to people or property resulting from any ideas, methods, instructions or products referred to in the content.

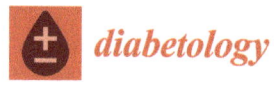

Article

The Quality of Life of Caregivers of People with Type 2 Diabetes Estimated Using the WHOQOL-BREF Questionnaire

Vilma Kolarić [1,2], Valentina Rahelić [3,4,5] and Zrinka Šakić [1,*]

1. Vuk Vrhovac University Clinic for Diabetes, Endocrinology, and Metabolic Diseases, Merkur Clinical Hospital, 10000 Zagreb, Croatia; vilma.kolaric6@gmail.com
2. School of Medicine, Catholic University of Croatia, 10000 Zagreb, Croatia
3. Department of Nutrition and Dietetics, University Hospital Center Zagreb, 10000 Zagreb, Croatia; valentina.rahelic@kbc-zagreb.hr
4. Department of Nursing Care, University of Applied Health Sciences, 10000 Zagreb, Croatia
5. Department of Food Technology, University North, 48000 Koprivnica, Croatia
* Correspondence: sakic.zrinka@gmail.com

Abstract: Type 2 diabetes (T2D) poses a growing global health challenge, impacting patients' and their caregivers' well-being. This study investigates the influence of T2D complications on caregivers' quality of life (QoL) using the WHOQOL-BREF questionnaire, accounting for factors like age, disease duration, and control. The research involved 382 T2D patients and 300 caregivers from Vuk Vrhovac University Clinic for Diabetes, Endocrinology, and Metabolic Diseases. The WHOQOL-BREF questionnaire assessed caregivers' QoL across physical, psychological, social, and environmental domains. Complications, including retinopathy, neuropathy, and kidney disease, were examined for their effects on QoL. Patients' age impact, gender differences, and disease duration were analyzed. T2D complications had varying impacts on different QoL domains. Caregivers of patients with multiple complications showed significant social functioning impairment. Those without complications reported lower psychological health. Age correlated with poorer physical health scores. Female caregivers rated higher in psychological and environmental health. Disease duration and T2D control had no significant impact on caregiver QoL. Caregivers' concerns included medication adherence and worry about their partner's health. This study illustrates the delicate interplay between T2D patients and caregivers, highlighting the multifaceted effects of chronic illness. Comprehensive healthcare techniques that address emotional and social components in addition to medical care are critical for improving the well-being of both patients and their caregivers. The findings contribute to a broader understanding of T2D care dynamics, advocating for empathetic and all-encompassing healthcare practices.

Keywords: type 2 diabetes; quality of life; caregiver; diabetes complications

Citation: Kolarić, V.; Rahelić, V.; Šakić, Z. The Quality of Life of Caregivers of People with Type 2 Diabetes Estimated Using the WHOQOL-BREF Questionnaire. *Diabetology* **2023**, *4*, 430–439. https://doi.org/10.3390/diabetology4040037

Academic Editor: Andrej Belančić

Received: 29 August 2023
Revised: 7 October 2023
Accepted: 9 October 2023
Published: 11 October 2023

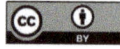

Copyright: © 2023 by the authors. Licensee MDPI, Basel, Switzerland. This article is an open access article distributed under the terms and conditions of the Creative Commons Attribution (CC BY) license (https://creativecommons.org/licenses/by/4.0/).

1. Introduction

Type 2 diabetes (T2D) is a complex metabolic condition characterized by an interplay of genetic and environmental factors. According to the International Diabetes Federation (IDF), 537 million individuals over the age of 18 have diabetes in 2021, with a predicted increase to 643 million by 2030. The number of patients with T2D is increasing in all parts of the world, and it is increasing the fastest in poorly or moderately developed countries with a lower national income. Diabetes is the main cause of blindness, end-stage renal disease, stroke, heart attack, and lower limb amputations [1]. Quality of life (QoL) has emerged as a prominent concept and research focus in the domains of health and medicine [2]. There is no universal definition of the term, however, the World Health Organization (WHO) defines QoL as: "An individual's perception of their position in life in the context of the culture in which they live and concerning their goals, expectations, standards, and concerns" [3,4]. Furthermore, the WHO developed the WHOQOL-BREF questionnaire, which is a condensed version of the WHOQOL-100 questionnaire, and is a widely used method for assessing an individual's overall quality of life. The abbreviation "BREF" refers to "Brief Version", suggesting that it contains fewer questions than the lengthier version. The questionnaire is intended to provide a thorough picture of a person's well-being and general quality of life. It is divided into four major domains, each reflecting a critical part of life's happiness and functioning. The physical domain examines a person's perception of their physical health, which includes characteristics such as energy level, pain, discomfort, sleep, mobility, and daily activities. The psychological domain investigates psychological well-being, such as sentiments of optimism, self-esteem, body image, and overall life satisfaction. The social domain assesses an individual's social connections, such as friendship and family support, personal relationships, and ability to participate in social activities. In contrast, the environmental domain is concerned with a person's contentment with their living conditions, access to health care, financial security, safety, and the entire environment in which they live. The WHOQOL-BREF questionnaire normally has 26 items covering the four aforementioned domains. In addition to these questions, there are two general questions about a person's overall quality of life and health. Individuals rate their level of agreement, contentment, or frequency of experiences on a Likert scale while responding to inquiries. The questionnaire is intended to be flexible to various cultural and linguistic situations, making it appropriate for usage in various countries and populations. It has been widely used in clinical and research contexts to assess the impact of health issues, therapies, and other factors on a person's quality of life. Social support given by immediate family, partners, or spouses has shown positive effects in patients with cardiac disease or cancer [5]. The psychological state of spouses has been shown to play a role in their ability to provide support and affect the physical HRQOL in patients with prostate cancer [6,7]. Several prior studies have evaluated caregiver QoL in different contexts and are discussed later, however, none have evaluated the effects of specific T2D complications on caregiver QoL. Considering the role of social support in the QoL of patients with T2D, an investigation of factors affecting it may be necessary for creating new approaches in the overall treatment of T2D and improving the QoL of these patients.

In this study, we aimed to determine the effect of T2D complications on the different aspects of the caregiver's QoL as determined by the WHOQOL-BREF questionnaire. Additionally, we aimed to investigate other additional factors that may contribute to decreased QoL, primarily age and disease duration.

2. Materials and Methods
2.1. Setting and Study Protocol

The study was designed as a quantitative study using the WHOQOL-BREF questionnaire and available medical data. The research was conducted at the "Vuk Vrhovac" University Clinic for Diabetes, Endocrinology, and Metabolic Diseases at Merkur Clinical Hospital from June 2019 to March 2020. This study was part of a doctoral thesis that involved researching the quality of life of patients with T2D, their caregivers, and the opinions of medical staff involved in the care of T2D patients. Caregivers were defined as persons sharing the household with the patient, regardless of relationship or marital status, who take care of the patient and are responsible for helping the patient adhere to treatment. The first part of the study involved T2D patients completing the WHOQOL-BREF questionnaire, followed by mailed questionnaires to partners. For patients whose caregivers came to their scheduled hospital visit, the questionnaire was given during the visit. Patients with T2D treated at the Clinic were included in the study. The study protocol planned the inclusion of 77 participants in each group classified by the comorbidity present. The number was determined based on an earlier pilot study investigating patient QoL, with standard power (80%) and significance (5%). The caregivers were separated into groups based on the comorbidity of the patient, namely: diabetic retinopathy, symptomatic diabetic polyneuropathy, patients with diabetic kidney disease (DKD) stage 4 or 5, second- and third-degree diabetic foot ulcers according to the Texas classification or with amputated extremities. For some patients, several comorbidities were expected and those patients were classified in the multiple complications group, and one group involved patients with T2D without complications. After completion of their questionnaires, patients were given caregiver questionnaires with stamped envelopes containing a letter of invitation to the study, informed consent, and the questionnaire form. All questionnaires were coded to enable pairing of the patient and caregiver questionnaires. Patients without T2D complications and their caregivers were used as the control group. Single or widowed patients or those without caregivers were included in the patient analysis, however, they were not given caregiver questionnaires.

2.2. Tools and Data Acquisition

The questionnaire used was the WHOQOL-BREF designed by the World Health Organization (WHO), which was translated into Croatian and validated in earlier research by Pibernik Okanović [8]. Written permission was obtained from the author for the use of the questionnaire. The questionnaire contains 26 original questions grouped into four domains: physical health (7 items), psychological health (6 items), social relationships (3 items), and environmental health. Each question in the WHOQOL-BREF is rated on a Likert scale, ranging from 1 (very dissatisfied/very poor) to 5 (very satisfied/very good). The scores for each domain are transformed into a linear scale from 0 to 100 [9]. Higher scores in a domain indicate a better quality of life in that specific area. Several additional questions on T2D were added to the patient questionnaire, specifically our added questions about the time of T2D diagnosis, complications of the disease, complication onset, and whether the complication ever required hospital admission. At the end of the questionnaire, we added questions that evaluated the patient's adherence to the instructions they received from the nurses and why (we offered several answers) they did so. We also offered potential explanations for not following the instructions. In question 39, we also asked them to rate the information they received from doctors and nurses on a scale from 1 to 10, where a rating of 1 means that they did not receive any information, and a rating of 10 means that they received all the necessary information. In question 40, we asked them what they would carry out to prevent chronic complications if they had all the necessary information about them. In question 41, we wanted to obtain patients' recommendations on what they now consider important in the care of people with diabetes. In the end, we provided a space for additional text if patients would like to write something else about the care of people with diabetes.

In the first three questions of the caregiver questionnaire, we asked for information on gender, age, and education. Questions 4 to 29 were questions from the WHOQOL-BREF questionnaire. We supplemented the original questionnaire with questions regarding the perceived burdens to caregivers related to the illness of their partners. The last added question was meant to investigate the opinions of caregivers and their recommendations about taking care of people with T2D.

Additionally, medical record data regarding complications of the disease and disease management, including laboratory results, were collected for each patient on a predetermined form.

2.3. Statistical Analysis

Numerical values were presented with average and standard deviation or median and interquartile ranges (IQR), where appropriate. Categorical values were presented as absolute values and proportions (%). The normality of data distribution was analyzed using the Shapiro–Wilk test. For the comparison of numerical data, the Mann–Whitney test was used, for the analysis of several groups the Kruskal–Wallis test was applied, and, where appropriate, for multiple comparisons, Dunn's post hoc test with Bonferroni correction was performed. For categorical variables, we used the Chi-squared test, with Yates correction where appropriate. For the determination of the correlation of numerical variables, the

Spearman rank correlation test was used. Data distribution was presented in graphical and tabular form. Data were presented in tables and text.

The primary goal of this study was to evaluate the QoL of caregivers of patients with T2D and its complications. The secondary goals were to evaluate the correlation of patient age, disease duration, T2D regulation, and the presence of comorbidities on the partner's QoL.

3. Results

3.1. Patient Characteristics

For participation in the study, 434 people with T2D were invited, 382 (84.9%) of whom signed informed consent and submitted a completed questionnaire. Of the 52 respondents who were not included in the research, 8 of them refused to participate, and 44 did not return the completed questionnaire. Overall, 382 patients were included in the study. The majority of participants were female (67.3%) and younger than 60 years of age (57%). Demographic data are presented in Table 1.

Table 1. Demographic characteristics of individuals with T2D.

Demographic Characteristics		N = 382	%
Sex	Male	236	61.8
	Female	146	38.2
Age	Under 40	3	0.8
	41 to 50	37	9.7
	51 to 60	77	20.2
	61 to 70	167	43.7
	Over 71	98	25.7
Education	Unfinished primary school	54	14.1
	High school	226	59.2
	College	51	13.4
	University	49	12.8
	Doctorate	2	0.5
Living with	Alone	88	23.0
	Partner	128	33.5
	Partner and children	122	31.9
	Children	19	5.0
	Parents	5	1.3
	In extended family	20	5.2
Number of family members	1 person	84	22.0
	2 persons	140	36.6
	3 persons	65	17.0
	4 persons	48	12.6
	5 or more persons	45	11.8

One-fifth (20.2%) of the included patients had no complications of the disease, a third (33.5%) had several complications, 9.9% had isolated DKD, 15.7% had isolated diabetic neuropathy, 10.2% had an isolated diabetic foot ulcer, and 10.5% had isolated diabetic retinopathy.

The most frequent comorbidity was arterial hypertension (85.6% of patients), followed by dyslipidemia (41.6%), coronary artery disease (CAD) or heart failure (HF) (36.6%), thyroid disease (23.3%), obesity (23%), and neoplastic diseases (2.6%). Other diseases were present in 25.4% of patients.

There were 123 (32.2%) patients treated with oral antihyperglycemics, 50 (13.1%) with insulin, 96 (25.1%) were on intensive insulin regimens, 9 (2.4%) on GLP-1 analogs, and 2 (0.5%) were treated with insulin pumps. The remainder (18.8%) were on conservative management without specific medication. Combined insulin and oral antihyperglycemic drugs were used by 29 (7.6%) of patients and a combination of insulin, GLP-1 analog, and oral antihyperglycemics by one patient.

In patients with disease complications, 34 had the first occurrence in the past year, 82 within 1–5 years, 68 6–10 years ago, and 121 more than 10 years ago. T2D complications necessitated up to two hospital admissions in 82 patients, three–four in 68 patients, five–six in 62 patients, and more than seven in 59 patients.

3.2. Caregiver Characteristics

A total of 344 caregivers of people with T2D were invited to participate in the research, 44 of which did not return a completed questionnaire, and for the remaining 300 partners and/or close family members, the survey was conducted during the visit, delivered by mail or brought by patients to the next check-up (87.2%). Most caregivers were female (67%), aged 51–70 (56%), and had a high school level education (55%). More detailed data are presented in Table 2.

Table 2. Demographic characteristics of caregivers of individuals with T2D.

Demographic Characteristics		N = 300	%
Sex	Male	98	32.7
	Female	202	67.3
Age	Under 40	34	11.3
	41 to 50	56	18.7
	51 to 60	81	27.0
	61 to 70	87	29.0
	Over 71	42	14.0
Education	Unfinished primary school	43	14.3
	High school	166	55.3
	College	29	9.7
	University	60	20.0
	Doctorate	2	0.7

Analyzing the answers of the caregivers in which they stated what burdens them in connection with the illness of their partner/family member, they were able to choose several answers. A total of 88 (29.3%) of them stated that they were burdened by the care of medication taking and 84 (28.0%) by the diet. A total of 56 (18.7%) of them worried about frequent check-ups and 94 (31.3%) about their partner not following the advice they received. Uncertainty regarding a family member falling seriously ill burdens 185 (61.7%) partners and financial problems 49 (16.3%) of them. A total of 136 (45.3%) of them worry about who will take care of the sick respondent if they become seriously ill and transportation burdens 31 (10.3%) caregivers.

The caregivers were asked to recommend or suggest what should be carried out regarding the care of people with diabetes, so 102 of them (34.0%) recommended more frequent check-ups, 108 (36%) advised hospital stay during the work-up and treatment of complications, 165 (55.0%) of them believe that all patients must attend educational classes, and 158 (52.7%) caregivers pointed out that chronic complications should be taught about at the beginning of the disease, while 215 (71.7%) believe that patients should have mandatory check-ups to detect complications as early as possible. A total of 76 (25.3%) caregivers believe that all patients should be educated in the day hospital, 101 (33.7%) suggest that there should be programs and tests on everything patients need to know regarding their illness, and 106 (35.3%) believe that a psychologist should be included in the treatment process.

3.3. Quality of Life of Caregivers of Individuals with Type 2 Diabetes

A further analysis of the correlation between T2D complications and their effects on the caregivers' quality of life was performed.

Table 3 presents a comprehensive comparison of caregiver groups based on the presence or absence of specific T2D complications and their corresponding dimensions of caregiving burden, including physical functioning, psychological functioning, social functioning, and environmental health. Our analysis revealed statistically significant differences among the caregiver groups. Specifically, we found a significant difference in social functioning (Kruskal–Wallis test, $p = 0.017$), indicating that this dimension varied significantly across caregiver groups based on the presence of complications. However, to provide a clearer understanding of these differences, we conducted post hoc multiple comparison tests. Upon closer examination, caregivers of patients with several complications reported significantly more impaired social functioning compared to caregivers of patients without T2D complications (post hoc multiple comparisons test, $p = 0.022$). This suggests that caregivers of patients facing multiple complications may experience a greater challenge in the social functioning dimension of caregiving compared to those without T2D complications. Additionally, it is worth noting that caregivers' perceptions of various dimensions varied across different complication types. For instance, caregivers of patients with diabetic retinopathy consistently rated social functioning as the lowest among all dimensions, while caregivers of patients without T2D complications gave the lowest rating to psychological health. Conversely, environmental health received the highest ratings from caregivers of patients with diabetic neuropathy and DKD and those without T2D complications.

Table 3. Quality of life of caregivers of individuals with T2D based on the presence or absence of specific chronic complications ($n = 300$).

Complication Type	Physical Functioning (Interquartile Range)	Psychological Functioning (Interquartile Range)	Social Functioning (Interquartile Range)	Environmental Functioning (Interquartile Range)
Diabetic retinopathy	64.29 (57.14–75.00)	62.50 (54.16–83.33)	58.33 (50.00–75.00)	70.31 (53.12–78.12)
Diabetic neuropathy	71.43 (60.71–82.14)	75.00 (66.66–83.33)	66.67 (50.00–75.00)	75.00 (62.50–81.25)
Diabetic kidney disease	75.00 (64.28–85.71)	75.00 (62.50–83.33)	75.00 (58.33–83.33)	75.00 (71.87–84.37)
Diabetic foot ulcers	71.43 (60.71–83.92)	72.92 (62.50–83.33)	70.83 (62.50–83.33)	71.88 (64.06–76.56)
No chronic complications	75.00 (60.71–89.28)	70.83 (62.50–83.33)	75.00 (58.33–83.33)	75.00 (68.75–84.37)
Multiple complications	71.43 (50.00–78.57)	66.67 (54.16–75.00)	66.67 (50.00–75.00)	68.75 (59.37–84.37)

3.4. The Effect of Risk Factors and Comorbidities on Caregivers' QoL

Examination of the association of patients' age, sex, disease duration, current T2D regulation, and caregivers' quality of life has shown a correlation between increased age and worse physical health ($p = 0.004$), but no associations between age and other domains. Disease duration was not associated with changes in QoL in any domain (Table 4). However, some sex differences were noted, notably, that caregivers of female patients had higher scores in psychological health ($p = 0.005$) and environmental health ($p = 0.036$). The domains of physical and social health were rated higher in caregivers of female patients than in caregivers of male patients, however, these were not statistically significant.

Current disease regulation, as estimated by the HbA1c, did not affect any of the domains of QoL. A weak but statistically significant difference was observed for social health, environmental health, and HbA1c (Table 5).

Table 4. Association of functioning domains with the duration of T2D.

Functioning Domains	Duration of T2D	Mean Value	p	H
Physical functioning	Less than 10 years	75.00	0.380	5.304
	11 to 20 years	71.43		
	21 to 30 years	71.43		
	31 to 40 years	71.43		
	More than 40 years	62.50		
Psychological functioning	Less than 10 years	72.92	0.978	0.788
	11 to 20 years	70.83		
	21 to 30 years	70.83		
	31 to 40 years	66.67		
	More than 40 years	75.00		
Social functioning	Less than 10 years	66.67	0.331	5.753
	11 to 20 years	66.67		
	21 to 30 years	66.67		
	31 to 40 years	70.83		
	More than 40 years	58.33		
Environmental functioning	Less than 10 years	75.00	0.351	5.564
	11 to 20 years	75.00		
	21 to 30 years	68.75		
	31 to 40 years	75.00		
	More than 40 years	76.56		

H = Kruskal–Wallis Test; p = Statistical significance.

Table 5. Relationship between HbA1c and quality of life of partners, and correlation coefficients for individual components (n = 300).

HbA1c	Physical Functioning	Psychological Functioning	Social Functioning	Environmental Functioning
Correlation coefficient	−0.013	−0.098	−0.133	−0.168
p	0.821	0.089	0.021	0.004

4. Discussion

Our study involved 300 caregivers of patients with T2D with or without complications of the disease. The results indicate a decreased QoL in different domains in caregivers of T2D patients, particularly in those with multiple complications. The QoL domain most affected is social health, which was rated the lowest by all patients with complications, while caregivers of patients without disease complications rated psychological health the lowest. The older age of patients was associated with worse scores in physical health. Interestingly, disease duration and current T2D control have shown no associations with the caregivers' QoL. The psychological and environmental health domains were rated higher in caregivers of female patients, probably indicating gender differences in coping. These results are consistent with the study by Hooker et al. focusing on spouse caregivers for patients with Alzheimer's disease (AD) and Parkinson's disease (PD), which found that wives caring for AD patients reported significantly worse mental health outcomes than husbands. This evidence suggests that gender differences can significantly impact the caregiving experience. Therefore, it is plausible that the gender-based disparities we observed in psychological and environmental health domains may be influenced by distinct coping strategies among caregivers of female patients. These findings highlight the importance of recognizing and addressing gender-related factors in caregiving support and interventions [10].

A Sudanese study carried out by Awadalla et al. examined the QoL of the caregivers of patients with type 1 and type 2 diabetes by using the WHOQOL BREF questionnaire [11]. Overall, caregivers of patients with type 1 diabetes had lower scores than T2D caregivers and the general population, while the caregivers of patients with T2D had similar scores in all categories as the general population. Furthermore, in that study, the patient's age and duration of illness were positively associated with caregiver QoL domain scores. However, this study did not evaluate disease severity or the presence of complications of diabetes. In another similar Mexican study that used a different questionnaire, the domains of social and physical functioning were the highest rated [12]. Additionally, the study demonstrated that increased caregiver overload was associated with decreased caregiver QoL. In a study of a large sample of US caregivers by Secinti et al., caregivers of patients of all chronic diseases reported worse mental health when compared to a population of non-caregivers. Studies investigating the effects of complications of T2D on the caregivers' QoL are few. A Turkish study evaluated the QoL of caregivers of patients with diabetic foot ulcers by comparing them to the QoL of caregivers of psychotic patients and patients with an inguinal hernia [13]. Caregiver burden level was similar for both psychotic and diabetic foot ulcer patients and significantly higher than for hernia patients. The depression and anxiety scales of the diabetic foot ulcer group were significantly high and some points of the quality of life scales were determined to be significantly low. A correlation between the duration of caregiving and the burden was determined in the diabetic foot ulcer group. QoL was assessed using the SF-36 questionnaire, and caregivers of patients with diabetic foot ulcers scored lower than the other two groups for the domains of physical difficulties, vitality, emotional difficulties, and mental health. Notably, the number of participants in this study was low. Portuguese researchers investigated caregiver QoL over 10 months after amputation due to a diabetic foot ulcer and have found that the mean score of caregiving stress and mental and physical quality of life decreased over time [14]. Providing support to caregivers, particularly during periods of increased burden and stress, may be important to improve the overall physical and mental health of the caregiver, which may indirectly improve the patient's QoL. Other factors that may influence QoL in the mental health domain of caregivers of diabetic foot amputees are the practice of physical activity, lower caregiver burden, better functionality in the family, and a lower number of reported traumatic symptoms. Better physical QoL was associated with a lack of other chronic diseases and fewer reported physical symptoms [15]. The involvement of family and caregivers and its effect on the patient's QoL was indirectly shown in a study by Ebrahimi et al., where an educational program about diabetes resulted in larger increases in the patient's QoL when attended by family members and caregivers rather than by patients alone [16].

The study's main advantages are that it investigates the effects of T2D complications and provides a comprehensive understanding of how being a caregiver of someone with T2D affects various domains of QoL, such as physical health, psychological well-being, social relationships, and environmental factors. Understanding the partners' QoL could also help healthcare practitioners understand the stressors and obstacles that caregivers encounter. This can result in more customized interventions and better healthcare services. The study has the potential to raise awareness about the emotional and psychological toll that caring for someone with T2D may have on spouses. This could lead to more public awareness and support for caregivers.

On the other hand, the drawbacks of this study include the lack of examination of additional caregiver characteristics that may have influenced their QoL. Furthermore, the data acquired through the WHOQOL-BREF questionnaire are based on self-reported responses, which can be influenced by individual biases, emotions, and perceptions, potentially leading to mistakes in the results. Additionally, while the study may uncover connections between caregiving and quality of life, it may not establish causality. Other factors, such as pre-existing well-being or personal circumstances, may influence partners' quality of life.

Additionally, the study did not include the financial and economic status of the patient and their caregiver, which may confound the results. Another limitation is possible selection bias. Partners who agreed to participate may have different features or experiences than those who declined, thus resulting in potential bias and affecting the generalizability of the findings. The study was limited by not reaching the planned number of participants. The study was abrupted in March 2020, at the onset of the COVID-19 pandemic, and was not continued as the pandemic has altered all aspects of everyday life and was considered a confounder to QoL measurement.

By addressing the specific issues of partners, healthcare practitioners can aim to improve the overall quality of life for this essential group within the diabetic ecosystem. Nonetheless, further research is needed to have a better knowledge of the individual aspects influencing partners' quality of life and to design tailored therapies that address their unique needs. Longitudinal studies could provide insights into the changing nature of partners' experiences over time, as well as the potential usefulness of various support interventions.

5. Conclusions

In conclusion, this study has shed light on the intricate relationship between T2D and the QoL of caregivers, primarily partners, who play a crucial role in supporting individuals with this condition. The research has unveiled several significant findings. Caregivers of individuals with T2D, particularly those with multiple complications, experience a notable decrease in their QoL. The domain most affected is social health, indicating the challenges faced by caregivers in maintaining their social connections and support networks. Furthermore, older caregivers tend to report lower physical health scores, suggesting that age may play a role in the physical strain experienced by caregivers. However, age does not significantly impact other domains of QoL. Next, female caregivers of T2D patients tend to rate their psychological and environmental health domains more positively. This may reflect gender-specific coping strategies and lifestyle changes adopted by female caregivers, which influence their perception of QoL. Surprisingly, neither the duration of the disease nor the current regulation of T2D in patients had significant associations with caregivers' QoL in this study. However, the burden on caregivers is influenced by factors such as medication management, diet, adherence to medical advice, financial concerns, and the fear of the patient's condition worsening. Providing support and resources for caregivers during these challenging times may contribute to improved overall QoL. Finally, caregivers emphasize the importance of regular check-ups, patient education programs, and early awareness of chronic complications as essential components of effective T2D management. The inclusion of psychologists in the treatment process is also suggested.

These findings underscore the critical role of caregivers in the lives of individuals with T2D and highlight the need for tailored support and interventions to enhance their QoL. Addressing the emotional and psychological aspects of caregiving, as well as providing practical resources and education, can significantly improve the well-being of caregivers. Furthermore, this research contributes to a broader understanding of the complexities of T2D management and its impact on the entire ecosystem surrounding the patient. While this study provides valuable insights, further research is warranted to explore the nuanced factors influencing caregivers' QoL comprehensively. Longitudinal studies and a more extensive exploration of additional caregiver characteristics could offer a deeper understanding of their unique experiences and needs. Ultimately, these efforts can lead to more effective support systems and improved healthcare services for individuals with T2D and their caregivers.

Author Contributions: The authors confirm their contribution to the paper as follows: Conceptualization, V.K.; Methodology, V.K.; Validation, V.K.; Formal analysis, V.K. and Z.Š.; Investigation, V.K.; Data curation, V.K. and Z.Š.; Writing—original draft, V.R. and Z.Š.; Writing—review and editing, V.K.,

V.R. and Z.Š.; Visualization, Z.Š.; Supervision, V.K. and Z.Š. All authors have read and agreed to the published version of the manuscript.

Funding: This research received no external funding.

Institutional Review Board Statement: The study was conducted in accordance with the Declaration of Helsinki and approved by the Ethics Committee of Merkur Clinical Hospital (protocol code 0351-4947 and date of approval 20 June 2018).

Informed Consent Statement: Informed consent was obtained from all subjects involved in the study.

Data Availability Statement: Data are available on reasonable request due to ethical restrictions. The data presented in this study are available on request from the first author, Vilma Kolarić.

Conflicts of Interest: The authors declare no conflict of interest.

References

1. Melmed, A.; Richard, J.; Goldfine, A.B.; Koenig, R.R.; Clifford, J.; Williams, R.H.S. *Williams Textbook of Endocrinology*; Elsevier: Philadelphia, PA, USA, 2019.
2. Fayers, P.M.; Machin, D. *Quality of Life: The Assessment, Analysis and Reporting of Patient-Reported Outcomes*, 3rd ed.; Wiley Blackwell: Hoboken, NJ, USA, 2016.
3. The World Health Organization Quality of Life assessment (WHOQOL): Position paper from the World Health Organization. *Soc. Sci. Med.* **1995**, *41*, 1403–1409. [CrossRef] [PubMed]
4. Mayo, N.E. *ISOQOL Dictionary of Quality of Life and Health Outcomes Measurement*; International Society for Quality of Life Research (ISOQOL): Milwaukee, WI, USA, 2015.
5. Carlsson, M.; Hamrin, E. Psychological and psychosocial aspects of breast cancer and breast cancer treatment. A literature review. *Cancer Nurs.* **1994**, *17*, 418–428. [CrossRef] [PubMed]
6. Chien, C.H.; Chuang, C.K.; Liu, K.L.; Pang, S.T.; Wu, C.T.; Chang, Y.H. Prostate cancer-specific anxiety and the resulting health-related quality of life in couples. *J. Adv. Nurs.* **2019**, *75*, 63–74. [CrossRef] [PubMed]
7. Kim, Y.; Carver, C.S.; Spillers, R.L.; Love-Ghaffari, M.; Kaw, C.K. Dyadic effects of fear of recurrence on the quality of life of cancer survivors and their caregivers. *Qual Life Res. Int. J. Qual Life Asp. Treat Care Rehabil.* **2012**, *21*, 517–525. [CrossRef] [PubMed]
8. Pibernik-Okanović, M. Psychometric properties of the World Health Organisation quality of life questionnaire (WHOQOL-100) in diabetic patients in Croatia. *Diabetes Res. Clin. Pract.* **2001**, *51*, 133–143. [CrossRef] [PubMed]
9. World Health Organization. *WHO-BREF: Introduction, Administration, Scoring and Generic Version of the Assessment*; WHO: Geneva, Switzerland, 1996. Available online: http://www.who.int/mental_health/media/en/76.pdf (accessed on 1 August 2023).
10. Hooker, K.; Manoogian-O'Dell, M.; Monahan, D.J.; Frazier, L.D.; Shifren, K. Does type of disease matter? Gender differences among Alzheimer's and Parkinson's disease spouse caregivers. *Gerontologist* **2000**, *40*, 568–573. [CrossRef] [PubMed]
11. Awadalla, A.W.; Ohaeri, J.U.; Al-Awadi, S.A.; Tawfiq, A.M. Diabetes mellitus patients' family caregivers' subjective quality of life. *J. Natl. Med. Assoc.* **2006**, *98*, 727–736. [PubMed]
12. Vega-Silva, E.L.; Barrón-Ortiz, J.; Aguilar-Mercado, V.V.; Salas-Partida, R.E.; Moreno-Tamayo, K. Quality of life and caregiver burden in caregivers with patients with complications from type 2 diabetes mellitus. *Rev. Med. Inst. Mex. Seguro Soc.* **2023**, *61*, 440–448. [PubMed]
13. Yazla, E.; Karadere, M.E.; Terzi, Ö.; Dolapçı, M.; Yastı, A. Caregiving burden and quality of life in diabetic foot patients & caregivers. *Fam. Pract. Palliat. Care.* **2017**, *2*, 28–37.
14. Costa, M.S.A.; Machado, J.C.; Pereira, M.G. Longitudinal changes on the quality of life in caregivers of type 2 diabetes amputee patients. *Scand. J. Caring Sci.* **2020**, *34*, 979–988. [CrossRef] [PubMed]
15. Alves Costa, M.S.; Pereira, M.G. Predictors and moderators of quality of life in caregivers of amputee patients by type 2 diabetes. *Scand. J. Caring Sci.* **2018**, *32*, 933–942. [CrossRef] [PubMed]
16. Ebrahimi, H.; Ashrafi, Z.; Rudsari, D.M.; Parsayekta, Z.; Haghani, H. Effect of Family-Based Education on the Quality of Life of Persons with Type 2 Diabetes: A Randomized Clinical Trial. *J. Nurs. Res.* **2018**, *26*, 97–103. [CrossRef] [PubMed]

Disclaimer/Publisher's Note: The statements, opinions and data contained in all publications are solely those of the individual author(s) and contributor(s) and not of MDPI and/or the editor(s). MDPI and/or the editor(s) disclaim responsibility for any injury to people or property resulting from any ideas, methods, instructions or products referred to in the content.

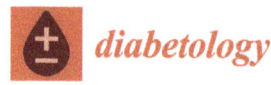

Article

3D-Printed Insoles for People with Type 2 Diabetes: An Italian, Ambulatory Case Report on the Innovative Care Model

Marco Mancuso [1], Rocco Bulzomì [2], Marco Mannisi [3], Francesco Martelli [1] and Claudia Giacomozzi [1,*]

[1] Istituto Superiore di Sanità, 00161 Rome, Italy; mancusopodologia@gmail.com (M.M.); francesco.martelli@iss.it (F.M.)
[2] Regional Healthcare Agency ASL ROMA2, 00159 Rome, Italy; rocco.bulzomi@aslroma2.it
[3] MEDERE s.r.l., 00118 Rome, Italy; marco.mannisi@medere.it
* Correspondence: claudia.giacomozzi@iss.it

Abstract: 3D-printed insoles are increasingly used for the management of foot pathologies, and the recent literature reports on various experimental studies dealing with either whole foot orthoses or pads fabricated through 3D-printing processes. In the case of diabetic foot disease, the main aim is to deliver more effective solutions with respect to the consolidated processes to reduce compressive risk forces at specific plantar foot sites. Clinical studies are, however, still limited, at least in peer-review journals. Additionally, in Italy, the manufacturing process of these medical devices has not been formally integrated yet into the list of care processes approved for reimbursement by the public healthcare service. Within the Italian DIAPASON project (DIAbetic PAtients Safe ambulatiON), a feasibility pilot study has been conducted in the territory on 21 patients with diabetic foot complications to assess the pros and cons of an innovative process. The process, which relies on in-shoe pressure measurements and on a patented 3D modeling and printing procedure, includes the prescription, design, manufacturing and testing of 3D-printed personalized insoles. The process has been tested in an ambulatory setting and showed the potential to be also implemented in community settings. In this paper, we report a case study on a single volunteer, and we describe and comment on how the whole process has been proven safe and suitable for the purpose.

Keywords: diabetic foot complications; plantar ulcers; 3D-printed personalized insoles; prevention; prescription; reimbursement; public healthcare system

1. Introduction

Diabetes mellitus (DM) is currently affecting 537 million people worldwide, and its already high prevalence, nearly 10%, is continuously increasing, especially in developing countries. Despite their different pathogenic mechanisms, both type 1 and type 2 DM show similar complications, among which diabetic foot syndrome is one of the most severe complications of diabetes and the most common cause of hospitalization in diabetic patients. Patients with diabetic foot syndrome have a risk of developing diabetic foot ulcers (DFU) up to 25%, and too often, DFU entails limb amputation. Further, diabetic foot complications are associated with a higher mortality rate than diabetes alone. Thus, diabetic foot syndrome is associated with very high public health and economic burdens, a very relevant impact on the quality of life for patients and their families, and can represent a major burden for healthcare professionals and institutions [1].

On average, the prevalence of DFU in people with diabetes reaches 6.3% worldwide; in Italy, it is in the range of 5.4–6.2% and raises to 20% in patients over 75 years [2]. According to the International Working Group on the Diabetic Foot (IWGDF) [3], therapeutic footwear is effective for primary and secondary ulcer prevention, even though its efficacy is often limited by poor adherence [4], despite valuable randomized controlled trials proving the effectiveness of offloading and ulcer healing techniques [5].

A 2020 systematic review [6] synthesized the following concepts: neuropathic DFU, which occurs mostly at the plantar forefoot and is very often associated with areas of peak plantar pressure; limited joint mobility, which likely contributes to the observed forefoot peak pressures. Furthermore, plantar pressure patterns are used to guide footwear and insole selections, adaptation and manufacturing, and to assess their effectiveness. Lowering plantar pressures represents a key factor for wound healing and ulcer prevention, where footwear and insoles are essential treatments for offloading pressures, with the desired reduction of dynamic in-shoe plantar pressure being >30% of the baseline or <200 kPa at the forefoot [6].

Despite, cautiously, the recommended thresholds in [6] should be intended as referred to specific measurement instrumentation and setup [7], the key-message of redistributing plantar pressure has a general validity.

The standard of care (SoC) for managing diabetic foot plantar pressures is represented by customized insoles [8,9], which exploit soft, accommodating material in the shape of open and closed cell foams, for example, polyurethane foam, to absorb compressive stress. These insoles, which are usually covered with a weight-bearing surface congruent with the patient's foot, have been reported as mechanically effective, even in the presence of active ulcers [8]. The SoC insoles' manufacturing process often requires hand craftsmanship, which may entail variability in the insole's design and therapeutic impact [9]. Those fabrication processes, which in some cases have been judged as inefficient and outdated, also heavily rely on clinical expertise and manual post-manufacturing adjustments (i.e., the creation of a manufactured depression, insertion of low-density foam disks, material removal from the base of the insole) to accommodate various patient-specific conditions and to ensure a proper fit to the patient's foot and shoes [10]. Further, they likely require more than one visit at the outpatients' service, eventual additional visits at the manufacturer, and quite long delivery times.

Advances in 3D-printing, materials science and software seem promising for significantly improving the offloading performance of the insoles and to optimize the whole fabrication process. While, in fact, the SoC insoles for the diabetic foot, though customized to the patient-specific geometry and conditions, rely on generic material properties, the 3D-printing approach is based on the concept of personalized materials to also address patient-specific stiffness and structural behavior [10,11]. Of course, biocompatible materials are mandatory for manufacturing 3D-printed insoles, which are intended to come in touch with human skin. As such, among the several printing techniques and materials, a suitable solution appears in the use of the fused deposition molding (FDM) technique to print polylactic acid (PLA) filaments. PLA is, in fact, a biodegradable thermoplastic polyester derived from natural resources that complies with the required biocompatibility and can be printed at a low temperature. A wide discussion on 3D-printing techniques and materials for constructing plastic materials can be found in Nguyen et al. [12], where infill printing and mechanical properties of PLA-printed models were investigated in detail, with a focus on investment casting. Another relevant, constructive issue to take into consideration when using the FMD technique and PLA material is the warpage of the model, which may occur in large-size models, as in the case of insoles. Huynh et al. [13] addressed this issue and showed that warpage can be reduced after consideration of the thermal effects and adhesion force.

Evidence from robust clinical studies is still lacking in the literature; however, pioneering papers confirm the mandatory safety and the potential effectiveness of personalized materials and graded stiffness and of the overall innovative approach, either specifically for diabetic foot management or with reference to other foot pathologies, such as a flat foot or the high-arched foot [8–11,14–28]. A more detailed digression of the relevant literature is reported in the Discussion section.

Despite technological advances, the prescription of 3D-printed insoles for diabetic foot syndrome is not yet reimbursed by the Italian public healthcare service. However, a decree by the Italian Minister of Health has been recently (April 2023) approved by the

State-Regions Conference, which establishes that the insoles for diabetic feet fabricated by using 3D-printing technologies, will also be reimbursable by the Public Healthcare Service, similarly to the SoC insoles. The updated document is expected to come officially into force in April 2024 [29].

Within the Italian project DIAPASON, regarding an innovative, multidimensional model of care for diabetic foot complications in very old people with diabetes and neuropathy, an ongoing pilot study in territorial healthcare facilities is exploring the feasibility and the potentiality of a novel insole fabrication process. Briefly, the process, which is based on a patented process for 3D personalized insoles modeling and manufacturing (Patents EP3916346A4, IT201900006076A1, IT201800010667A1) [11], has been integrated with measurements from a consolidated in-shoe pressure assessment [7], and from the patient's functional and behavioral assessment. In agreement with the diabetic foot-related issues listed in this introduction, the focus of the DIAPASON investigation was on: the appropriateness and safety of 3D-printed insoles for diabetic foot management; the feasibility of a novel 3D-printing-based workflow in an ambulatory setting; its portability in primary care settings, long-term care facilities or other community settings; the possible clinical relevance of the custom 3D-printed insoles; and the overall impact of the entire manufacturing process and its refundability by the Italian National Healthcare Service. Prior to the pilot implementation, which involved 20 outpatients aged 75 and over and one younger patient who volunteered as the first on-the-field tester, the present paper reports on the single case study of this younger patient as a vehicle to explore the core topics of the DIAPASON investigation.

Outline of the Paper

The present paper is articulated according to the conventional paper sections, namely the Introduction, Materials and Methods, Results, Discussion and Conclusions.

The Materials and Methods section addresses three main topics, namely: the context, scope and main objectives of the DIAPASON Project, i.e., the project within which the case study has been designed and executed; the fabrication process of the 3D-printed insoles, based on the 3D-printing workflow of a patented process integrated with new elements purposely developed within the DIAPASON Project; and relevant information on the case study.

The Results section is articulated in three paragraphs that report on the main outcomes of the instrumental and functional assessment of the case study's volunteers on Visit 1, whose suitable subset was sent to the 3D-insoles manufacturer; the fabrication process of the custom 3D insoles for the volunteers; the testing of the custom 3D insoles at Visit 2; and the data analysis and interpretation of the case study's main outcomes.

The Discussion section is articulated in the following three paragraphs: a brief digression on the relevant recent literature on the use of 3D-printed insoles for diabetic foot management and for other foot pathologies; the interpretation and potential impact of the case study's outcomes, dealing with the outcomes impact within the DIAPASON project and in the clinics, the portability of the reported solution, and its possible refundability within the Italian National Health Service; and a brief discussion of the main limitations of the study.

Finally, the Conclusions section summarizes the impact of the presented case study, in general, and in the peculiar Italian scenario.

2. Materials and Methods

2.1. The DIAPASON Project

The project proposal won an internal application for a small grant from the Italian National Institute of Health (ISS) as a two-year experimental pilot project, running from July 2021 to July 2023. The full name of the project is "DIAPASON: DIAbetic PAtients Safe ambulatiON. Enhancing resilience of very old patients with Diabetes and Neuropathy to maintain safe ambulation: an innovative multidimensional care model integrating new orthotics technology and new metabolic biomarkers". The research topic of the new metabolic biomarkers is outside the scope of this paper and will no longer be discussed. To address the topic of the novel care model exploiting new orthotics technology, ISS has been working in collaboration with the territorial primary care premises of the ASL ROMA2 Lazio Region healthcare service and with the Medere s.r.l. Company (Rome, Italy)—the owner of the patented process. The following key topics of the project were addressed:

- Integration of the ISS instrumental assessment protocol [7] with the existing diabetic foot care processes (foot screening, footwear prescription, manufacturing, testing, approval and reimbursement). The protocol, as detailed in [7], is based on the in-shoe pressure assessment measurement based on the Pedar-X system (novel$_{GmbH}$, Munich, Germany) and on the ad hoc risk thresholds, which are slightly more restrictive than the 200 kPa threshold [6,7]. Three additional functional tests have been integrated into the DIAPASON protocol namely the HHD (Hand-Held Dynamometry), the HRT (Heel Raise Test) and the TUG (Timed-Up-and-Go test) [30–32];
- Use, feasibility and optimization of the patented process to deliver 3D-printed personalized insoles; the insoles were meant to be inserted in proper, pre-selected home shoes to implement foot care prevention at home;
- Assessment of the appropriateness of the 3D-printed personalized insoles, especially in terms of safety and effectiveness;
- Information, education and enhanced motivation of patients and caregivers to reach higher adherence to the foot care interventions.

The DIAPASON project could be implemented on the basis of a scientific agreement already in force between ISS and ASL ROMA2 and of the ethical approval provided by the ASL ROMA2 Committee in 2019 and renewed in 2022 (ASL ROMA2 Resolution, number 1948 (20 September 2019); ASL ROMA2 Resolution, number 1570 (18 October 2022)). All study documents and actions were prepared and conducted in compliance with the Helsinki Declaration and with the GDPR (General Data Protection Regulation). For the DIAPASON pilot study (which is still ongoing and will be reported in future publications), twenty people of 75 years or more with type 2 diabetes and neuropathy were enrolled among those referring to the outpatients' Diabetic Foot Service of the ASL ROMA2 territorial facilities. Due to their foot complications (either in primary or secondary prevention), they were already in charge of the Diabetic Foot Service; thus, they were informed of the study (together with their relatives or caregivers) when they came to the service for their periodic examination. For those who agreed to participate, the clinical history was reviewed and completed so as to assess the presence of possible serious exclusion reasons, among which, scheduled hospitalization for any reason, locomotion prevented also at home, hostile approach towards using the prescribed footwear, home-shoes and the 3D-printed insoles. Written informed consent was gathered from those who agreed to participate. They did not receive any compensation. Two of them refused to participate since they were not available to wear prescribed footwear and insoles. Two of them abandoned the study for other complications requiring long hospitalizations. Those patients were highly representative of the people leaving with diabetes in the ASL ROMA2 healthcare district since up to 20% of people with type 2 diabetes and more than 50% of people with type 2 diabetes and neuropathy in the district have age and main clinical features comparable with the enrolled patients. The sample size was established on the basis of previous knowledge about ulcer rates and injuries from falls (20% and 45%, respectively, in the population from which we extracted our sample over a 12-month period), and also taking into consideration the project scheduling (12 months of intervention and follow-up) and resources (human resources and a budget for assessment and for 3D insoles fabrication). The sample size was adequate to detect an improvement in the two mentioned clinical outcomes of $\geq 6\%$ (G*Power 3.1.9.7, $\alpha = 0.05$, $1 - \beta = 0.8$).

One younger patient was also enrolled to volunteer as the first ambulatory tester, whose only difference from the DIAPASON sample consisted of her age (50 years old).

She received the information on the study and signed the informed consent. While the characterization of the DIAPASON sample has been detailed here to introduce the aim and the clinical scenario that also originated the case study, the outcomes associated with the 20 patients will not be further mentioned in the present paper, which only focuses on the outcomes from the younger volunteer.

2.2. The 3D Insoles Fabrication Process

The Medere patented process (Figure 1) allows the collection of the patient's anatomical data by means of a proprietary App (Medere) available for both IOS and Android mobile operating systems. At regimen, healthcare professionals can be easily trained to use the App. During the DIAPASON project, to ensure procedure repeatability, the PI (Principal Investigator) of the DIAPASON project acted as the measurements manager and collected the data in person. The anatomical data acquisition includes the use of the smartphone to 3D scan the foot and to acquire a sequence of foot images under loaded and unloaded predefined conditions (unilateral half-loaded internal sagittal view; unilateral half-loaded internal sagittal view with maximum dorsi-flexion of the 1st metatarso-phalangeal joint; bilateral frontal view with joined heels; bilateral rear view with parallel feet). The App also asks for basic anthropometrics (height and body mass) and a picture and some details of the shoes where the insoles should be inserted; in the DIAPASON project, this section was integrated with additional accurate measurements of the home-shoes previously selected to host the 3D insoles and of their commercial insoles to replace. Further, additional information was also delivered to Medere to optimize the modeling process, among which:

- plantar pressure measurements: at least 12 at regimen footprints for each foot were extracted from the three repetitions of the TUG and averaged to calculate the map of the peak pressures and the map of the pressure impulses (dedicated novel software packages by novel$_{GmbH}$, Munich, Germany; OriginPro 2022, OriginLab Corp, Northampton, MA, USA);
- anthropometric asymmetry, if present (especially in case of clinically relevant asymmetry in the lower limb length);
- semi-quantitative (normal; reduced; increased) joint mobility and muscle performance, based on video recordings during HHD, unloaded HRT and loaded HRT, and on force measurements by the wireless Biometrics Myometer (Biometrics Ltd., Nine Mile Point Industrial Estate, Ynysddu, UK) during MTT; video semi-quantitative analysis was done by using Kinovea 0.8.15 tools (Joan Charmant developer; https://www.kinovea.org/) (2 July 2023)
- history of falls and ulcers;
- behavioral information about daily activity and habits.

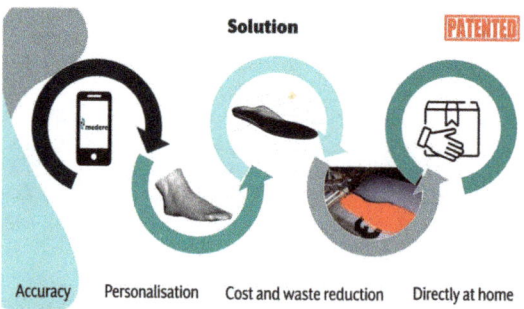

Figure 1. Synthesis of the patented process's phases to fabricate the Medere 3D-printed personalized insoles (source: Medere s.r.l.).

Following all those data acquisitions, Medere then proceeded to model the insole according to the patented workflow, as summarized in the following steps:

- The video and image datasets are used to accurately reconstruct the anatomy of the feet. The second stage involves the automatic creation of the 3D model of the foot using a photogrammetric algorithm based on the Structure From Motion (SFM) technique. This computer vision-based approach, validated as reliable and accurate in numerous fields (e.g., geosciences, cultural heritage, digital object reconstruction), significantly reduces both the modeling time and material waste. The algorithm works via SIFT (scale-invariant characteristic transform) and SURF (accelerated robust transform) to accurately identify foot geometries and their relative orientation in space. A point cloud is generated and finally converted into a mesh object. Dedicated filtering procedures are implemented to reduce inaccuracies when detected.
- The creation of the 3D model of the footbed is then performed using the computer-aided drafting (CAD) modeling technique. CAD modeling is the gold standard tool for prototype creation and optimization. This technique provides a high level of customization since, following the guidelines of a clinician, it is possible to modify the personalized footplate model to achieve the desired result. The method validated and patented by Medere consists of the creation of a starting model based on the patient's shoe geometry to create the best-fitting outline. A few transversal lines are then added following each foot geometry and modified to create the final plantar surface of the custom-made insoles. A more detailed description can be found in the patents [33–35]. The final model is then divided into regions to be printed with different density and mechanical properties.
- In the final stage of the process, insoles are produced using an additive manufacturing process (3D printing) based on the fused material deposition approach (FDM). FDM is a method that allows users to make almost any type of design while optimizing material waste with respect to standard production methods. The inner part of the insoles has an internal structure (infill) that can be adjusted and modified. Changing the geometric characteristics of the filler has a direct impact on the properties of the insoles and the mechanical behavior of the final object. Different shapes and densities of internal structures are used to maximize the required mechanical response (e.g., shock absorption and the required level of elasticity).
- The plantar surface of the insoles is covered with antibacterial ethylene vinyl acetate (EVA) sheet with a Shore A 35 to maximize smoothness and reduce the friction of the foot.

Within the DIAPASON project, the model was further refined before printing on the basis of the additional information (pressure maps, destination home shoes, patient's clinical history and behavioural habits, and any other relevant information) (Figure 2).

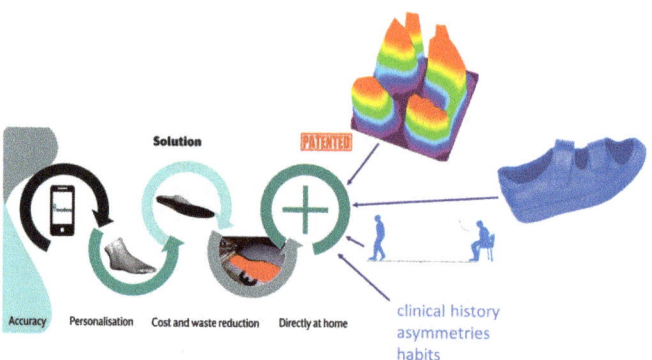

Figure 2. Synthesis of the integration of the 3D-printed personalized insoles fabrication process within the DIAPASON project (permission of adaptation by Medere s.r.l.).

Once manufactured, the 3D insoles were shipped to the ASL ROMA2 ambulatory, where the patient underwent the same instrumental assessment protocol as for the SoC insoles testing. Approval of the 3D insoles was thus based on a visual examination by the reference diabetologist and by the expert health professional who managed the patient's whole screening and assessment on instrumental testing outcomes (pressure patterns within the acceptable ranges, acceptable stability and balance during the TUG test), and on feedback from the patient. In case of criticalities, similar to the SoC procedure, the 3D insoles were sent back to the manufacturer for remodeling and reprinting.

2.3. The Case Study

The woman who first volunteered for the feasibility study was younger with respect to the 20 enrolled patients of the DIAPASON Project and had the following clinical, biological and behavioral features collected during the anamnesis and the podiatric screening:

- The patient was a woman;
- 50 years old, 1.62 m, 85 kg;
- Mild obesity (BMI: 32.4 kg·m^{-2});
- Type 2 diabetes mellitus (first diagnosed in 2019);
- Neuropathy: Vibration Perception Threshold (VPT) > 25 V; Michigan Neuropathy Score Index (MNSI) = 6 (normal reference < 1);
- No peripheral arterial disease (ankle–brachial index (ABI) > 0.90); with
- Normal vascular stiffness and peripheral pulses;
- Diabetic foot disease in primary prevention (no history of DFU);
- Bilateral flatfoot, hallux valgus and overlapping toes;
- Self-reported imbalance and postural instability but no history of falls;
- Left ankle osteotomy for Achilles tendon pain in 2018; the same problem is currently suspected for the right ankle;
- Acquired hypothyroidism since 2019 (treated with radiometabolic therapy for thyrotoxicosis);
- No history of smoking;
- No regular sports activity practiced;
- Needs to walk and stand for daily activities (housework, job, family).

3. The Case Study Results

3.1. Instrumental Assessment and Data Collection at Visit 1

On Visit 1, after the clinical anamnesis and the podiatry screening (the most relevant data are summarized in Section 2.3), the woman underwent the following protocol:

- HHD at each foot, under a maximum push-and-pull task against the resistance of the trained healthcare professional, three repetitions each, with the patient supine and the feet perpendicular to the ground (the force data were acquired by using the Biometrics Myometer and a video recording in the sagittal view, Figure 3). The maximum right push-and-pull reached 8.6 kg (10.1% of body mass) and 6.4 kg, respectively; the maximum left push-and-pull reached 7.2 kg (8.5% of body mass) and 5.6 kg, respectively;
- Barefoot standing for 10 s (the pressure data were from Pedar-X; wide insoles' size VW; the video recordings (webcams) were taken in the rear and sagittal views, Figure 4a); "barefoot" means wearing special socks purposely hand-made to host the Pedar insoles and to keep them solid with the foot, and to fix three markers roughly on the fifth metatarsal head, the lateral malleolus and along the ideal line joining the lateral malleolus with the head of the fibula. During barefoot standing, the rearfoot resulted more loaded than the forefoot, and the right more than the left, with a maximum average pressure of 245 kPa;
- The HRT (barefoot condition) of both feet, simultaneously while sitting (unloaded conditions), included 10 consistent repetitions (the pressure data were from Pedar-X; the video recordings (webcams) were taken in the rear and sagittal views, Figure 4b). The task lasted 15 s and showed the simultaneous raising of the heels, with greater force on the left and at the central repetitions;
- The HRT (barefoot condition) of both feet, simultaneously while standing (loaded conditions), included 10 consistent repetitions (the pressure data were from Pedar-X; the video recordings (webcams) were taken in the rear and sagittal views, Figure 4c). The task lasted 26 s (73% longer than the HRT while sitting) and showed asynchronous and variable raising patterns of the two heels, with comparable force, higher at the central repetitions;
- The TUG test (barefoot condition), comprising three repetitions (the pressure data were from Pedar-X; the video recordings (webcams) were taken in the rear and sagittal views, Figure 5). The total task lasted 44.4 s, and the average duration of each repetition was 14.1 s; maximum peak pressures of >200 kPa were found: at the heel (638 kPa) and hallux (238 kPa) on the left foot; at the heel (465 kPa), midfoot (280 kPa), forefoot (275 kPa) and hallux (285 kPa) on the right foot;
- Video recordings, alternatively, of the right and the left foot while sitting with the foot perpendicular to the ground and the hallux dorsiflexed were recorded. (the video acquired through the Medere app on an iPhone 8, Figure 6a,b);
- The sequence of pictures of the barefoot feet is described in paragraph 2.2 (the pictures were acquired through the Medere app on an iPhone 8, Figure 6c–h).

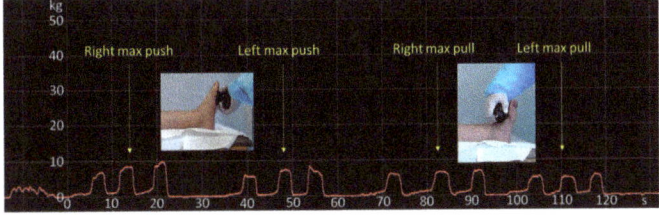

Figure 3. HHD test of the volunteer, measured by using the Biometrics Myometer. The volunteer was asked to perform and maintain the maximum ankle push-and-pull for roughly 3 s, counted loud by the health professional, with three repetitions for each foot and task.

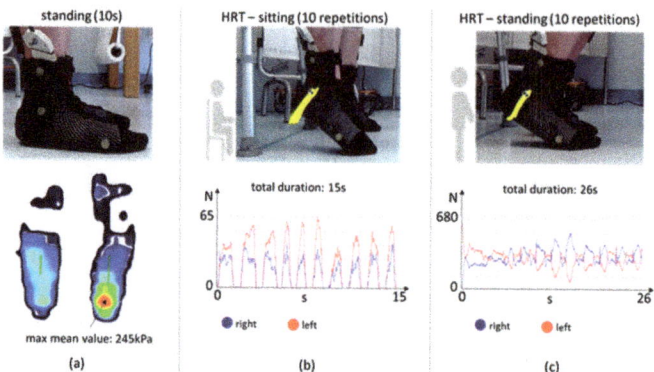

Figure 4. Volunteer's functional tests outcomes: (**a**) 10 s of upright standing; pressure map at the bottom (Pedar-X system, insole size VW) shows values averaged over the standing period; (**b**) HRT under unloaded condition (sitting); (**c**) HRT under loaded condition (upright, with hands on a front support). In (**b**) and in (**c**), the plot at the bottom shows right and left forces (Pedar-X system) during the 10 repetitions, while the yellow track on the top image (snapshot at the maximum ankle plantarflexion) shows the cumulative quasi-sagittal trajectory of the lateral malleolus.

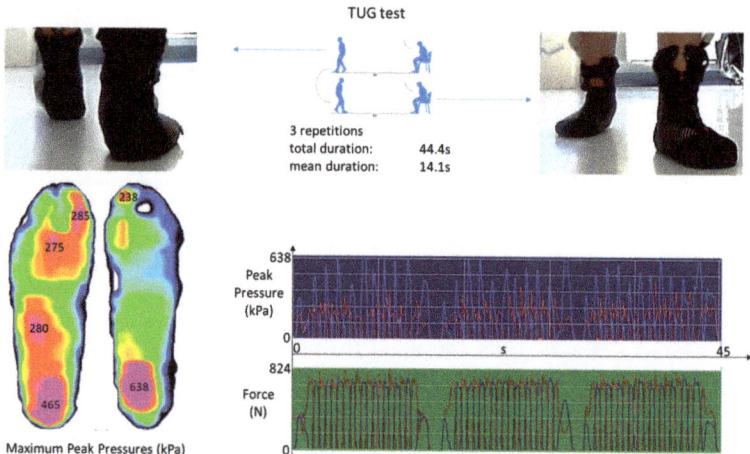

Figure 5. TUG test outcomes: the top part of the figure shows two exemplificative snapshots of the video recording in the frontal plane during the three repetitions of the volunteer's TUG; the peak pressure map, with the superimposed values > 200 kPa, is reported at the bottom left, while time processes of peak pressure (blue background) and vertical force (green background) are plotted at the bottom right of the figure (data from the Pedar-X system, insole size VW).

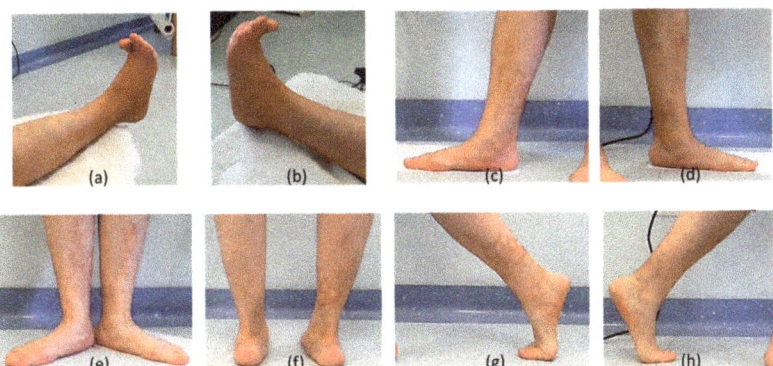

Figure 6. Volunteer's data acquisition through the Medere app: snapshot from 360° video acquisition of the right (**a**) and of the left (**b**) foot; sagittal view of the half-loaded right (**c**) and left (**d**) foot; frontal view of the feet, open toes and heels in contact (**e**); rear view of the feet, parallel position (**f**); sagittal view of the maximum heel-raise of the right (**g**) and of the left (**h**) foot.

The whole ambulatory visit lasted roughly one hour, during which one expert health professional and one engineer worked to collect all the needed data and information.

At the end of the instrumental assessment, the diabetologist was involved in preliminary data analyses and, together with the health professional, authorized and started the consolidated prescription procedure (SoC shoes and insoles) and identified the off-the-shelf home shoe to host the 3D insoles (MAC2 Fanny home shoe, (Optima Molliter s.rl., Civitanova Marche, Italy), an MD-certified shoe for the prevention of diabetic foot complications). The selection was conducted among a certain number of MD-certified home shoes made available at the healthcare premises for the DIAPASON feasibility study and whose commercial standard insoles had been previously scanned in the sizes from EU 36 to EU 45. The final decision was taken after the volunteer's agreement.

The data collected through the Medere app were immediately sent to Medere; some additional processing time was required to prepare the synthesis of the additional data and information.

3.2. 3D Insoles Fabrication Process

The 3D-insoles manufacturer received the data collected through the Medere app and the following additional information to model the insoles:

- A woman, 50 years, 1.62 m, 85 kg;
- Type 2 DM with neuropathy;
- Bilateral flatfoot, hallux valgus and overlapping toes;
- Achilles tendon pain at right (solved at left after ankle osteotomy);
- Active at home (walking and standing);
- Self-reported unbalance and postural instability;
- Ankle joint mobility was slightly reduced when unloaded and compromised when loaded;
- Ankle dorsi-flexion was slightly weaker than plantarflexion; the left leg was slightly weaker than the right;
- Barefoot pronation and hallux scarcely loaded during gait;
- Very high plantar pressure (peaks and impulses) at the hindfoot, more on the right foot; abnormally high pressures on the left foot; unexpected offload of the forefoot (Figure 7, containing peak pressure maps and pressure impulse maps);
- The selected home shoe was a Molliter Fanny, EU size 38 (the technical details of the shoe and insole were already available in the Medere DIAPASON database).

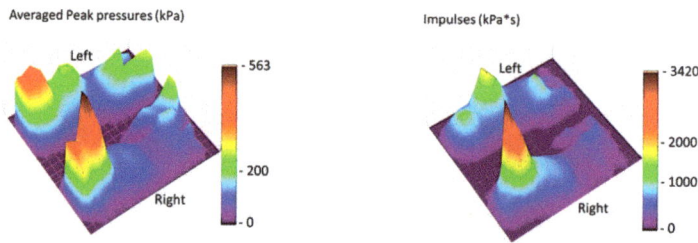

Figure 7. Volunteer's peak pressure map (**left**) and pressure impulse map (**right**) averaged over the at-regimen footprints extracted from the three repetitions of the TUG and sent to Medere for insoles modeling and manufacturing. Data were acquired by the Pedar-X system and insole size VW, acquired and processed by novel$_{GmbH}$ software and OriginPro2022.

Based on the received data, Medere modeled the insoles based on the patented process (as previously described) and integrated the received additional information.

The model was created to maximize the contact between the plantar surface of the insole and the foot of the patient, with the aim of distributing the pressure evenly across the foot and increasing the level of stability. The arch support was modeled to reduce barefoot pronation.

The foot pressure map was aligned with the CAD model of the insoles to identify the area of interest (e.g., peak pressure regions) and to subdivide the insoles into different parts. Using a parametrization method based on the anthropometric and pressure data, the density of the different parts of the insoles was calculated. The initial step was to calculate the density of the main part and then the density of the parts where the pressure needed to be reduced.

The model was imported into a slicing software (Simplify3D V4.1.2—Simplify3D, LLC.). The parts were aligned and positioned on the printing bed surface, and the previously calculated parameters for the density were assigned to each part. For this case study, the regions of max pressure were identified in correspondence with the heels only. Therefore, the model was divided into two parts, which were printed with the following parameters:

- Infill type: Full honeycomb;
- Infill density: 29% for the main part, 25% for the heel region.

A flexible filament with Shore A 82 was used for the printing process (Filaflex82A-RECREUS INDUSTRIES S.L., Elda (Alicante) Spain). The insoles were then covered with EVA Shore A 35 sheet.

The 3D insoles were then shipped to the project PI, who preliminarily checked them for congruency and alerted the ASL ROMA2 ambulatory of Visit 2 for the volunteer.

3.3. 3D-Insoles Testing at Visit 2

The whole 3D fabrication process took one week (standard fabrication time, no priority was asked to the Manufacturer). Three weeks were however needed to have the SoC footwear ready and to allow the volunteer to go to the shoemaker to gather them. During visit 2 both products were tested, to optimise the number of visits.

The instrumental assessment protocol at visit 2 was much simpler than visit 1, and only consisted of the following steps (testing of the SoC footwear, very similar to this, is not reported since it falls outside the scope of this paper):

- With the home shoes and their commercial insoles: standing for 10 s and three repetitions of the TUG test (the pressure data were from Pedar-X; wide insoles size VW; the video recordings (webcams) were taken in the rear and sagittal views, Figure 8a). The

TUG test lasted 41.7 s in total (barefoot total duration: 44.4 s); the mean TUG duration was 13.2 s (barefoot mean TUG duration: 14.1 s);
- With the home shoes and the 3D-printed personalized insoles: standing for 10 s and three repetitions of the TUG test (the pressure data were from Pedar-X; wide insoles size VW; the video recordings (webcams) were taken in the rear and sagittal views, Figure 8b). The TUG test lasted 38.9 s in total, and the mean TUG duration was 12.5 s.

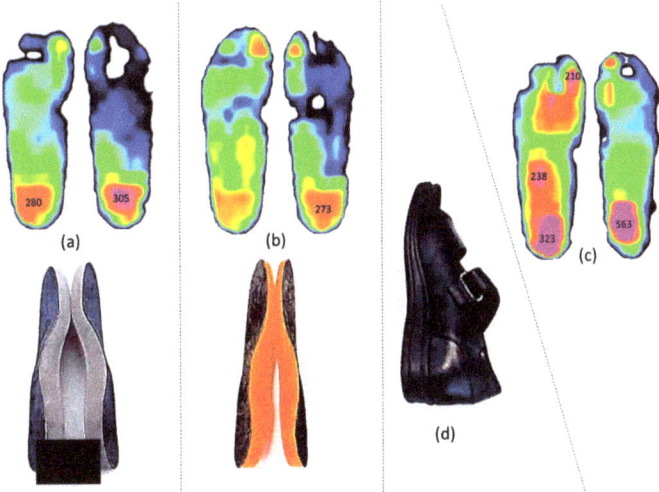

Figure 8. Volunteer's testing of 3D-printed insoles. Peak pressure map and values >200 kPa over at-regimen footprints of the three repetitions of TUG while wearing the selected home shoes (**d**) and their commercial insoles (**a**) or the 3D-printed personalized insoles (**b**). Reference, barefoot Peak pressure map is reported in (**c**) for a qualitative comparison. Data were acquired by the Pedar-X system and the insole size VW.

The pressure data were processed to investigate the appropriateness of the 3D insoles with respect to the risk thresholds and gait balance (only data from at-regimen footprints) and their eventual advantage with respect to the commercial accommodative insoles of the home shoes. Briefly: the peak pressures were greatly reduced by the home shoes and their commercial insoles with respect to the barefoot conditions, with the maximum peak at the right hindfoot being reduced by roughly 45% (Figure 8a); the 3D-printed personalized insoles, together with the home shoes, performed even better, with the maximum peak pressure at the right hindfoot—the only remaining area with pressures above the 200 kPa threshold—reduced by >50% (Figure 8b). The overall assessment, including visual examinations from the clinician and health professional, feedback from the volunteer, comparisons with Visit 1's barefoot assessment and a review of the video recordings, fetched a positive evaluation of the 3D insoles.

4. Discussion

4.1. 3D-Printed Insoles: Feedback from the Recent Literature

Advances in 3D technology may represent a promising, significant improvement in the optimization of the therapeutic performance of plantar orthoses.

In the specific field of diabetic foot care, robust clinical studies are still needed to provide evidence either of a comparable clinical efficacy of 3D-printed insoles, with respect to custom conventional insoles (SoC solutions), or even of their superiority. However, several preliminary studies have reported on the potentialities of 3D-printed insoles for diabetic foot management or with respect to other relevant foot and musculoskeletal pathologies.

Zuniga et al. [15] reported a proof-of-concept of 3D-printed insoles for patients with diabetes and tested it on one volunteer only. Their developed 3D-printed insoles used two polymers, thermoplastic polyether-polyurethane and thermoplastic polyurethane polyester-based polymer, and they assessed their performance through measurements of plantar pressure distribution during walking. The two 3D-printed insoles performed as well as a standard insole, with no significant difference in the average peak pressures. They concluded that 3D-printed insoles have the potential for diabetic foot management and that the digital manufacturing workflow of customized insoles can be helpfully implemented in middle-income countries.

Chhikara et al. [16] recently conducted a valuable review on the effectiveness of 3D-printed orthoses for diabetic foot management. They reported on the following human subject studies: Telfer et al. [17] compared standard milled insoles with 3D-printed insoles in 20 patients with type 2 diabetes and proved that the former performed better than the latter in improving plantar offloading. Anggoro et al. [18] conducted a preliminary study on the expectations and satisfaction of two patients with a long history of diabetes after having used the 3D-printed insoles for 6 weeks and obtained high satisfaction and expectation scores and overall satisfactory performance and good comfort. Tang et al. [19] conducted an exploratory study on one healthy volunteer, and the supplied 3D-printed insoles showed an effective reduction in the peak plantar pressures (>33%) compared to SoC insoles. Hudak et al. [10] enrolled one patient with diabetes to compare an SoC insole, a hybrid 3D-printed insole with a bi-laminate foam top, and a fully 3D-printed insole: the latter showed improved durability, reduced shear stiffness and lower plantar pressures. The authors of review [16] concluded that: the available literature on development of 3D-printed orthosis for patients with Diabetes is still limited; more generally, the 3D-printed orthoses demonstrated equivalent performance in clinical aspect; 3D-printing process may bring to biomechanical changes in the foot, however further validation is required to confirm that these changes can indeed be associated with clinically relevant outcomes; additive manufacturing applied to the diabetic foot management may benefit of the integration with Finite Elements Analysis (FEA), biomechanical measurements and modelling; there is still a lack of orthoses for post-ulcer diabetic foot and 3D-printed insoles impact as an intervention against the foot ulcer progression is yet to be tested [20]; patients with partial foot amputations can also be managed using 3D-printed partial foot orthosis [21,22].

Shaikh et al. [23] conducted quite an extensive, experimental study involving 200 patients suffering from various foot-related problems and joint pain; 18 of them (38–69 years old) suffered from diabetic foot complications. Their 3D-printed insoles were designed using plantar pressure systems and a clinical practitioner's assessment and, for patients with diabetes, also providing additional podiatry elements. In particular, diabetic 3D-insole fabrication exploited the slicing options, which allowed for variable density printing and the possibility to add elements for corn pressure relief, metatarsal bar and pads since the insole design phase. The insoles were tested under walking and other relevant motion tasks, with only two dropouts (with active ulcers and obesity) among patients with diabetes. The authors found that the custom 3D-printed insoles provided biomechanical correction whenever required, contributed to alleviating pain and relief from high peak pressures, and showed the potential of being long-lasting (still well-performing after 21 months for the patients who participated in the follow-up).

Daryabor et al. [24] recently published a systematic review aimed at evaluating custom 3D-printed insoles for flat feet. As the main outcome of their narrative analysis, based on 10 studies, including 225 subjects with flexible flatfeet, the evidence from the literature was found to be weak; however, it emerged that using custom 3D-printed insoles may positively affect pain and foot function, with no significant change in the vertical loading rate during walking or running. However, the authors reported insufficient evidence to conclude the comparison between 3D-printed insoles and other types of insoles.

Xu et al. [25] compared custom 3D-printed insoles with traditional prefabricated rehabilitation insoles in 80 patients with bilateral symptomatic flatfoot. After 8 weeks, their RCT showed that the 3D-printed insoles reduced the pressure on the metatarsals and redistributed it over the midfoot significantly more than the prefabricated insoles.

Jandova et al. [26] showed that, in both flatfoot and high-arched feet, 3D-printed insoles perform as comparably well as traditional, customized insoles. The study relied on 51 adults, and comparisons were conducted on the basis of plantar pressure distribution. The authors concluded that in the case of a high-arched foot, where peak pressures are higher and more difficult to compensate for, 3D-printed insoles might reach even better results than traditional customized insoles.

Jin et al. [27] tested a customized 3D-printed heel support insole on a sample of 30 healthy male participants. The authors found that the biomechanical properties of the customized 3D-printed heel support may be better than those of the traditional heel support insole, especially when there is a need for an additional increase in heel height. Their volunteers did not decrease midfoot motion function while using the insoles.

Prakotmongkol et al. [28] compared custom 3D-printed insoles with regard to custom conventional insoles for flatfeet, focusing on foot and ankle function, navicular height, patient satisfaction and insole durability. Their RCT (60 patients in total) lasted for three months and revealed that the scores of foot and ankle functions and insole use significantly improved at three months in both the intervention and the control group; deformation of insoles was found in both groups with no significant difference between them, and durability and patient-reported satisfaction were significantly higher for the intervention group.

4.2. Interpretation and Potential Impact of the Case Study Outcomes

When dealing with patients, the adoption of this new technology mandatorily requires an investigation of the feasibility of the whole fabrication process, thus also including those phases of the workflow which mostly impact the patient, namely the acquisition of the input data, the identification of the most suitable shoes to use and/or adapt the final product testing.

The hereby reported case study showed that an integrated process to obtain 3D-printed personalized insoles for patients with diabetic foot disease may be feasible, safe and effective in delivering an appropriate offloading device while also optimizing the number and duration of the patient's visits. Specifically, the case study was conducted by rigorously applying the procedure designed and approved within an Italian project, the DIAPASON project, where the SoC process for diabetic ulcer prevention in the territorial healthcare facilities of the ASL ROMA2 Regional Health Agency had been integrated (i) with an instrumental assessment of the in-shoe plantar pressure profile at the SoC footwear prescription and testing phases and (ii) with functional tests (HHD, HRT and TUG) at the prescription phase only. Additional data collection was required, specifically for the 3D fabrication process, consisting of a 3D scan of the foot and a sequence of foot images under pre-established loading conditions, all acquired by means of a dedicated app. Gathering a few models and sizes of home shoes marketed as MD-certified for the diabetic foot and scanning their commercial insoles (to be replaced by the 3D-printed personalized insoles), represented the remaining preliminary actions needed to complete the input dataset of the 3D workflow. Key findings from the case study may thus be summarized as follows: the 3D insoles fabrication process was feasible and required only two visits by the patient to the diabetic foot outpatient service (ambulatory setting): Visit 1 lasted about one hour and it involved one health professional and one technology expert to gather and process data, and one diabetologist to approve the data synthesis and home shoes selection, while Visit 2 lasted <20 min and involved the same personnel as Visit 1. The experimental setup for quantitative and semi-quantitative data collection was safe and adequate for the purpose, with no risks of adverse events for the volunteer.

In agreement with [10], the proposed integrated fabrication process resulted in effectively optimizing the resources, delivery times and burden on the patient. According to the Italian SoC process, in fact, at least two additional visits are needed at the manufacturer's premises: the first for the imprint collection and the shoe selection, and the second to test the insole fit with the patient's foot and the selected shoe before the delivery for clinical testing.

Results of the case-study were well in agreement with Hudak et al [10], who described a comparable approach to deliver 3D-fabricated personalized insoles for the diabetic foot. Differently from the foot data acquisition method used in the hereby described case-study (foot 3D scan and images), they started their fabrication workflow by scanning the foam crush box impression of the patient's foot. However, to define the 3D model of the foot, they similarly collected the patient-specific plantar pressure distribution using the same in-shoe Pedar-X device. They defined the offloading regions using the 200 kPa threshold value [6], and manually identified anatomical landmarks of the foot (heel and first and fifth metatarsal heads) to facilitate proper insole positioning and sizing. Finally, they modelled the insole to match the geometry of the patient's scanned foot, and defined the offloading segments on the basis of the plantar pressure map. The reported results of the technical assessment showed a matched or improved durability, a reduced shear stiffness, and a reduction in plantar pressure of their 3D insoles compared to SoC insoles. Further, the Authors stressed the advantage of the new process when compared with the SoC one, where: manually performed modifications are usually done to the plaster model; layers of foam of different compositions are usually glued together; the pressure-relieving region is based on clinical judgments and obtained by adding material to the positive plantar model, or using disks of low-density foam, or by removing material from the base of the insole in the desired region; the insole is finally manually shaped to ensure proper fit to the patient's foot and shoes; last but not least, the entire fabrication process typically requires patient visits over multiple days and may last for weeks.

Despite the fact that therapeutic personalized insoles based on 3D technology are not yet refundable in Italy, a regulatory official act already exists [29], which is expected to enter into force by April 2024. The current approved budget for SoC personalized insoles reimbursement may be adequate for the 3D-printed personalized insoles. Of course, manufacturers should reorganize their workflow. In the case of a remote process, which is more convenient for the patient, it will be necessary that the clinical foot service reorganizes itself so as to acquire all the needed measurements and scans and to have a set of shoes and home shoes available to allow for on-site identification as the best solution for the specific patient. The reported case study, and the pilot study, which is ongoing within the DIAPASON project on very old and fragile patients, may thus result as valuable for the spread of 3D-printing techniques in the Italian scenario of diabetic foot management, and similar feasibility and experimental studies are needed and welcome.

The case study also allowed us to explore the portability of the proposed novel care model in other healthcare structures or even in long-term care facilities or community settings, so as to reach those fragile and disadvantaged patients who have serious limitations to reach dedicated labs, shoemaker settings or outpatient's clinics. The assessment phases of the whole process showed the potential to be moved from the ambulatory to other local settings; however, this means that the portable equipment and the expert personnel shall move twice for each patient to reach the local setting. Reasonably, the process might become feasible and sustainable if groups of patients are scheduled for assessment on the same day.

4.3. Limitations of the Study

The outcomes of the reported case study, though encouraging, remain valid within the specific, adopted 3D fabrication process, including materials, algorithms and modeling features. The case study relied on a patented process integrated with a consolidated assessment protocol; however, to generalize the feasibility and effectiveness of 3D-printing technology with respect to diabetic foot management, many experimental studies are still needed. Insole effectiveness was tested with respect to plantar pressure distribution and the quantified outcomes of the functional tests addressing balance and force, as well as on visual inspection from an expert podiatrist and diabetologist and on the patient's feedback;

however, shear stress measurements would have completed the overall insole assessment. Further, the study did not contain information on the durability and follow-up outcomes; the patient is, however, followed, and the eventual relevant outcomes will be documented in future works.

Transferability of the results to other patients might represent another limitation. The volunteer in this case study was quite young (50 years old); however, all tasks and measurements had already been validated on cohorts of very old and fragile patients, and they had been found safe and feasible, even in the case of partially impaired patients, where the use of walking aids and the assistance from healthcare personnel was included (and properly accounted for) in the functional assessment.

5. Conclusions

Despite the limited evidence from the literature, custom 3D-printed insoles seem to have the potential for diabetic foot management, their effectiveness appearing as at least comparable or even greater than custom conventional insoles, with an expected longer durability. Further validation is, however, still required to confirm that these high-level performances can indeed be translated into clinically relevant outcomes.

The hereby reported case study proved the feasibility and safety of an integrated workflow, including in-shoe pressure measurements and the outcomes from functional tests to obtain 3D-printed insoles for patients with diabetic foot disease. The insoles were found effective in delivering the appropriate offloading while also optimizing the number and duration of the patient's visits: specifically, only two visits at the diabetic foot outpatient service were needed, with no additional visits at the manufacturer's premises (as it happens in the case of SoC insoles manufacturing). The workflow, successfully tested during the case study, can thus be used to implement a pilot study—the ongoing DIAPASON project—at the territorial healthcare facilities of the Italian ASL ROMA2 Regional Health Agency, dealing with very old patients with type 2 diabetes and foot complications. The workflow also has the potential to be used in long-term care facilities or community settings, with an expected relevant impact on diabetic foot management, the burden of care for fragile or disadvantaged patients and healthcare resources. The essential requirement is, of course, that the portable equipment and expert, trained personnel are available to reach local settings twice for each patient. Italian legislation has already officially approved the reimbursement of 3D-printed insoles for diabetic foot management; the law is expected to enter into force within the spring of 2024.

Author Contributions: Conceptualization, C.G., M.M. (Marco Mancuso) and R.B.; methodology, C.G. and M.M. (Marco Mancuso); software and validation, C.G., M.M. (Marco Mannisi) and F.M.; investigation, C.G., M.M. (Marco Mancuso) and R.B.; resources, C.G.; data curation, C.G., M.M. (Marco Mancuso), M.M. (Marco Mannisi) and F.M.; writing—original draft preparation, C.G., M.M. (Marco Mancuso) and M.M.(Marco Mannisi); writing—review and editing, all authors; supervision, C.G. and R.B.; project administration, C.G.; funding acquisition, C.G. All authors have read and agreed to the published version of the manuscript.

Funding: This research was funded by the Italian National Institute of Health (ISS), grant number ISS2020-DIAPASON. The APC was funded by ISS.

Institutional Review Board Statement: This study was conducted in accordance with the Declaration of Helsinki and approved by the Institutional Review Board of the Regional Health Service ASL ROMA2 (Resolution number 1948/2019 and Resolution number 1570/2022).

Informed Consent Statement: Informed consent was obtained from all subjects involved in the study.

Data Availability Statement: The data presented in this study are available on request from the corresponding author. The data are not publicly available due to ongoing patent submissions.

Acknowledgments: The authors acknowledge Matilde Bocci for administrative support; the ASL ROMA2 personnel for administrative and technical support; all the patients who volunteered for the study; Molliter s.r.l. and Podartis s.r.l. for the donation of home shoes to partly cover the DIAPASON needs.

Conflicts of Interest: The authors M.M., R.B., F.M. and C.G. declare no conflicts of interest. One of the authors, Ma.M., who actively participated in the research study, also holds a position as the co-founder of Medere s.r.l. The utmost care has been taken to ensure the integrity and objectivity of the research presented in this paper. The funders had no role in the design of the study; in the collection, analyses, or interpretation of data; in the writing of the manuscript; or in the decision to publish the results.

References

1. Matijević, T.; Talapko, J.; Meštrović, T.; Matijević, M.; Erić, S.; Erić, I.; Škrlec, I. Understanding the multifaceted etiopathogenesis of foot complications in individuals with diabetes. *World J. Clin. Cases* **2023**, *11*, 1669–1683. [CrossRef]
2. Bonora, E.; Sesti, G. (Eds.) Società Italiana di Diabetologia. In *Il Diabete in Italia*; Bononia University Press: Bologna, Italy, 2016; ISBN 978-88-6923-146-9.
3. International Working Group on Diabetic Foot (IWGDF). IWGDF 2019 Guidelines. 2019. Available online: www.iwgdfguidelines.org (accessed on 2 July 2023).
4. Crews, R.T.; King, A.L.; Yalla, S.V.; Rosenblatt, N.J. Recent Advances and Future Opportunities to Address Challenges in Offloading Diabetic Feet: A Mini-Review. *Gerontology* **2018**, *64*, 309–317. [CrossRef]
5. Piaggesi, A.; Macchiarini, S.; Rizzo, L.; Palumbo, F.; Tedeschi, A.; Nobili, L.A.; Leporati, E.; Scire, V.; Teobaldi, I.; Del Prato, S. An Off-the-Shelf Instant Contact Casting Device for the Management of Diabetic Foot Ulcers. *Diabetes Care* **2007**, *30*, 586–590. [CrossRef]
6. Ahmed, S.; Barwick, A.; Butterworth, P.; Nancarrow, S. Footwear and insole design features that reduce neuropathic plantar forefoot ulcer risk in people with diabetes: A systematic literature review. *J. Foot Ankle Res.* **2020**, *13*, 30. [CrossRef] [PubMed]
7. Giacomozzi, C.; Uccioli, L. Learning from experience: A simple effective protocol to test footwear prescriptions for the Diabetic foot by using the Pedar system. *J. Biomed. Sci. Eng.* **2013**, *6*, 45–57. [CrossRef]
8. Muir, B.C.; Li, J.-S.; Hudak, Y.F.; Kaufman, G.E.; Cullum, S.; Aubin, P.M. Evaluation of novel plantar pressure-based 3-dimensional printed accommodative insoles—A feasibility study. *Clin. Biomech.* **2022**, *98*, 105739. [CrossRef]
9. Leung, M.S.-H.; Yick, K.-L.; Sun, Y.; Chow, L.; Ng, S.-P. 3D printed auxetic heel pads for patients with diabetic mellitus. *Comput. Biol. Med.* **2022**, *146*, 105582. [CrossRef] [PubMed]
10. Hudak, Y.F.; Li, J.-S.; Cullum, S.; Strzelecki, B.M.; Richburg, C.; Kaufman, G.E.; Abrahamson, D.; Heckman, J.T.; Ripley, B.; Telfer, S.; et al. A novel workflow to fabricate a patient-specific 3D printed accommodative foot orthosis with personalized latticed metamaterial. *Med. Eng. Phys.* **2022**, *104*, 103802. [CrossRef]
11. Ferro, N.; Perotto, S.; Bianchi, D.; Ferrante, R.; Mannisi, M. Design of cellular materials for multiscale topology optimization: Application to patient-specific orthopedic devices. *Struct. Multidiscip. Optim.* **2022**, *65*, 79. [CrossRef]
12. Nguyen, T.T.; Tran, V.T.; Pham, T.H.N.; Nguyen, V.-T.; Thanh, N.C.; Thi, H.M.N.; Duy, N.V.A.; Thanh, D.N.; Nguyen, V.T.T. Influences of Material Selection, Infill Ratio, and Layer Height in the 3D Printing Cavity Process on the Surface Roughness of Printed Patterns and Casted Products in Investment Casting. *Micromachines* **2023**, *14*, 395. [CrossRef] [PubMed]
13. Huynh, T.T.; Nguyen, T.V.T.; Nguyen, Q.M.; Nguyen, T.K. Minimizing Warpage for Macro-Size Fused Deposition Modeling Parts. *Comput. Mater. Contin.* **2021**, *68*, 2913–2923. [CrossRef]
14. Shaulian, H.; Gefen, A.; Biton, H.; Wolf, A. Graded stiffness offloading insoles better redistribute heel plantar pressure to protect the diabetic neuropathic foot. *Gait Posture* **2023**, *101*, 28–34. [CrossRef]
15. Zuñiga, J.; Moscoso, M.; Padilla-Huamantinco, P.G.; Lazo-Porras, M.; Tenorio-Mucha, J.; Padilla-Huamantinco, W.; Tincopa, J.P. Development of 3D-Printed Orthopedic Insoles for Patients with Diabetes and Evaluation with Electronic Pressure Sensors. *Designs* **2022**, *6*, 95. [CrossRef]
16. Chhikara, K.; Singh, G.; Gupta, S.; Chanda, A. Progress of additive manufacturing in fabrication of foot orthoses for diabetic patients: A review. *Ann. 3D Print. Med.* **2022**, *8*, 100085. [CrossRef]
17. Telfer, S.; Woodburn, J.; Collier, A.; Cavanagh, P. Virtually optimized insoles for offloading the diabetic foot: A randomized crossover study. *J. Biomech.* **2017**, *60*, 157–161. [CrossRef] [PubMed]
18. Anggoro, P.W.; Tauviqirrahman, M.; Jamari, J.; Bayuseno, A.P.; Bawono, B.; Avelina, M.M. Computer-aided reverse engineering system in the design and production of orthotic insole shoes for patients with diabetes. *Cogent Eng.* **2018**, *5*, 1470916. [CrossRef]
19. Tang, L.; Wang, L.; Bao, W.; Zhu, S.; Li, D.; Zhao, N.; Liu, C. Functional gradient structural design of customized diabetic insoles. *J. Mech. Behav. Biomed. Mater.* **2019**, *94*, 279–287. [CrossRef]
20. Choo, Y.J.; Boudier-Revéret, M.; Chang, M.C. 3D printing technology applied to orthosis manufacturing: Narrative review. *Ann. Palliat. Med.* **2020**, *9*, 4262–4270. [CrossRef] [PubMed]
21. Desmyttere, G.; Leteneur, S.; Hajizadeh, M.; Bleau, J.; Begon, M. Effect of 3D printed foot orthoses stiffness and design on foot kinematics and plantar pressures in healthy people. *Gait Posture* **2020**, *81*, 247–253. [CrossRef]
22. Cha, Y.H.; Lee, K.H.; Ryu, H.J.; Joo, I.W.; Seo, A.; Kim, D.-H.; Kim, S.J. Ankle-Foot Orthosis Made by 3D Printing Technique and Automated Design Software. *Appl. Bionics Biomech.* **2017**, *2017*, 9610468. [CrossRef] [PubMed]

23. Shaikh, S.; Jamdade, B.; Chanda, A. Effects of Customized 3D-Printed Insoles in Patients with Foot-Related Musculoskeletal Ailments—A Survey-Based Study. *Prosthesis* **2023**, *5*, 550–561. [CrossRef]
24. Daryabor, A.; Kobayashi, T.; Saeedi, H.; Lyons, S.M.; Maeda, N.; Naimi, S.S. Effect of 3D printed insoles for people with flatfeet: A systematic review. *Assist. Technol.* **2022**, *35*, 169–179. [CrossRef]
25. Xu, R.; Wang, Z.; Ren, Z.; Ma, T.; Jia, Z.; Fang, S.; Jin, H. Comparative Study of the Effects of Customized 3D printed insole and Prefabricated Insole on Plantar Pressure and Comfort in Patients with Symptomatic Flatfoot. *Experiment* **2019**, *25*, 3510–3519. [CrossRef] [PubMed]
26. Jandova, S.; Mendricky, R. Benefits of 3D Printed and Customized Anatomical Footwear Insoles for Plantar Pressure Distribution. *3D Print. Addit. Manuf.* **2022**, *9*, 547–556. [CrossRef] [PubMed]
27. Jin, H.; Xu, R.; Wang, S.; Wang, J. Use of 3D-Printed Heel Support Insoles Based on Arch Lift Improves Foot Pressure Distribution in Healthy People. *Experiment* **2019**, *25*, 7175–7181. [CrossRef]
28. Prakotmongkol, V.; Chaemkhuntod, C.; Nutchamlong, Y.; Charoenvitvorakul, T.; Tongsai, S.; Janvikul, W.; Thavornyutikarn, B.; Kosorn, W.; Praewpipa, B. Comparison of Effectiveness, Patient Satisfaction, and Durability between 3D-Printed Customized Insoles and Conventional Custom-Made Insoles for Flat Feet: A Randomized Controlled Trial. *ASEAN J. Rehabil. Med.* **2023**, *33*, 2–9.
29. Italian Minister of Health; Italian Minister of Economy and Finance. Schema Decreto LEA 2023. Available online: https://www.simfer.it/approvato-il-nomenclatore-tariffario-dei-nuovi-livelli-essenziali-di-assistenza-lea/ (accessed on 28 June 2023).
30. Pfister, P.B.; de Bruin, E.D.; Sterkele, I.; Maurer, B.; de Bie, R.A.; Knols, R.H. Manual muscle testing and hand-held dynamometry in people with inflammatory myopathy: An intra- and interrater reliability and validity study. *PLoS ONE* **2018**, *13*, e0194531. [CrossRef]
31. Bohannon, R.W. The heel-raise test for ankle plantarflexor strength: A scoping review and meta-analysis of studies providing norms. *J. Phys. Ther. Sci.* **2022**, *34*, 528–531. [CrossRef] [PubMed]
32. Kim, H.-I.; Kim, M.-C. Physical Therapy Assessment Tool Threshold Values to Identify Sarcopenia and Locomotive Syndrome in the Elderly. *Int. J. Environ. Res. Public Health* **2023**, *20*, 6098. [CrossRef] [PubMed]
33. Patent EP3916346A4: Method for the Production of Customised Orthotics. Available online: https://worldwide.espacenet.com/patent/search/family/073498107/publication/EP3916346A1?q=EP3916346A1 (accessed on 29 June 2023).
34. Patent IT201900006076A1: Procedimento per la Produzione di Plantari Personalizzati su Misura, con Acquisizione da Remoto e Stampa Tridimensionale. Available online: https://worldwide.espacenet.com/patent/search/family/067660635/publication/IT201900006076A1?q=IT201900006076A1 (accessed on 29 June 2023).
35. Patent IT201800010667A1: Metodo per la Produzione di Ortesi Personalizzate Basate Sulla Stampa 3D. Available online: https://worldwide.espacenet.com/patent/search/family/073698258/publication/IT201800010667A1?q=IT201800010667A1 (accessed on 29 June 2023).

Disclaimer/Publisher's Note: The statements, opinions and data contained in all publications are solely those of the individual author(s) and contributor(s) and not of MDPI and/or the editor(s). MDPI and/or the editor(s) disclaim responsibility for any injury to people or property resulting from any ideas, methods, instructions or products referred to in the content.

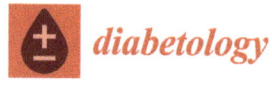

Article

Biological Evidence of Improved Wound Healing Using Autologous Micrografts in a Diabetic Animal Model

Mariza Brandão Palma [1,2,*], Elisa Paolin [3,4], Ismaela Maria Ferreira de Melo [1], Francisco De Assis Leite Souza [1], Álvaro Aguiar Coelho Teixeira [1,2], Leucio Duarte Vieira [5], Fabio Naro [6], Antonio Graziano [4] and Anísio Francisco Soares [1,2]

[1] Department of Morphology and Physiology, Anatomy Unit, Rural Federal University of Pernambuco, Recife 52171-900, Brazil; ismaelamelo@yahoo.com.br (I.M.F.d.M.); francisco.alsouza@ufrpe.br (F.D.A.L.S.); alvaro.teixeira@ufrpe.br (Á.A.C.T.); anisio.soares@ufrpe.br (A.F.S.)

[2] Postgraduate Program in Animal Bioscience, Rural Federal University of Pernambuco, Recife 52171-900, Brazil

[3] Department of Public Health, Experimental and Forensic Medicine, Human Anatomy Unit, University of Pavia, 27100 Pavia, Italy; elisa.paolin01@universitadipavia.it or elisa.paolin@hbwsrl.com

[4] Human Brain Wave, 10128 Turin, Italy; lab@hbwsrl.com

[5] Department of Physiology and Pharmacology, Biosciences Center, Federal University of Pernambuco, Recife 50670-901, Brazil; leucio.vieirafo@ufpe.br

[6] Department of Anatomical, Histological, Forensic Medicine and Orthopedic Science, Sapienza University of Rome, 00185 Roma, Italy; fabio.naro@uniroma1.it

* Correspondence: mariza.palma@ufrpe.br; Tel.: +55-81-999671506

Abstract: Background: Tissue healing consists of four main phases: coagulation, inflammation, proliferation, and remodeling. In diabetic patients, this process is stagnant in the inflammatory stage, leading to chronic wounds. The aim of this study is to evaluate in an animal model the biological evidence related to the use of the Rigenera® technology (Turin Italy), an innovative mechanical procedure to isolate autologous micrografts (AMG). Methods: Fifty male Wistar rats were divided into four groups: control (C), control treated with micrografts (CM), diabetic (DB), and diabetic treated with micrografts (DBM). The experimental setup involved: the quantification of the total collagen and elastic fibers; histopathological analysis; immunohistochemical analysis for collagen type I (COL1), collagen type III (COL3), vascular endothelial growth factor (VEGF-A), and interleukin 4 (IL4) and 10 (IL10); evaluation of the oxidative stress; measurement of gluthatione (GSH); and, finally, an enzyme-linked immunosorbent assay (ELISA) on tumor necrosis factor-α (TNF-α). Results: The AMG technology induces a faster healing process: VEGF-A, IL4, IL10, and GSH increased, while TNF-α and oxidative stress decreased. Conclusions: Animals treated with micrografts showed more favorable results for healing compared to those that did not receive treatment, demonstrating a positive participation of the micrografts in the treatment of difficult-to-heal wounds.

Keywords: regenerative medicine; chronic wounds; diabetes; cytokines; skin healing; impaired healing

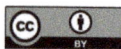

1. Introduction

The skin is considered the largest organ in the human body. In an adult, it represents about 16% of the total body weight, and, when distended, it occupies an area of approximately two square meters. Histologically, it is divided into the epidermis, dermis, and hypodermis (also known as the subcutaneous fat layer) [1]. The epidermis is the superficial layer of the skin, and it is composed of keratinized, stratified, and squamous epithelial tissue (Figure 1). It is avascular and receives nutrients by diffusion through the layer just below it, the dermis. In the epidermis, there are distinct layers arranged from the outermost to the innermost region, including the stratum corneum, stratum lucida, stratum granulosum, and stratum spinosum [2]. The deepest layer, known as the basal layer, is situated adjacent to the dermis, with finger-like projections towards it, referred to as the dermal papillae. The presence of these projections, known as rete ridges, is absent in the early stages of wound healing, which renders the wound more vulnerable to injury if exposed to trauma [3].

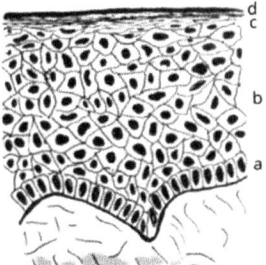

Figure 1. Schematic illustration depicting the stratification of the epidermis. The diagram showcases the different layers of the skin, arranged in a hierarchical manner from the deepest to the most superficial regions, namely: (a) the basal layer; (b) the spinous layer; (c) the granular layer; and (d) the stratum corneum. It should be noted that the lucid layer is situated above the granulosa layer, but it is only present in specific areas of the body, such as the tips of the fingers, the soles of the feet, and the palms of the hands.

The basal layer is formed by a single row of cuboidal or columnar keratinocytes, interspersed with stem cells responsible for the renewal of resident cells; it has a great ability to proliferate, and daughter cells migrate towards the skin surface. That suprabasal migration is accompanied by cell maturation until the formation of corneocytes on the skin surface [4]. Their cytoskeleton contains intermediate filaments formed by keratin that attach to desmosomes. In this way, the cells of the basal layer attach to each other and to the adjacent spinous layer [5]. When attached to hemidesmosomes, actin filaments allow the attachment of keratinocytes to the basement membrane, located between the epidermis and the dermis [6].

There are four main types of cells in the epidermis: keratinocytes, melanocytes, Langerhans cells, and Merkel cells. Keratinocytes make up about 90% of the epidermis, and the source of replacement of these cells is the basal layer; they produce the keratin protein that provides protection to the skin and the underlying tissues against heat, chemical agents, and microorganisms [7].

Keratinocytes are identified as the primary cell responsible for the healing of wounds of the epidermis and for maintaining tissue integrity. A stratified keratinized epithelium undergoes constant turnover, regenerating completely in 48 h. Keratinocytes originating from the basal layer are devoid of keratin and begin to accumulate more and more of this protein as they pass from one epidermal layer to another. This process is accelerated in the case of injuries, such as abrasions and burns [8].

Melanocytes are cells with long and thin processes, called dendrites, placed between the keratinocytes. They correspond to 8% of skin cells and release melanin pigment granules that are absorbed by the keratinocytes. Once in keratinocytes, melanin forms a barrier around the core on the side facing the skin surface. In this way, melanin protects cellular DNA against the deleterious effects of ultraviolet radiation [9].

The Langerhans cells migrate to the epidermis from the bone marrow. They represent a small percentage of the total epidermis cells and participate in the immune response.

Merkel cells are located deeper in the epidermis, where they come into contact with sensory neurons; together with them, they participate in the sense of touch [10].

The dermis is the layer that lies just below the epidermis and receives the increased blood supply to the skin. Most skin appendages are in the dermis: apocrine glands, eccrine glands, and hair follicles. The dermis is a connective tissue containing collagen and elastic fibers. Fibroblasts, macrophages, and adipocytes constitute the cellular component from the dermis. It has two layers: superficial or papillary and deep dermis or reticulate [11].

The superficial layer corresponds to only one-fifth of the total dermis. It contains fine elastic fibers. Its total area is increased by the presence of dermal papillae, which are finger-like projections towards the epidermis. In some dermal papillae, corpuscles of Meissner (touch-sensitive nerve endings) and also free nerves (responsible for sensations of heat, cold, pain, tickling, and itching) are present [12].

In the deepest layer of the dermis, the reticular region, tissue is observed as dense, irregular connective tissue, with bundles of collagen fibers and thicker elastic fibers. Among the bundles of collagen fibers, follicles, hair, sweat, and sebaceous glands, nerves and fat cells can be observed. The combination of collagen fibers and elastic fibers gives the dermis the properties of elasticity, strength, and extensibility. When tissue damage reaches the reticular dermis, grafts are usually necessary [13].

The deepest layer of the skin is called the hypodermis or subcutaneous layer. It contains a large amount of adipose tissue, sensitive receptors pressure (Pacinian corpuscles), and large blood vessels that supply the dermis. Fibers that come from the dermis cross the hypodermis and attach to tissues and underlying organs [14].

The skin possesses an excellent regenerative capacity due to the presence of various mesenchymal stem cells (MSCs) located in its appendages (hair follicles, sebaceous glands, and sweat glands) as well as in the basal layer [15]. These cells exhibit a high degree of plasticity and are arranged in distinct compartments known as niches, where they interact with neighboring cells and a specific extracellular matrix to determine their functions [16–18]. In the skin, three different niches of MSC have been identified: (i) the basal layer of the epidermis, (ii) the hair follicle bulb (present in mice, but not in humans), and (iii) the base of the sebaceous gland duct, which suggests the existence of a niche also in the duct of the sweat glands [19–21].

A wound is defined as damage to or discontinuity of the structural anatomy of the skin and the consequent loss of its normal functions. It can be a simple interruption of the epithelial integrity or it can be deeper, extending to the subcutaneous tissue, with damage to various structures, such as tendons, muscles, vessels, nerves, organs' parenchyma, and bones [22].

Healing consists of the reestablishment of the continuity of the epidermis, so that the tissue that differentiates it acts as a physical, chemical, and bacterial barrier, which is one of the skin's vital functions [1]. The healing process requires an integrated expression of several chemokines, cytokines, growth factors, and cell types that are present in the wound from tissue injury to the final healing events. Throughout this process, their expression varies temporally and quantitatively. They are produced by cells present at the wound site and act in paracrine and autocrine signaling [23].

Wound healing can happen by regeneration or through the reparation process. When regeneration occurs, the tissue for reconstruction is the same as that of the healthy tissue. This can be observed in the superficial epidermis, in the mucous membranes, or in fetal skin. In tissue repair, the wound is filled with fibrotic tissue and presents with scars [11,24].

Tissues have different healing times. Wounds can be classified as acute or chronic according to the way they establish and evolve. Acute wounds heal within the period expected and in a way that is hassle-free. Chronic wounds are those that do not fulfill the progression of the normal healing stages, and the damage established is not repaired in the expected order and time. Many factors can contribute to the interruption and consequent damage of normal healing: infection, tissue hypoxia, necrosis, and exudates. Excessive amounts of inflammatory cytokines can prolong one or more phases of the healing time, leading to wound chronicity [23].

After the injury has occurred, to reestablish the anatomical condition and function (that is, healing), the following steps are necessary in the affected tissues: coagulation and hemostasis, the inflammatory phase, the proliferative phase, and the remodeling phase. These phases are sequential, overlapping, and interdependent such that in different areas of the same wound, distinct phases of the healing process can be observed. Thus, deficiency in any of the healing stages determines the failure of the event [25–27] (Figure 2).

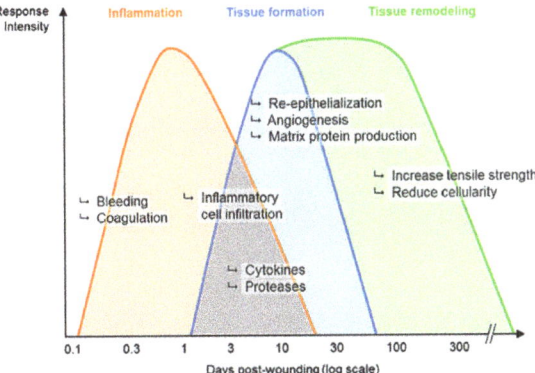

Figure 2. Temporal sequence illustrating the phases of epithelial healing. The diagram showcases the different phases that occur during the process of tissue regeneration and how they are interposed with one another.

Diabetes mellitus (DM) is an important global health problem caused by changes in nutritional habits, sedentary lifestyle, overweight, population growth and aging, increasing urbanization, and the greater survival of diabetic patients. It has a cost of billions of annual dollars that impacts the health systems of all countries, but it is more representative in underdeveloped countries. Type 1 diabetes is the carrier of exogenous insulin, while type 2 diabetes is more common and accounts for 85–90% of cases. Diabetes is characterized by disturbances in the secretion and action of insulin and can be managed with food control and physical exercise. Other less common types of diabetes have been reported, such as genetic defects of beta cells and of the insulin, degenerative diseases of the pancreas, diabetes related to other endocrinopathies, and drug diabetes. Complications include cardiovascular and cerebrovascular diseases, retinopathy, nephropathy, and ulcers and skin conditions [28]. Diabetic individuals have difficulty healing wounds in the extremities, especially in the feet. Diabetic foot (DF) wounds are caused by neuropathy and vascular insufficiency, with 20% having previous arterial occlusive disease, 50% having peripheral neuropathy, and 80% having both conditions. Any trauma leading to the formation of skin ulcers predisposes patients to complications [29,30]. Treatments for DF ulcers aim to increase vascularity and to break down physiological barriers that prevent healing, but the success of treatment depends on several factors. Chronic wounds of diabetic feet have their healing interrupted in the inflammatory phase due to deficiencies in cells involved in the process, as well as of chemokines, cytokines, and growth factors.

A possible countermeasure to treat chronic wounds in diabetic patients is the use of adult stem cells for tissue maintenance and repair [31]. Among them, mesenchymal stem cells (MSCs) are present throughout the organism and in the perivascular region of adult tissues. They are multipotent and capable of forming ectoderm, mesoderm, and endoderm cells [32], and they release exosomes to stimulate tissue regeneration and to regulate the immune system [33,34]. However, an important limitation of using MSCs lies in the necessity to cultivate cells, which involves enzymatic manipulation, leading additionally to an increase in the time to obtain them and the financial cost [35,36].

Rigenera® technology (Human Brain Wave, Turin, Italy) is now a currently available alternative technology for obtaining micrografts (namely progenitor cells (PCs) within their own extracellular matrix) involving disposable medical devices as mechanical disruptors of biological tissues [37–45]. It allows for obtaining micrografts in an autologous, homologous, and minimally invasive manner, and these can be used immediately without the need for culture cells. Scientific studies have shown that the cellular population obtained after the mechanical disaggregation is positive for mesenchymal stem cells, with markers identifying those cells as PCs, and they have shown a viability ranging between 70 and 90%. AMTs have the ability to act both through cellular differentiation and in a paracrine manner through the release of secretomas containing various molecules that will act on neighboring cells; they have the potential to stimulate multiple events at once, allowing interdependent phases to be resolved endogenously [46].

In this study, diabetic foot wounds were used as an experimental model in order to verify the performance of AMTs in the evolution of the healing process in skin wounds. Fifty male Wistar rats were involved and divided into four groups: "control (C)"; "control treated with micrografts (CM)"; "diabetic (DB)"; and "diabetic treated with micrografts (DBM)".

2. Results

2.1. Histopathological Analysis

Research findings on hematoxylin-eosin-stained slides revealed an extensive inflammatory infiltration among the granulation tissue seen in all groups at the start of healing (3 days). Nevertheless, the number of neutrophils in the CM group is substantially smaller (Figure 3). The images were acquired from samples collected 3 days after the creation of the artificial wound.

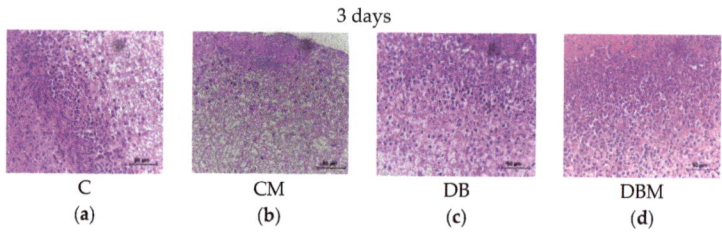

Figure 3. Photomicrograph showcasing the animals' skin on the third day of treatment. The image features the four different groups, namely (**a**) C "control", (**b**) CM "control treated with micrografts", (**c**) DB "diabetic", and (**d**) DBM "diabetic treated with micrografts". It is observed that all groups display an abundance of inflammatory cells, particularly degenerated neutrophils, within the granulation tissue. However, the CM group (**b**) exhibits a lower quantity of inflammatory cells compared to the C group. The staining utilized in the image is hematoxylin eosin (HE).

Despite the progression of the healing process, inflammatory cells remained in the diabetes groups (DB and DBM) longer than in the non-diabetic groups (C and CM) (Figure 4).

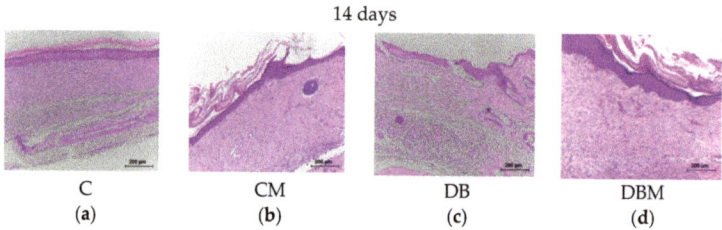

Figure 4. Photomicrograph displaying the animals' skin on the fourteenth day of treatment, featuring (**a**) C "control", (**b**) CM "control treated with micrografts", (**c**) DB "diabetic", and (**d**) DBM "diabetic treated with micrografts" groups. The image shows that the wound is completely re-epithelialized in all four groups. However, in the diabetic group (**c**), the lining epithelium is thinner and contains fewer layers in the stratum corneum. Additionally, collagen appears less organized in this group as compared to the others. Notably, the presence of persistent inflammatory cells is observed in the diabetic and diabetic groups treated with the micrograft.

According to histological studies, the CM group is in the healing phase after 3 days, which is equal to the C group after 7 days of recovery. At 7 days, the proliferation phase begins, leading to fibroblasts migration, angiogenesis, and the commencement of epithelialization (Figure 5).

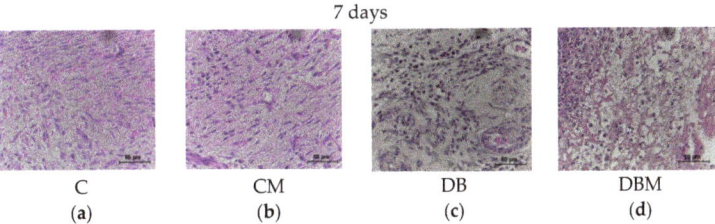

Figure 5. Photomicrograph displaying the animals' skin on the seventh day of treatment, featuring (**a**) C "control", (**b**) CM "control treated with micrografts", (**c**) DB "diabetic", and (**d**) DBM "diabetic treated with micrografts" groups. The image highlights the presence of hemorrhage and the formation of blood vessels in the C group. In the CM group, a greater quantity of fibroblasts and collagen fibers are observed in comparison to the C group. However, the presence of blood vessels and hemorrhage is lower in this group. In the DB group, an expressive presence of inflammatory cells is observed, which is also present in the DBM group. The staining utilized in the image is hematoxylin eosin (HE).

The epidermal tissue was detected at 3 days in the treatment groups (Figure 6), indicating a faster epithelialization in the micrograft groups.

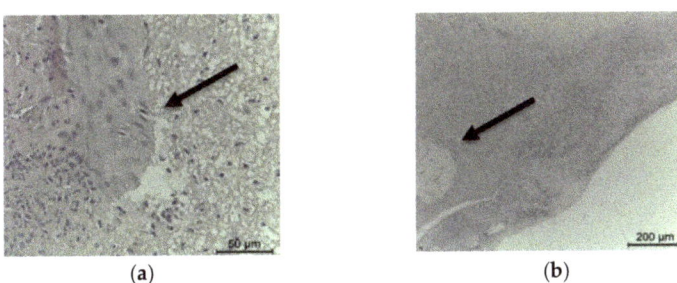

Figure 6. Photomicrograph showcasing the presence of lingual epithelial (indicated by an arrow) at three days in the CM "control treated with micrografts" group (**a**) and in the DBM "diabetic treated with micrografts" group (**b**). The staining technique employed in the image is hematoxylin eosin (HE).

Angiogenesis occurs in all groups; however, it takes longer to begin in the diabetic group, with detection occurring after just 7 days. Active fibroblasts were likewise discovered only after 7 days of recovery. The CM group has much more fibroblasts and collagen fiber production than the C group. Although there are still disordered regions, collagen is thicker than in the control group.

Granulation tissue with many newly formed capillaries and fibroblasts is present in the DBM group in the middle of the extracellular matrix formed by the newly formed fibrillar collagen synthetized. By 14 days (Figure 7), there was a full region of healing in all groups, with no discontinuity of the epidermis, and the healing was in the final phase of proliferation and the beginning of remodeling. Every layer of the epidermis is visible, from the stratum basale to the stratum cornea; however, the epidermis is thinner and has fewer keratin layers in the diabetic group. The formation of epidermal attachments has begun in the groups treated with the micrograft, but it is still lacking in the untreated groups. Granulation tissue has already been totally replaced by collagen, although collagen remains fibrillar, with thin and disordered fibers, with an appearance of newly formed collagen in the diabetic group. The majority of fibroblasts have already been replaced by fibrocytes.

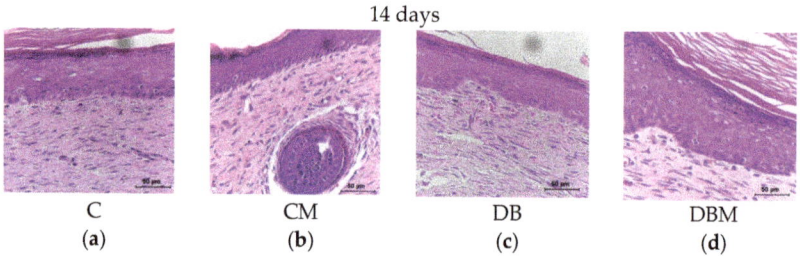

Figure 7. Photomicrograph displaying the animals' skin on the fourteenth day of treatment, featuring (**a**) C "control", (**b**) CM "control treated with micrografts", (**c**) DB "diabetic", and (**d**) DBM "diabetic treated with micrografts" groups. The image demonstrates complete epithelialization of the wound in all groups. In the CM group (**b**), the formation of an epidermal annex is observed. In the DB group (**c**), a reduction in the thickness of the epidermis and keratin layers is observed. Conversely, in the DBM group (**d**), the epidermis is fully re-epithelialized, with several layers of keratin and keratohyalin granules. The staining technique employed in the image is hematoxylin eosin (HE).

2.2. Collagen and Elastic Fibers Quantification

The animals in the C group had less collagen at 7 and 14 days of evolution than the DBM group, which was still at 3 days of healing. As a result, the DBM group produced more collagen in a shorter healing time than the C groups with longer healing times (Figure 8).

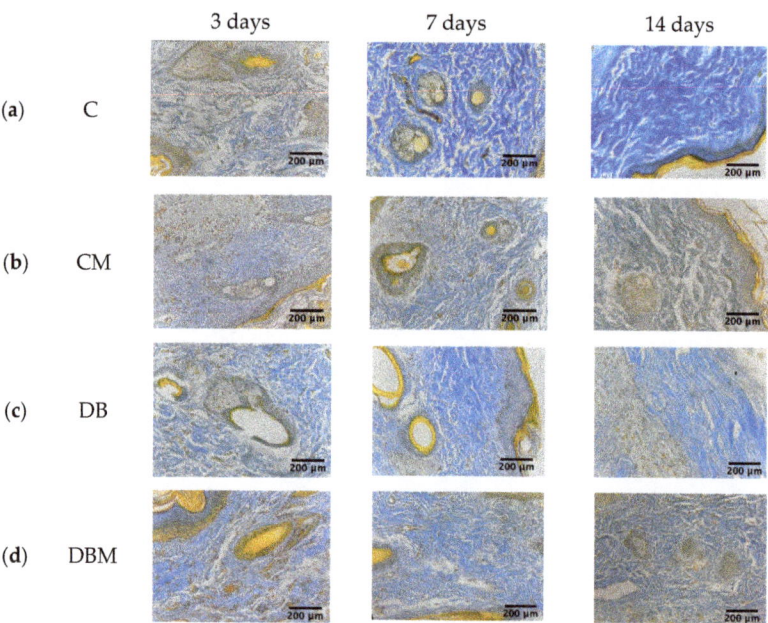

Figure 8. Photomicrograph displaying the rat skin with Mallory's trichrome for collagen quantification at 3, 7, and 14 days of healing evolution of (**a**) C "control", (**b**) CM "control treated with micrografts", (**c**) DB "diabetic", and (**d**) DBM "diabetic treated with micrografts" groups. The blue color represents collagen.

The morphometric analysis for elastic fibers quantification revealed no statistically significant differences between the groups (Figures 9 and 10).

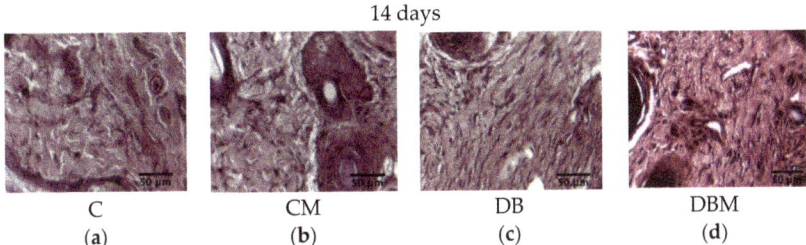

Figure 9. Microscopic images of nitric-orcein-stained mouse skin depicting elastic fiber quantification during the 14-day healing progression. (**a**) C "control", (**b**) CM "control treated with micrografts", (**c**) DB "diabetic", and (**d**) DBM "diabetic treated with micrografts".

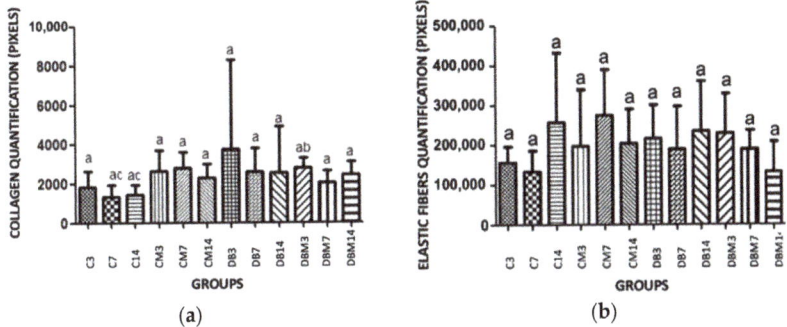

Figure 10. Statistical analysis of collagen production (**a**) and quantification of elastic fibers (**b**), measured using the Gimp 2.0 software. Statistical analyses were performed using the Kruskal–Wallis test with post hoc Dunn. Means denoted by the same letter do not exhibit significant differences ($p < 0.05$). The different groups analyzed include the C group (control), CM group (control treated with micrografts), DB group (diabetic), and DBM group (diabetic treated with micrografts).

From the statistical analysis conducted to quantify collagen production and elastic fibers, it was found that there is a statistical difference between C (7 days) and C (14 days) compared to DBM (3 days) for collagen (Figure 10a). However, no statistically significant differences were observed among the groups for elastic fibers (Figure 10b).

2.3. Immunohistochemical Analysis for COL1, COL3, VEGF-A, IL4, and IL10

Throughout the 3-day assessment, there were no significant changes in collagen I labeling. At 7 days, the CM group had more COL1 marking than the C group. The animals in the DB and DBM groups had the lowest marking and did not distinguish from one another. At 14 days, the same behavior was seen (Figure 11a).

At the 3-day assessment, there were no significant changes in collagen III labeling. At 7 days, tissues in the C and CM groups had more marking in their fragments, followed by the animals in the DBM group. The animals in the DB group had the least amount of staining. The animals in the CM and DBM groups had more marking at 14 days than the C and DB groups, with the latter having the lowest average (Figure 11b).

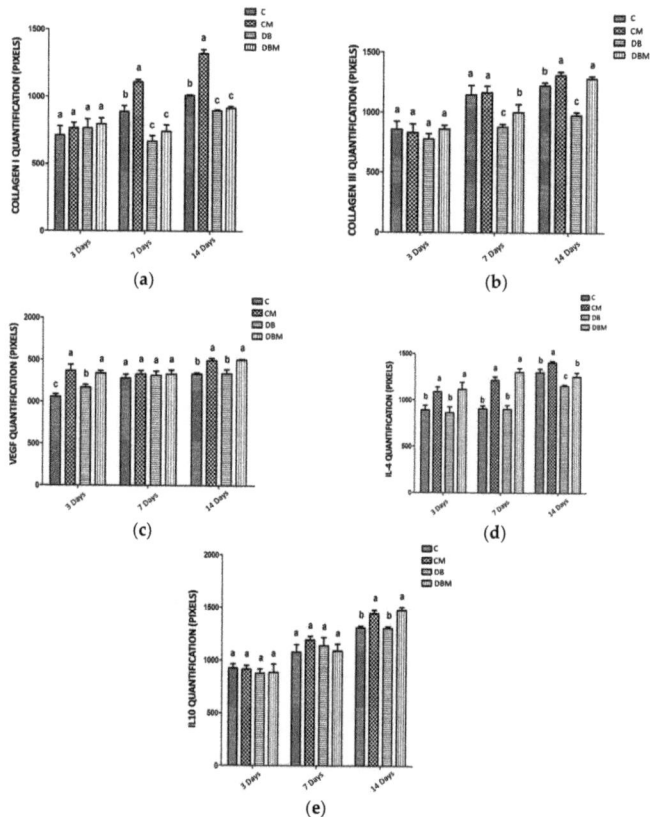

Figure 11. The different groups statistically analyzed include C "control", CM "control treated with micrografts", DB "diabetic", and DBM "diabetic treated with micrografts". (**a**) Pixel-based quantification of collagen I in skin tissue samples obtained from experimental animal groups. Tukey and Kramer Multiple Comparisons tests revealed no significant differences ($p > 0.05$) among means marked with the same letter. (**b**) Pixel-based quantification of collagen III in skin tissue samples obtained from experimental animal groups. Tukey and Kramer Multiple Comparisons tests revealed no significant differences ($p > 0.05$) among means marked with the same letter. (**c**) Pixel-based quantification of VEGF in skin tissue samples obtained from experimental animal groups. Tukey and Kramer Multiple Comparisons tests revealed no significant differences ($p > 0.05$) among means marked with the same letter. (**d**) Pixel-based quantification of IL4 in skin tissue samples obtained from experimental animal groups. Tukey and Kramer Multiple Comparisons tests revealed no significant differences ($p > 0.05$) among means marked with the same letter. (**e**) Pixel-based quantification of IL10 in skin tissue samples obtained from experimental animal groups. Tukey and Kramer Multiple Comparisons tests revealed no significant differences ($p > 0.05$) among means marked with the same letter.

At 3 days, there were significant variations in the evaluation of VEGF, with skin samples from the CM and DBM groups demonstrating higher marking than the DB and C groups, with the latter showing the lowest markup. There were no variations in marking between the experimental groups after 7 days. By 14 days, however, the animals in the CM and DBM groups had more markings than the C and DB groups, which did not differ from each other (Figure 11c).

We observed the same trend at the 3- and 7-day evaluations, characterized by increased marking in the skin pieces of the CM and DBM animals, whereas the C and DB groups showed less staining without significant differences. The animals in the CM group, on the other hand, had more marking at 14 days. The animals in the C and DBM groups did not vary from one another, but the DB had less marking (Figure 11d).

During 3 and 7 days, there was no significant change in the labeling of this cytokine. By 14 days, however, the animals in the CM and DBM groups had more marking. The animals in the C and DB groups had less marking but did not vary from one another (Figure 11e).

2.4. Evaluation of the Oxidative Stress—Measurement of Gluthatione (GSH)

Tissue assessment of GSH levels at three points in the groups' studies revealed that the groups treated with the micrograft had greater levels than the diabetic group (Figure 12a). In terms of tissue concentrations of skin lipid peroxidation (TBARS) levels, the DB group showed a substantial rise, but the DBST group showed a decrease when compared to the diabetic and control groups (Figure 12b).

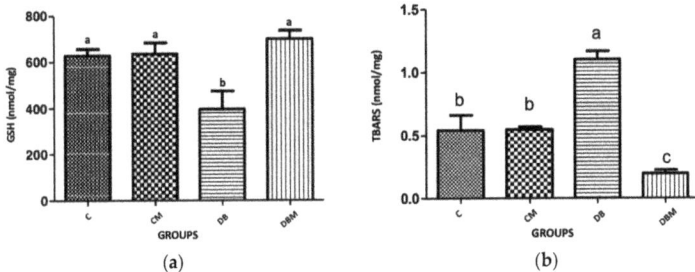

Figure 12. Graphs showing GSH and TBARS values in the skin of animals belonging to different experimental groups (nmol/mg of protein) on the 14th day of treatment. The experimental groups include the C (control group), the CM (control group treated with AMGs), the DB (diabetic group), and the DBM (diabetic group treated with AMTs). Statistical significance was determined by the Kruskal–Wallis test with Dunn's post hoc analysis. Means sharing the same letter are not significantly different from each other. (**a**) GSH; (**b**) TBARS.

2.5. Evaluation of Tumor Necrosis Factor-α (TNF-α)

In terms of TNF-α dose, the control group (C) had a greater concentration than the other experimental groups on the third day. However, on the seventh and fourteenth days, the diabetic (DB) group had a greater concentration, contrasting with the other groups' findings (Figure 13).

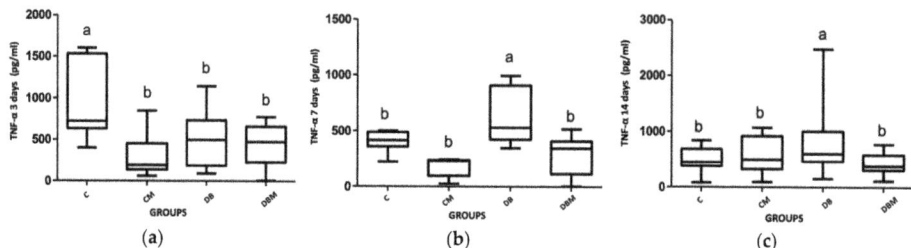

Figure 13. The graphs display the TNF-α values in the skin of animals belonging to different experimental groups (pg/mL), including the C (control group), the CM (control group treated with AMGs), the DB (diabetic group), and the DBM (diabetic group treated with AMTs). The y axis shows the different treatment times, which are labeled as the 3rd treatment time, 7th treatment time, and 14th treatment time. The statistical analysis was performed using the Kruskal–Wallis test with Dunn's post hoc test. Means with the same letter are not significantly different from each other. (**a**) TNF-α 3 days; (**b**) TNF-α 7 days; (**c**) TNF-α 14 days.

3. Discussion

The process of tissue healing involves a series of events that are interdependent and involve various chemokines, cytokines, and growth factors produced by cells that participate in tissue repair [11,23–25]. This process goes through phases of coagulation and hemostasis, inflammation, proliferation, and tissue remodeling [24]. In extremity wounds of diabetic individuals, the healing process is interrupted in the inflammatory phase due to a large amount of cytokines, chemokines, and pro-inflammatory factors that prevent progression to the proliferation phase and result in chronic wounds [47].

Stem cells are seen as a possible solution to this problem as they can release exosomes containing factors that positively interfere in healing and also differentiate into other cell types, which can act on stagnant healing and act on several factors simultaneously [48].

Micrografts containing progenitor cells have been shown to induce a faster evolution of the wound healing process [49]. Animals treated with micrografts present at 3 days a histological appearance similar to those at 7 days that did not receive the micrograft.

The presence of neutrophils in the proliferation and remodeling phases has been shown to be a characteristic of diabetic animals, which was different from the control group. This finding may be due to the greater number of inflammatory cytokines in diabetics, which attract a greater number of neutrophils to the lesion.

The skin wound samples for histopathological analysis were collected three, seven, and fourteen days after creating the artificial wounds for several reasons, which can be justified based on the wound healing process and recent scientific studies. Firstly, this multi-time-point approach allows for a more comprehensive assessment of the dynamic changes that occur during different phases of wound healing. The three-day time stop captures the early inflammatory phase, characterized by acute inflammation, immune cell infiltration, and the initiation of tissue repair processes. By collecting samples at this time point, the initial response to the wound and the early cellular and molecular events can be monitored. The seven-day time stop represents the proliferative phase, during which granulation tissue formation, angiogenesis, and collagen synthesis occur. It is a crucial period for cell proliferation, migration, and extracellular matrix deposition. Collecting samples at this time point enables the evaluation of tissue regeneration and the progression of healing. The fourteen-day mark corresponds to the remodeling phase, characterized by collagen remodeling, wound contraction, and the maturation of the newly formed tissue. By collecting samples at this time point, the structural and functional changes that occur during this critical phase of wound healing can be assessed [25,50,51].

The quantification of collagen production through staining showed that collagen production was more effective in animals treated with micrografts at 3 days of healing compared to those at 7 and 14 days of evolution of control animals. The elastic fibers present in the skin showed no significant difference among the groups studied with regard to fiber production elasticity.

Angiogenesis is the process by which new blood vessels are formed from preexisting vessels in the tissue. VEGF is a potent stimulator of this process, and increased expression of VEGF indicates that blood vessel formation is active, which is important for cell growth and proliferation as well as the formation of granulation tissue. In this study, it was found that at 3 days of healing, VEGF was increased in the groups treated with micrografts compared to the untreated groups, indicating an earlier recovery of vascularization in the CM and DBM groups and favoring faster healing.

Overall, micrografts containing progenitor cells have been shown to accelerate and produce collagen in greater quantities than the control group with longer healing time, resulting in scar tissue with better collagen organization.

Cytokines are proteins that bind to cell membrane receptors and induce their biological effects. The action of cytokines can be autocrine, paracrine, or endocrine. TNF-α is a cytokine produced by macrophages, lymphocytes, and monocytes. Its main physiological effect is to promote immune and inflammatory responses through the recruitment of neutrophils and monocytes to the site of infection and the activation of these cells [52]. TNF-α is present in chronic wounds, such as those present in diabetic feet. In wounds that heal under normal conditions, TNF-α decreases as the cells that produce it are eliminated from the inflammatory process. However, in the wounds of diabetic feet, TNF-α tends to remain at high levels. The treatment with micrografts showed a reduction in TNF-α in diabetic animals compared to those who were also diabetic but did not receive treatment. Thus, the applied micrograft helped to reduce this cytokine, and, consequently, its inflammatory effects.

In addition to pro-inflammatory cytokines, anti-inflammatory cytokines are also important regulators of healing. IL-4 is a cytokine with anti-inflammatory characteristics that is produced mainly by mast cells, eosinophils, Th2 cells, and basophils. IL-4 works in tissue homeostasis by changing macrophages from the M1 profile (pro-inflammatory) to the M2 profile (anti-inflammatory) [53]. Up to 7 days of healing, IL-4 maintained its highest levels in the groups treated with the micrograft. In this phase, inflammatory cells were present from the wound, including macrophages. Therefore, IL-4 may have activated the macrophage alternative pathway for the M2 profile, contributing to the reduction of inflammation. IL-4 is also able to promote the repair of epithelial wounds in vitro by reducing the cytokine-induced epithelial barrier defects.

The importance of IL-10 in wound healing lies in its limitation and termination of inflammatory responses. IL-10 inhibits the infiltration of neutrophils and macrophages into the lesion, as well as the expression of various pro-inflammatory chemokines and cytokines [54]. In this study, at 3 and 7 days after injury, there was no significant difference in IL-10 production among the groups studied. Only at 14 days of healing was IL-10 increased in the groups treated with micrografts compared to the untreated groups. The two together, IL-4 and IL-10, being anti-inflammatory in nature, maintain a favorable environment for healing throughout the healing process. IL-10 is also capable of inhibiting TNF-α. In fact, IL-10 was higher at 14 days in the micrograft-treated groups at the same time that TNF-α was lower in these same groups.

Oxidative stress is the result of an increase in reactive oxygen species (ROS) and/or reactive nitrogen species (RNS) as a result of a constant imbalance between the production of reactive molecules (mainly ROS and RNS) and antioxidant agents [55]. The level of TBARS is pointed out as an effective method to identify these radicals, and high levels of TBARS are present in patients with complications of diabetes mellitus. The level of TBARS was shown to be significantly increased in the DB group compared to the DBM and CM groups.

4. Materials and Methods

4.1. Animal Model

Fifty male Wistar rats (90 days old, weighing around 300 ± 30 g) from the Department of Animal Morphology and Physiology, Rural Federal University of Pernambuco, were involved in this study. The project was submitted to the institutional ethics committee and approved under protocol number 23082.014335/2018–85 and license No. 89/2018.

These animals were kept in cages, with food and water ad libitum, at a temperature of 22 ± 1 °C and with artificial lighting that established a photoperiod of 12 h of light and 12 of dark hours, considering the light period from 06:00 to 18:00 h. The animals were randomly divided into 4 groups, namely: control (C) ($n = 10$); control treated with micrografts (CM) ($n = 10$); diabetic (DB) ($n = 15$); and diabetic treated with micrografts (DBM) ($n = 15$).

4.2. Diabetes Induction

Diabetes was induced in the animals of the DB and DBM groups by intraperitoneal administration of Streptozotocin solution (Sigma Chemical Co., St. Louis, MO, USA) after a 14 h fasting period. Diabetes was confirmed on the seventh day after the application. Streptozotocin was diluted in 10 mM sodium citrate buffer (pH 4.5) and administered in a single dose of 60 mg/kg of animal weight. The C and CM groups received, in the same way, equivalent doses of saline solution. After 30 min from administration, all animals were fed normally [56].

Only animals with blood glucose above 200 mg/dL (Accu-Chek Activ Kit Glucometer, Roche Diabates Care, Indianapolis, IN, USA) were included in this study, except for the control groups.

4.3. Wound Preparation

The lesions were performed on the backs of the left hind legs of the rats, with a sterile scalpel, in order to remove the skin and subcutaneous tissue until exposure of the muscle tendons (Figure 14).

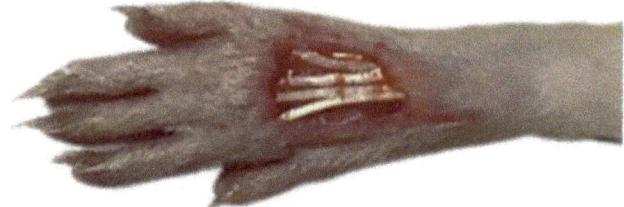

Figure 14. A lesion was performed on the left hind legs of the animals, which involved the removal of the overlying skin and subcutaneous tissue to expose the underlying muscle tendons. The resulting lesion area measured approximately 1 cm^2.

4.4. Autologous Micrografts Rigenera® Technology

AMGs were obtained utilizing a Class II medical device, called Rigeneracons, that consists of a grid with six micro-blades encircling hundreds of holes that are 80 µm in diameter, allowing the selection of AMGs with exact sizes using a dimensional exclusion method. An electrical motor, known as Sicurdrill, drives the mechanical fragmentation (Figure 15). Many soft and hard tissues, including the dermis, cartilage, bone, fat, and heart tissues, may be swiftly and effectively broken down using the technology. The AMG solution can be injected around the margins and the bed of a wound or used to imbibe a dermal substitute. Because the AMG technology does not require the use of enzymes or other chemicals, the operation takes only 30 min to complete.

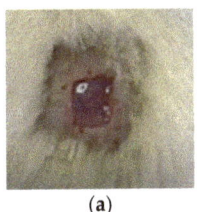
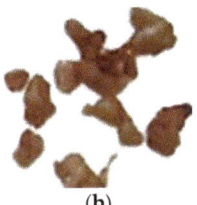

(a)   (b)

Figure 15. After shaving, a skin incision was made on the animal's back (**a**). The skin fragment was subsequently cut into smaller pieces, as shown in image (**b**), before being placed into the Rigeneracons device for processing.

4.5. Histopathological Analysis

The animals in both the experimental and control groups were sedated with ketamine hydrochloride (80 mg/kg) and xylazine (6.0 mg/kg) intramuscularly three, seven, and fourteen days after the artificial wounds creation. The wound skin was collected by a rectangular incision around the lesion (Figure 16). The rats were then euthanized with 100 mg/kg sodium thiopental.

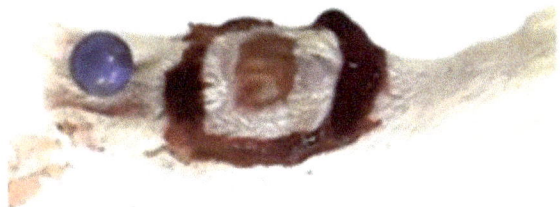

Figure 16. A skin fragment was collected for analysis, ensuring a sufficient safety margin around the wound. Half of the fragment was fixed in buffered formalin, while the other half was frozen at $-20\ °C$ for subsequent analysis.

Half of the material was fixed in buffered formalin for 48 h before being paraffin embedded. The sections were stained with hematoxylin and eosin, Mallory's trichrome, and nitric orcein for histological investigation using a light microscope (OLYMPUS BX-50, Tokyo, Japan). The other half was frozen at $-20\ °C$ in a freezer.

Samples for histological analysis were collected at three, seven, and fourteen days following the injury.

4.6. Collagen and Elastic Fibers Quantification

Histological slices were stained with Mallory's trichrome and nitric orcein, respectively, to quantify the collagen and elastic fibers. For this purpose, three slides were utilized for each group, with five fields captured on each slide. The images were captured with a Sony® (Tokyo, Japan) video camera attached to an Olympus® (Tokyo, Japan) Bx50 microscope and submitted to the Gimp 2.0 application for quantification using the RGB Histogram (Red-Green-Blue), which is based on luminescence intensity and where the tones of the image pixels vary from 0 to 255, with tone 0 representing absolute darkness (lowest luminescence) and tone 255 representing absolute white (higher luminescence) [57].

4.7. Immunohistochemical Analysis for COL1, COL3, VEGF-A, IL4, and IL10

COL1A1 (sc-293182, Santa Cruz Biotechnology, Santa Cruz, CA, USA), COL3A1 (sc-271249, Santa Cruz Biotechnology, Santa Cruz, CA, USA), VEGF-A (MBS2540134, MyBioSource, San Diego, CA, USA), IL-4 (sc-53084, Santa Cruz Biotechnology, Santa Cruz, CA,

USA), and IL-10 (sc-365858, Santa Cruz Biotechnology, Santa Cruz, CA, USA) antibodies in a 1:100 dilution ratio were used.

The slides were deparaffinized and rehydrated in xylene and alcohols, respectively. The antigen recovery was carried out in the microwave for 5 min at high temperature with a citrate buffer solution (pH 8.0). Endogenous peroxidase was inhibited by a 3% hydrogen peroxide in methanol solution [58]. The nonspecific antigen–antibody interaction was inhibited by incubating the slides in PBS and 5% bovine serum albumin (BSA) for 1 h. All antibodies were diluted in PBS/BSA 1% overnight. The parts were then treated with Histofine® (Cod. 414191F—Nichirei Biosciences, Tokyo, Japan) for 30 min. The antigen–antibody reaction was detected as a brown precipitate after four minutes of treatment with 3,3 diaminobenzidine and counterstained with hematoxylin. A video camera (Sony) coupled with the Olympus BX-50 microscope was used to collect the images.

4.8. Evaluation of the Oxidative Stress—Measurement of Gluthatione (GSH)

The skin's oxidative stress was assessed by measuring lipid peroxidation and GSH levels. The quantities of acid reactive chemicals thiobarbiturate (TBARS) were used to estimate lipid peroxidation (Figure 17), whereas non-protein sulfhydryl groups were used to estimate reduced GSH (Figure 18) [59,60]. Skin pieces were macerated in 1.15% KCl in a proportion of 10 mL/1 g until completely homogenized. The homogenate was transferred to a test tube, and 2 mL of the reagent (0.375% thiobarbituric acid and 75% acid trichloroacetic acid) was added for every mL of the mixture. Duplicate tubes were sealed and heated in a water bath (100 °C) for 15 min. The supernatant was separated, and the absorbance was measured at 535 nm [61].

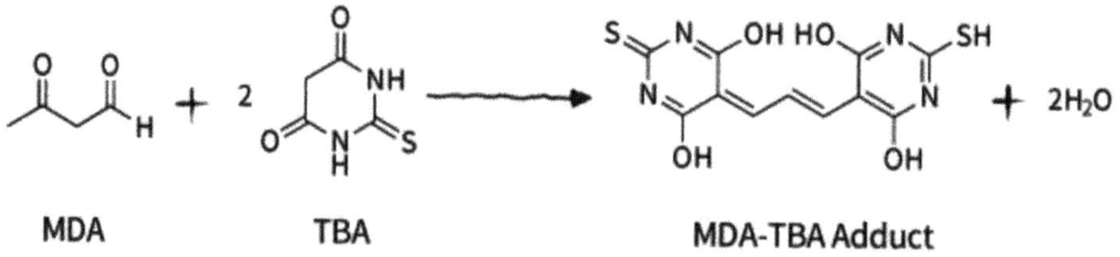

Figure 17. Lipid peroxidation is a widely recognized cellular injury mechanism in both plants and animals, often used as an indicator of oxidative stress in cells and tissues. Polyunsaturated fatty acids give rise to unstable lipid peroxides, which subsequently decompose to form a range of complex compounds, including reactive carbonyl compounds like malondialdehyde (MDA). Thiobarbituric acid reactive substances (TBARS) measurement is a well-established screening and monitoring method for lipid peroxidation. In this method, MDA in the sample reacts with thiobarbituric acid (TBA) to form the MDA–TBA adduct, which can be quantified colorimetrically at 532 nm. This analytical approach relies on the reaction of MDA with TBA, a chromogenic reagent, at a constant temperature of 25 °C.

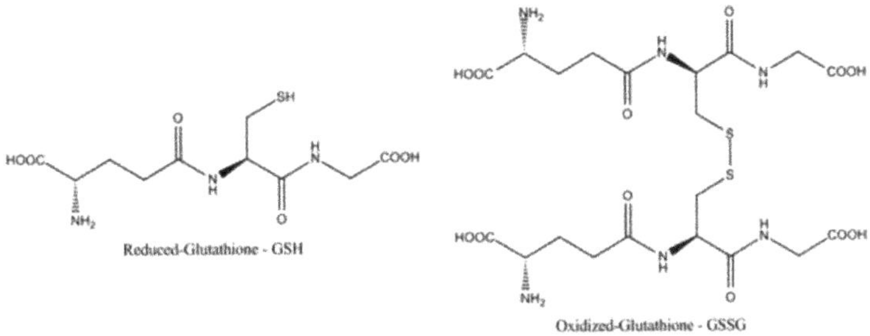

Figure 18. Glutathione is a tripeptide that exists in two forms: reduced (GSH) and oxidized (GSSG). The ratio of GSH to GSSG within cells is a widely used marker of cellular oxidative stress, as an increased GSSG-to-GSH ratio indicates greater oxidative stress. GSH acts as an important antioxidant by neutralizing (reducing) reactive oxygen species, protecting cells from oxidative damage.

4.9. Evaluation of Tumor Necrosis Factor-α (TNF-α)

TNF-α dose was determined using the ELISA method, according to the manufacturer's instructions (RAB0479-1KT—Sigma-Aldrich (St. Louis, MO, USA)) [62].

4.10. Statistical Analysis

Statistical analysis was conducted using the Kruskal–Wallis test with post hoc Dunn analysis to assess collagen production and quantification of elastic fibers utilizing Gimp 2.0 software. The significance level was set at $p < 0.05$.

Regarding collagen I quantification, pixel-based analysis was performed on skin tissue samples from the animal groups. Tukey and Kramer Multiple Comparisons tests showed no significant differences ($p > 0.05$) among means labeled with the same letter.

Similarly, pixel-based quantification of collagen III, VEGF, IL4, and IL10 in skin tissue samples showed no significant differences ($p > 0.05$) among means marked with the same letter.

For GSH and TBARS values, statistical significance was determined using the Kruskal–Wallis test with Dunn's post hoc analysis ($p < 0.05$). Means sharing the same letter were not significantly different from each other.

The analysis of TNF-α values in the skin of animals across different experimental groups and treatment times was performed using the Kruskal–Wallis test with Dunn's post hoc test ($p < 0.05$). Means with the same letter were not significantly different from each other.

The software used for statistical analysis was GraphPad Prism 9.0.0.

5. Conclusions

Autologous micrografts have demonstrated effectiveness in promoting healing of difficult-to-heal wounds by influencing epithelialization, angiogenesis, and collagen production. Treatment with AMG has been observed to reduce tissue inflammation, resulting in improved healing in animals with and without diabetes.

Author Contributions: Conceptualization, M.B.P., F.N., A.G. and A.F.S.; methodology, M.B.P. and I.M.F.d.M.; validation, M.B.P. and A.F.S.; formal analysis, M.B.P. and I.M.F.d.M.; investigation, M.B.P.; resources, F.D.A.L.S., Á.A.C.T. and L.D.V.; data curation, M.B.P. and I.M.F.d.M.; writing—original draft preparation, M.B.P. and E.P.; writing—review and editing, M.B.P., E.P. and A.F.S.; visualization, M.B.P. and E.P.; supervision, F.N. and A.F.S.; project administration, A.F.S.; funding acquisition, A.F.S. All authors have read and agreed to the published version of the manuscript.

Funding: This research was funded by CAPES (Coordenação de Aperfeiçoamento de Pessoal de Nível Superior), Brazil and Human Brain Wave, Italy.

Institutional Review Board Statement: The animal study protocol was approved by the Ethics Committee of the Rural Federal University of Pernambuco, protocol code 89/2018, process 23082.014335/2018-85, approval in 22 August 2018.

Informed Consent Statement: Not applicable.

Data Availability Statement: Not applicable.

Conflicts of Interest: E.P. belongs to the R&D department of HBW srl, the company owner of the Rigenera Micrografting Technology. A.G. holds the position of Chief Executive Officer at HBW srl. The remaining authors declare that the research was conducted in the absence of any commercial or financial relationships that could be construed as a potential conflict of interest.

References

1. Rittié, L. Cellular mechanisms of skin repair in humans and other mammals. *J. Cell Commun. Signal.* **2016**, *10*, 103–120. [CrossRef]
2. Blair, M.J.; Jones, J.D.; Woessner, A.E.; Quinn, K.P. Skin Structure–Function Relationships and the Wound Healing Response to Intrinsic Aging. *Adv. Wound Care* **2020**, *9*, 127–143. [CrossRef] [PubMed]
3. Shen, Z.; Sun, L.; Liu, Z.; Li, M.; Cao, Y.; Han, L.; Wang, J.; Wu, X.; Sang, S. Rete ridges: Morphogenesis, function, regulation, and reconstruction. *Acta Biomater.* **2023**, *155*, 19–34. [CrossRef] [PubMed]
4. Goleva, E.; Berdyshev, E.; Leung, D.Y.M. Epithelial barrier repair and prevention of allergy. *J. Clin. Investig.* **2019**, *129*, 1463–1474. [CrossRef] [PubMed]
5. Pontiggia, L.; Ahuja, A.K.; Yosef, H.K.; Rütsche, D.; Reichmann, E.; Moehrlen, U.; Biedermann, T. Human Basal and Suprabasal Keratinocytes Are Both Able to Generate and Maintain Dermo–Epidermal Skin Substitutes in Long-Term In Vivo Experiments. *Cells* **2022**, *11*, 2156. [CrossRef]
6. Nguyen, A.V.; Soulika, A.M. The Dynamics of the Skin's Immune System. *Int. J. Mol. Sci.* **2019**, *20*, 1811. [CrossRef]
7. Gantwerker, E.A.; Hom, D.B. Skin: Histology and Physiology of Wound Healing. *Clin. Plast. Surg.* **2012**, *39*, 85–97. [CrossRef] [PubMed]
8. Piipponen, M.; Li, D.; Landén, N.X. The Immune Functions of Keratinocytes in Skin Wound Healing. *Int. J. Mol. Sci.* **2021**, *21*, 8790. [CrossRef] [PubMed]
9. Yardman-Frank, J.M.; Fisher, D.E. Skin pigmentation and its control: From ultraviolet radiation to stem cells. *Exp. Dermatol.* **2020**, *30*, 560–571. [CrossRef]
10. Rippa, A.L.; Kalabusheva, E.P.; Vorotelyak, E.A. Regeneration of Dermis: Scarring and Cells Involved. *Cells* **2019**, *8*, 607. [CrossRef]
11. Woodley, D.T. Distinct Fibroblasts in the Papillary and Reticular Dermis. *Dermatol. Clin.* **2017**, *35*, 95–100. [CrossRef] [PubMed]
12. Piccinin, M.A.; Miao, J.H.; Schwartz, J. *Histology, Meissner Corpuscle*; StatPearls Publishing: Treasure Island, FL, USA, 2023.
13. Losquadro, W.D. Anatomy of the Skin and the Pathogenesis of Nonmelanoma Skin Cancer. *Facial Plast. Surg. Clin. N. Am.* **2017**, *25*, 283–289. [CrossRef] [PubMed]
14. Takeo, M.; Lee, W.; Ito, M. Wound Healing and Skin Regeneration. *Cold Spring Harb. Perspect. Med.* **2015**, *5*, a023267. [CrossRef] [PubMed]
15. Yuan, T.; Yang, T.; Chen, H.; Fu, D.; Hu, Y.; Wang, J.; Yuan, Q.; Yu, H.; Xu, W.; Xie, X. New insights into oxidative stress and inflammation during diabetes mellitus-accelerated atherosclerosis. *Redox Biol.* **2019**, *20*, 247–260. [CrossRef]
16. Wong, T.C.; Piehler, K.; Meier, C.G.; Testa, S.M.; Klock, A.M.; Aneizi, A.A.; Shakesprere, J.; Kellman, P.; Shroff, S.G.; Schwartzman, D.S.; et al. Association Between Extracellular Matrix Expansion Quantified by Cardiovascular Magnetic Resonance and Short-Term Mortality. *Circulation* **2012**, *126*, 1206–1216. [CrossRef]
17. Gattazzo, F.; Urciuolo, A.; Bonaldo, P. Extracellular matrix: A dynamic microenvironment for stem cell niche. *Biochim. Biophys. Acta* **2014**, *1840*, 2506–2519. [CrossRef]
18. Assis-Ribas, T.; Forni, M.F.; Winnischofer, S.M.B.; Sogayar, M.; Trombetta-Lima, M. Extracellular matrix dynamics during mesenchymal stem cells differentiation. *Dev. Biol.* **2018**, *437*, 63–74. [CrossRef] [PubMed]
19. Hsu, Y.-C.; Fuchs, E. A family business: Stem cell progeny join the niche to regulate homeostasis. *Nat. Rev. Mol. Cell Biol.* **2012**, *13*, 103–114. [CrossRef]
20. Hsu, Y.-C.; Li, L.; Fuchs, E. Emerging interactions between skin stem cells and their niches. *Nat. Med.* **2014**, *20*, 847–856. [CrossRef] [PubMed]
21. Fuchs, E.; Blau, H.M. Tissue Stem Cells: Architects of Their Niches. *Cell Stem Cell* **2020**, *27*, 532–556. [CrossRef]
22. Atiyeh, B.S.; Abbas, J.; Costagliola, M. Barreira cutânea para reconstrução mamária com prótese. *Rev. Bras. Cir. Plástica* **2012**, *27*, 630–635. [CrossRef]
23. Velnar, T.; Bailey, T.; Smrkolj, V. The Wound Healing Process: An Overview of the Cellular and Molecular Mechanisms. *J. Int. Med. Res.* **2009**, *37*, 1528–1542. [CrossRef]
24. Reinke, J.; Sorg, H. Wound Repair and Regeneration. *Eur. Surg. Res.* **2012**, *49*, 35–43. [CrossRef]
25. Eming, S.A.; Martin, P.; Tomic-Canic, M. Wound repair and regeneration: Mechanisms, signaling, and translation. *Sci. Transl. Med.* **2014**, *6*, 265–266. [CrossRef] [PubMed]
26. Forbes, J.M.; Cooper, M.E. Mechanisms of Diabetic Complications. *Physiol. Rev.* **2013**, *93*, 137–188. [CrossRef]

27. Boniakowski, A.E.; Kimball, A.S.; Jacobs, B.N.; Kunkel, S.L.; Gallagher, K.A. Macrophage-Mediated Inflammation in Normal and Diabetic Wound Healing. *J. Immunol.* **2017**, *199*, 17–24. [CrossRef]
28. GBD 2016 Disease and Injury Incidence and Prevalence Collaborators. Global, regional, and national incidence, prevalence, and years lived with disability for 328 diseases and injuries for 195 countries, 1990–2016: A systematic analysis for the Global Burden of Disease Study 2016. *Lancet* **2017**, *390*, 1211–1259. [CrossRef] [PubMed]
29. Bandyk, D.F. The diabetic foot: Pathophysiology, evaluation, and treatment. *Semin. Vasc. Surg.* **2018**, *31*, 43–48. [CrossRef]
30. Patel, S.; Srivastava, S.; Singh, M.R.; Singh, D. Mechanistic insight into diabetic wounds: Pathogenesis, molecular targets and treatment strategies to pace wound healing. *Biomed. Pharmacother.* **2019**, *112*, 108615. [CrossRef]
31. Wan, C.-D.; Cheng, R.; Wang, H.-B.; Liu, T. Immunomodulatory effects of mesenchymal stem cells derived from adipose tissues in a rat orthotopic liver transplantation model. *Hepatobiliary Pancreat. Dis. Int.* **2008**, *7*, 29–33.
32. Mafi, P. Adult Mesenchymal Stem Cells and Cell Surface Characterization—A Systematic Review of the Literature. *Open Orthop. J.* **2011**, *5*, 253–260. [CrossRef] [PubMed]
33. Waszak, P.; Alphonse, R.S.; Vadivel, A.; Ionescu, L.; Eaton, F.; Thébaud, B.; Abreu, S.C.; Weiss, D.J.; Rocco, P.R.M.; Rüdiger, M.; et al. Preconditioning Enhances the Paracrine Effect of Mesenchymal Stem Cells in Preventing Oxygen-Induced Neonatal Lung Injury in Rats. *Stem Cells Dev.* **2012**, *21*, 2789–2797. [CrossRef]
34. Phinney, D.G.; Pittenger, M.F. Concise Review: MSC-Derived Exosomes for Cell-Free Therapy. *Stem Cells* **2017**, *35*, 851–858. [CrossRef] [PubMed]
35. Ferrin, I.; Beloqui, I.; Zabaleta, L.; Salcedo, J.M.; Trigueros, C.; Martin, A.G. Isolation, Culture, and Expansion of Mesenchymal Stem Cells. In *Stem Cell Banking*; Humana Press: New York, NY, USA, 2017; pp. 177–190. [CrossRef]
36. Wang, C.; Börger, V.; Sardari, M.; Murke, F.; Skuljec, J.; Pul, R.; Hagemann, N.; Dzyubenko, E.; Dittrich, R.; Gregorius, J.; et al. Mesenchymal Stromal Cell–Derived Small Extracellular Vesicles Induce Ischemic Neuroprotection by Modulating Leukocytes and Specifically Neutrophils. *Stroke* **2020**, *51*, 1825–1834. [CrossRef]
37. Baena, R.R.Y.; D'Aquino, R.; Graziano, A.; Trovato, L.; Aloise, A.C.; Ceccarelli, G.; Cusella, G.; Pelegrine, A.A.; Lupi, S.M. Autologous Periosteum-Derived Micrografts and PLGA/HA Enhance the Bone Formation in Sinus Lift Augmentation. *Front. Cell Dev. Biol.* **2017**, *5*, 87. [CrossRef] [PubMed]
38. Ceccarelli, G.; Presta, R.; Lupi, S.M.; Giarratana, N.; Bloise, N.; Benedetti, L.; De Angelis, M.G.C.; Baena, R.R.Y. Evaluation of Poly(Lactic-co-glycolic) Acid Alone or in Combination with Hydroxyapatite on Human-Periosteal Cells Bone Differentiation and in Sinus Lift Treatment. *Molecules* **2017**, *22*, 2109. [CrossRef] [PubMed]
39. Marcarelli, M.; Zappia, M.; Rissolio, L.; Baroni, C.; Astarita, C.; Trovato, L.; Graziano, A. Cartilage Micrografts as a Novel Non-Invasive and Non-Arthroscopic Autograft Procedure for Knee Chondropathy: Three-Year Follow-Up Study. *J. Clin. Med.* **2021**, *10*, 322. [CrossRef]
40. Marcarelli, M.; Fiammengo, M.; Trovato, L.; Lancione, V.; Novarese, E.; Indelli, P.F.; Risitano, S. Autologous Grafts in the Treatment of Avascular Osteonecrosis of the Femoral Head. 1885. Available online: https://www.actabiomedica.it (accessed on 1 June 2023).
41. Hawwam, S.A.; Ismail, M.; Elhawary, E.E. The role of autologous micrografts injection from the scalp tissue in the treatment of COVID-19 associated telogen effluvium: Clinical and trichoscopic evaluation. *Dermatol. Ther.* **2022**, *35*, e15545. [CrossRef]
42. Niimi, Y.; Baba, K.; Tsuchida, M.; Takeda, A. A Histological Evaluation of Artificial Dermal Scaffold Used in Micrograft Treatment: A Case Study of Micrograft and NPWT Performed on a Postoperative Ulcer Formation after Tumor Resection. *Medicina* **2022**, *58*, 73. [CrossRef]
43. Andreone, A.; De Hollander, D. Case Report A Case Report on the Effect of Micrografting in the Healing of Chronic and Complex Burn Wounds. *Int. J. Burn. Trauma* **2020**, *10*, 15–20.
44. Aliberti, F.; Paolin, E.; Benedetti, L.; Cusella, G.; Ceccarelli, G. 3D bioprinting and Rigenera®micrografting technology: A possible countermeasure for wound healing in spaceflight. *Front. Bioeng. Biotechnol.* **2022**, *10*, 937709. [CrossRef]
45. Nummi, A.; Mulari, S.; Stewart, J.A.; Kivistö, S.; Teittinen, K.; Nieminen, T.; Lampinen, M.; Pätilä, T.; Sintonen, H.; Juvonen, T.; et al. Epicardial Transplantation of Autologous Cardiac Micrografts During Coronary Artery Bypass Surgery. *Front. Cardiovasc. Med.* **2021**, *8*, 726889. [CrossRef] [PubMed]
46. Trovato, L.; Monti, M.; del Fante, C.; Cervio, M.; Lampinen, M.; Ambrosio, L.; Redi, C.A.; Perotti, C.; Kankuri, E.; Ambrosio, G.; et al. A New Medical Device Rigeneracons Allows to Obtain Viable Micro-Grafts From Mechanical Disaggregation of Human Tissues. *J. Cell. Physiol.* **2015**, *230*, 2299–2303. [CrossRef]
47. Blakytny, R.; Jude, E. The molecular biology of chronic wounds and delayed healing in diabetes. *Diabet. Med.* **2006**, *23*, 594–608. [CrossRef] [PubMed]
48. Yu, J.R.; Navarro, J.; Coburn, J.C.; Mahadik, B.; Molnar, J.; Holmes, J.H.; Nam, A.J.; Fisher, J.P. Current and Future Perspectives on Skin Tissue Engineering: Key Features of Biomedical Research, Translational Assessment, and Clinical Application. *Adv. Healthc. Mater.* **2019**, *8*, 1801471. [CrossRef] [PubMed]
49. Andreone, A.; Hollander, D.D. A Retrospective Study on the Use of Dermis Micrografts in Platelet-Rich Fibrin for the Resurfacing of Massive and Chronic Full-Thickness Burns. *Stem Cells Int.* **2019**, *2019*, 8636709. [CrossRef]
50. Gurtner, G.C.; Werner, S.; Barrandon, Y.; Longaker, M.T. Wound repair and regeneration. *Nature* **2008**, *453*, 314–321. [CrossRef] [PubMed]
51. Diegelmann, R.F.; Evans, M.C. Wound healing: An overview of acute, fibrotic and delayed healing. *Front. Biosci.* **2004**, *9*, 283–289. [CrossRef]

52. Idriss, H.T.; Naismith, J.H. TNF alpha and the TNF receptor superfamily: Structure-function relationship(s). *Microsc. Res. Tech.* **2000**, *50*, 184–195. [CrossRef]
53. Tu, C.; Lu, H.; Zhou, T.; Zhang, W.; Deng, L.; Cao, W.; Yang, Z.; Wang, Z.; Wu, X.; Ding, J.; et al. Promoting the healing of infected diabetic wound by an anti-bacterial and nano-enzyme-containing hydrogel with inflammation-suppressing, ROS-scavenging, oxygen and nitric oxide-generating properties. *Biomaterials* **2022**, *286*, 121597. [CrossRef]
54. Ouyang, W.; Rutz, S.; Crellin, N.K.; Valdez, P.A.; Hymowitz, S.G. Regulation and Functions of the IL-10 Family of Cytokines in Inflammation and Disease. *Annu. Rev. Immunol.* **2011**, *29*, 71–109. [CrossRef]
55. Franco, R.; Panayiotidis, M.I.; Cidlowski, J.A. Glutathione Depletion Is Necessary for Apoptosis in Lymphoid Cells Independent of Reactive Oxygen Species Formation. *J. Biol. Chem.* **2007**, *282*, 30452–30465. [CrossRef] [PubMed]
56. Dall'Ago, P.; Silva, V.O.K.; De Angelis, K.L.D.; Irigoyen, M.C.; Fazan, R., Jr.; Salgado, H.C. Reflex control of arterial pressure and heart rate in short-term streptozotocin diabetic rats. *Braz. J. Med. Biol. Res.* **2002**, *35*, 843–849. [CrossRef] [PubMed]
57. Oberholzer, M.; Östreicher, M.; Christen, H.; Brühlmann, M. Methods in quantitative image analysis. *Histochem. Cell Biol.* **1996**, *105*, 333–355. [CrossRef] [PubMed]
58. Bussolati, G.; Radulescu, R.T. Blocking Endogenous Peroxidases in Immunohistochemistry. *Appl. Immunohistochem. Mol. Morphol.* **2011**, *19*, 484. [CrossRef]
59. Ohkawa, H.; Ohishi, N.; Yagi, K. Assay for lipid peroxides in animal tissues by thiobarbituric acid reaction. *Anal. Biochem.* **1979**, *95*, 351–358. [CrossRef] [PubMed]
60. Sedlak, J.; Lindsay, R.H. Estimation of total, protein-bound, and nonprotein sulfhydryl groups in tissue with Ellman's reagent. *Anal. Biochem.* **1968**, *25*, 192–205. [CrossRef]
61. Buege, J.A.; Aust, S.D. Microsomal lipid peroxidation. *Methods Enzymol.* **1978**, *52*, 302–310. [CrossRef] [PubMed]
62. Mohammad, H.M.; El-Baz, A.A.; Mahmoud, O.M.; Khalil, S.; Atta, R.; Imbaby, S. Protective effects of evening primrose oil on behavioral activities, nigral microglia and histopathological changes in a rat model of rotenone-induced parkinsonism. *J. Chem. Neuroanat.* **2023**, *127*, 102206. [CrossRef] [PubMed]

Disclaimer/Publisher's Note: The statements, opinions and data contained in all publications are solely those of the individual author(s) and contributor(s) and not of MDPI and/or the editor(s). MDPI and/or the editor(s) disclaim responsibility for any injury to people or property resulting from any ideas, methods, instructions or products referred to in the content.

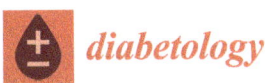

Review

Importance of Dyslipidaemia Treatment in Individuals with Type 2 Diabetes Mellitus—A Narrative Review

Dominik Strikić [1], Andro Vujević [1,*], Dražen Perica [2], Dunja Leskovar [2], Kristina Paponja [2], Ivan Pećin [3] and Iveta Merćep [3]

1. Division of Clinical Pharmacology, Department of Internal Medicine, University Hospital Centre Zagreb, 10000 Zagreb, Croatia; strikic.dominik@gmail.com
2. Division of Metabolic Diseases, Department of Internal Medicine, University Hospital Centre Zagreb, 10000 Zagreb, Croatia; drazen.perica1@gmail.com (D.P.); dunja.leskovar@gmail.com (D.L.); kpaponja505@gmail.com (K.P.)
3. Department of Internal Medicine, School of Medicine, University of Zagreb, 10000 Zagreb, Croatia; ipecin@kbc-zagreb.hr (I.P.); imercep@gmail.com (I.M.)
* Correspondence: androandro726@gmail.com

Abstract: Type 2 diabetes mellitus (T2DM) is a common metabolic disease characterised by insulin resistance and elevated blood glucose levels, affecting millions of people worldwide. T2DM individuals with dyslipidaemia have an increased risk of cardiovascular disease (CVD). A complex interplay of risk factors such as hyperglycaemia, dyslipidaemia, hypertension, obesity, inflammation, and oxidative stress favour the development of atherosclerosis, a central mechanism in the pathogenesis of cardiovascular disease. Dyslipidaemia, a hallmark of T2DM, is characterised by elevated triglycerides, decreased high-density lipoprotein (HDL) cholesterol and the presence of small, dense low-density lipoprotein (LDL) particles, all of which promote atherosclerosis. In this article, we have attempted to present various treatment strategies that include pharmacological interventions such as statins, ezetimibe, PCSK9 inhibitors, fibrates, and omega-3 fatty acids. We have also tried to highlight the pivotal role of lifestyle modifications, including physical activity and dietary changes, in improving lipid profiles and overall cardiovascular health in T2DM individuals. We have also tried to present the latest clinical guidelines for the management of dyslipidaemia in T2DM individuals. In conclusion, the treatment of dyslipidaemia in T2DM individuals is of great importance as it lowers lipid particle levels, slows the progression of atherosclerosis, and ultimately reduces susceptibility to cardiovascular disease.

Keywords: type 2 diabetes mellitus; dyslipidaemia; metabolic disorder; pharmaceutical treatment; nonpharmaceutical treatment

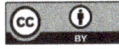

1. Introduction

Type 2 diabetes mellitus (T2DM) is a chronic metabolic disorder characterised by insulin resistance and high blood glucose levels. It is estimated that 462 million people are affected by this disease, which corresponds to a prevalence rate of 6059 cases per 100,000. T2DM is more common in developed regions (Europe, North America) with equal gender distribution [1]. T2DM is a significant risk factor for cardiovascular disease including coronary artery disease, myocardial infarction, stroke, peripheral artery disease, and heart failure. Cardiovascular comorbidities in T2DM patients impose high costs on both the population and individuals. Cardiovascular expenditure accounts for between 20% and 49% of the total direct costs of treating T2DM at the population level. In the 2016 analysis of the economic burden of T2DM complications in Sweden, the cost per person was EUR 1317. This comprehensive figure encompasses a complex interplay of factors, with a notable 25% of the total costs being due to absenteeism. The main contributors to these costs were macrovascular complications such as angina, heart failure, and stroke, and microvascular complications such as eye disease (e.g., retinopathy), kidney disease, and neuropathy. Furthermore, early mortality in the working-age population resulted in an additional cost of EUR 579 per person, while expenditure on drugs to treat risk factors amounted to EUR 418 per person [2]. The increased risk of CVD in individuals with T2DM is influenced by a complex interplay of risk factors that include hyperglycaemia, dyslipidaemia, hypertension, obesity, inflammation, and oxidative stress. These risk factors contribute to the development and progression of atherosclerosis, one of the major underlying processes in CVD [3,4]. The aim of this review is to shed light on the management of dyslipidaemia in people with type 2 diabetes mellitus, focusing on the underlying pathophysiology and the intricate web of interrelated metabolic disorders.

2. Pathophysiology

The pathophysiology of atherosclerosis in T2DM is a complex process, but it is important to understand its relationship to the increased risk of cardiovascular disease and mortality in people with T2DM. Atherosclerosis in T2DM is primarily caused by a combination of metabolic abnormalities, inflammation, oxidative stress, and endothelial dysfunction. The main pathophysiological mechanism is hyperglycaemia due to insulin resistance, which can damage blood vessels and increase the risk of atherosclerosis. People with T2DM have a significantly increased risk of developing cardiovascular disease, including coronary heart disease, stroke, and peripheral vascular disease. Cardiovascular disease is the leading cause of morbidity and mortality in this population, with T2D patients at similar risk to people who have already had a heart attack (coronary risk equivalent) [3,5,6]. The complicated pathophysiological processes described above contribute significantly to this increased risk. Dyslipidaemia, characterised by increased triglyceride levels, decreased high density lipoprotein (HDL) cholesterol levels and small, dense low-density lipoprotein (LDL) particles, is common in T2DM and promotes the development of atherosclerotic plaques. Chronic low-grade inflammation and oxidative stress are hallmarks of T2DM and play a critical role in the development and progression of atherosclerosis. These processes, in conjunction with endothelial dysfunction, lead to a proinflammatory and prothrombotic state in the blood vessels. The formation of atherosclerotic plaques with lipid deposits, inflammatory cells, smooth muscle cells, and fibrous tissue marks the beginning of the vicious circle [3,7,8]. Vulnerable plaques are prone to rupture, which can lead to thrombosis and cause acute cardiovascular events such as heart attacks and strokes. As atherosclerosis progresses, artery walls can remodel, leading to narrowing and reduced blood flow in the affected vessels. In summary, the pathophysiology of atherosclerosis in T2DM plays a critical role in the increased risk of cardiovascular disease and mortality in these patients. Understanding the intricate relationships between these factors is essential for effective management and risk reduction in people with T2DM [3,6,8].

3. Type 2 Diabetes Mellitus and Dyslipidemia Interconnection

Dyslipidaemia is one of the most common findings in people with type 2 diabetes, affecting about 72–85% of those affected [9]. It additionally increases cardiovascular risk, especially the risk of developing coronary heart disease. The most important lipid abnormalities in diabetics are increased levels of triacylglycerols and decreased HDL cholesterol. In addition to quantitative changes in lipoproteins, there are also qualitative and kinetic changes in lipoprotein metabolism that contribute to the development of atherosclerosis [10]. Prior to the development of manifest type 2 diabetes, increased insulin resistance affects the accumulation of triglycerides and small, dense LDL particles. Starting from the chylomicron level, diabetics experience increased production of chylomicrons as a result of insulin resistance, leading to postprandial hyperlipidaemia, although the complex pathway that triggers this phenomenon is not yet fully understood [11,12]. On the other hand, the clearance of chylomicrons is impaired due to the decreased activity of lipoprotein lipase (LPL), an enzyme necessary for the degradation of chylomicrons [13].

In addition, the production of large VLDL particles is increased, leading to an increase in plasma triacylglycerol levels. Studies have shown the link between VLDL production rates and fatty liver in people with type 2 diabetes [14]. Unlike other lipids, LDL cholesterol levels are not significantly increased in diabetics compared to the general population, but increased glycation of LDL leads to severe atherosclerosis. Glycated LDL cholesterol has a lower binding affinity to LDL receptors and is taken up by macrophages, leading to the formation of foam cells [15]. In addition, oxidised LDL particles increase the formation of cytokines (TNF-α, IL-1), adhesion molecules that promote the inflammatory atherosclerotic process. Diabetics also have reduced levels of HDL cholesterol, which plays a key role in the uptake and transport of lipoproteins. Studies have shown that HDL particles are more degraded in diabetics due to the accumulation of triacylglycerol [16]. HDL plays an important role in cardiovascular prevention due to its antioxidant and vasodilatory effects, so lower levels also increase overall cardiovascular risk. The most common quantitative changes in the lipid profile of diabetics are increased triglyceride levels, residual particles, and decreased HDL cholesterol levels. Qualitative and kinetic changes in the metabolism of LDL cholesterol have a major atherogenic effect, so that the treatment of dyslipidaemia should be taken very seriously.

4. Target Lipid Levels in Type 2 Diabetes Mellitus

The American Diabetes Association recently released updated guidelines for 2023 that include new recommendations for people with diabetes, including guidance on managing lipid levels. According to the current recommendations, it is advisable to prescribe high-intensity statin treatment for people with diabetes who are at increased risk for cardiovascular problems, especially those with one or more risk factors for atherosclerotic cardiovascular disease (ASCVD). The primary goal is to reduce LDL cholesterol levels by at least 50% from baseline, aiming for an LDL cholesterol level of less than 70 mg/dL (1.8 mmol/L) [17]. However, in clinical practise, it can be difficult to determine the exact baseline LDL cholesterol level before starting statin therapy. Therefore, for these individuals, it is recommended to focus on achieving a target LDL cholesterol of less than 70 mg/dL (1.8 mmol/L) rather than on the percentage reduction in LDL cholesterol. If appropriate, it may also be useful to supplement maximally tolerated statin therapy with ezetimibe or a proprotein convertase subtilisin/kexin type 9 (PCSK9) inhibitor to achieve the desired LDL cholesterol reduction of at least 50% and reach the recommended LDL cholesterol target of below 70 mg/dL (1.8 mmol/L). Although primary prevention trials have typically involved limited numbers of older people with diabetes, they have not shown significant differences in the relative benefits of lipid-lowering therapy between age groups. However, because older age is associated with a higher risk profile, the absolute benefit of lipid-lowering therapy is greater. Therefore, it is advisable to recommend moderate-intensity statin therapy to people with diabetes aged 75 years or older. High-intensity statin therapy is recommended for all people with diabetes who have a history of ASCVD. The goal is to achieve a significant reduction in LDL cholesterol levels of at least 50% from baseline, with a specific goal of maintaining LDL cholesterol levels below 55 mg/dL (1.42 mmol/L) [17]. If these targets are not met despite administration of the maximally tolerated statin, it is advisable to consider additional administration of ezetimibe or a PCSK9 inhibitor. The new guidelines do not include precise target values for other lipoproteins. Therefore, it is advisable to consider the following target values: HDL cholesterol levels should be above 40 mg/dL (1.02 mmol/L) and triglyceride levels should be below 150 mg/dL (1.7 mmol/L) [18] (Table 1).

Table 1. Statin treatment goal in T2DM individuals.

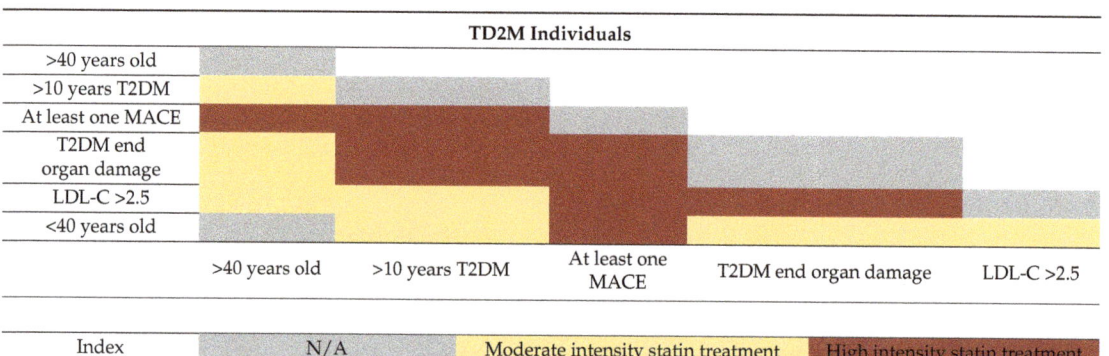

5. Treatment of Dyslipidaemia in Type 2 Diabetes Mellitus

The treatment of dyslipidaemia in individuals with type 2 diabetes mellitus (T2DM) can be divided into two categories: nonpharmacological and pharmacological. If we talk about pharmacological therapeutic strategies with regard to elevated lipid levels in individuals who have already been diagnosed Type 2 DM, the most important approach is treatment with statins. Other options include cholesterol absorption inhibitors, fibrates, PCSK9 inhibitors, and omega-3 fatty acids [19].

Despite the significant benefits of treatment strategies that reduce CVD risk factors, CVD remains the major cause of morbidity and mortality in individuals with T2DM. The risk of MACE in T2DM is strongly determined by the presence of target organ damage, with risks increasing with the number of diseases present. In light of this information, the main focus of treatment for dyslipidaemia in individuals with T2DM is early initiation of treatment [19]. According to the latest guidelines, individuals who have had diabetes for at least 10 years or less but have known cardiovascular disease and/or at least one target organ damage and elevated lipid levels should start statin treatment immediately [19,20]. If an early 50% reduction is achieved, further supplementation is not required but continuation of pharmacological and nonpharmacological treatment is. However, if the desired reduction is not achieved, the additional administration of ezetimibe or PCSK9 inhibitor is suggested depending on the primary or secondary prevention setting [19,20] (Figure 1).

5.1. Statins

Statins are the first treatment option for individuals with T2DM. Management of LDL cholesterol is of paramount importance in these individuals. The Cholesterol Treatment Trialists (CTT) study performed a comprehensive analysis of the data and uncovered 3247 serious vascular events in the diabetic cohort [21]. Strikingly, each one millimole per litre (mmol/L) reduction in LDL cholesterol was associated with a remarkable 9% proportional reduction in all-cause mortality in participants with diabetes. Remarkably, this reduction paralleled the 13% decrease observed in individuals without diabetes, underscoring the importance of LDL-C modulation in preventing mortality [21]. This positive trend was underlined by a statistically significant reduction in vascular mortality in the diabetic cohort, while no discernible effect on non-vascular mortality was observed. In addition, a substantial proportional reduction in major vascular events of 21% per mmol/L reduction in LDL cholesterol was observed in participants with diabetes, mirroring the effects in participants without diabetes [21]. The discernible effects of statin therapy also extended to specific cardiovascular outcomes in the diabetes population, including reductions in myocardial infarction or coronary death, coronary revascularisation, and stroke. Notably, these results held true regardless of whether participants had a history of vascular disease [22,23]. After 5 years, statin therapy had significant clinical benefit in the diabetic cohort, as evidenced by a reduction in major vascular events among participants receiving statin therapy [21]. Overall, these results highlight the compelling efficacy of statin therapy in reducing the burden of serious vascular events in people with diabetes mellitus and support the thesis that statins are a key therapeutic intervention for LDL-C management in the context of diabetes treatment. On the other hand, recent studies have brought to light a possible increase in the incidence of diabetes mellitus (DM) in individuals receiving statin therapy [24,25]. This trend has been supported by clinical trials, with the clearest effects observed in people who are already at increased risk of DM, such as those with prediabetes [26]. It is critical to emphasise that these results should not diminish our commitment to patient care, as the overarching benefits of reducing cardiovascular disease persist and far outweigh the increased incidence of DM. Conversely, a separate prospective study of T2DM individuals found no statistically significant difference in glycosylated haemoglobin (HbA1c) levels between statin-treated and non-statin-treated groups [27]. The safety profile of statins is well established, with adverse effects such as muscle pain and liver damage frequently reported [28]. These adverse effects may be the most important factor in the low adherence to statin treatment. However, newer approaches such as fixed-dose combination therapy with statins and other drugs such as antihypertensives or even antidiabetics are leading to better adherence and positive cardiovascular outcomes in individuals [29].

5.2. Ezetimibe

Ezetimibe, a lipid-lowering agent that acts as a cholesterol absorption inhibitor, is associated with a 19% reduction in LDL-C levels [30]. Although ezetimibe alone has no positive results in risk reduction MACE, when added to statin therapy, ezetimibe has shown remarkable ability to reduce the risk of serious vascular events. It is important to note that the magnitude of relative risk reduction in MACE is directly proportional to the absolute degree of LDL-C reduction, a relationship consistent with the observed effects of statins [31]. In the study IMPROVE-IT, which included a subgroup of individuals diagnosed with T2DM, it was expected that this subgroup would have a higher rate of major vascular events than individuals without DM. In fact, the placebo arm of the study showed that individuals with DM had a significantly increased rate of MACE, with a 7-year Kaplan–Meier rate of 46% compared to 31% in individuals without DM [32]. Of particular importance is the observation that ezetimibe proved to be particularly effective in individuals with DM in the IMPROVE-IT study. When ezetimibe was added to their treatment regimen, individuals with DM experienced a relative risk reduction of 15% in MACE, which corresponds to a substantial absolute risk reduction of 5.5% [32]. However, it is worth noting that the IMPROVE-IT study did not demonstrate a significant reduction in MACE with single-use ezetimibe [33]. The reduction in major vascular events was most notable when ezetimibe was used in conjunction with statin therapy, highlighting the synergy between these therapies in achieving significant clinical benefits in cardiovascular risk management. Importantly, the safety profile of the combined statin-ezetimibe treatment remained consistent regardless of the presence of DM, underscoring the tolerability of this therapeutic approach [32,33] (Table 2) Based on the observed results, ezetimibe is used as a second treatment option in combination with statins in individuals in whom LDL-C lowering cannot be achieved with statin treatment alone [19,20].

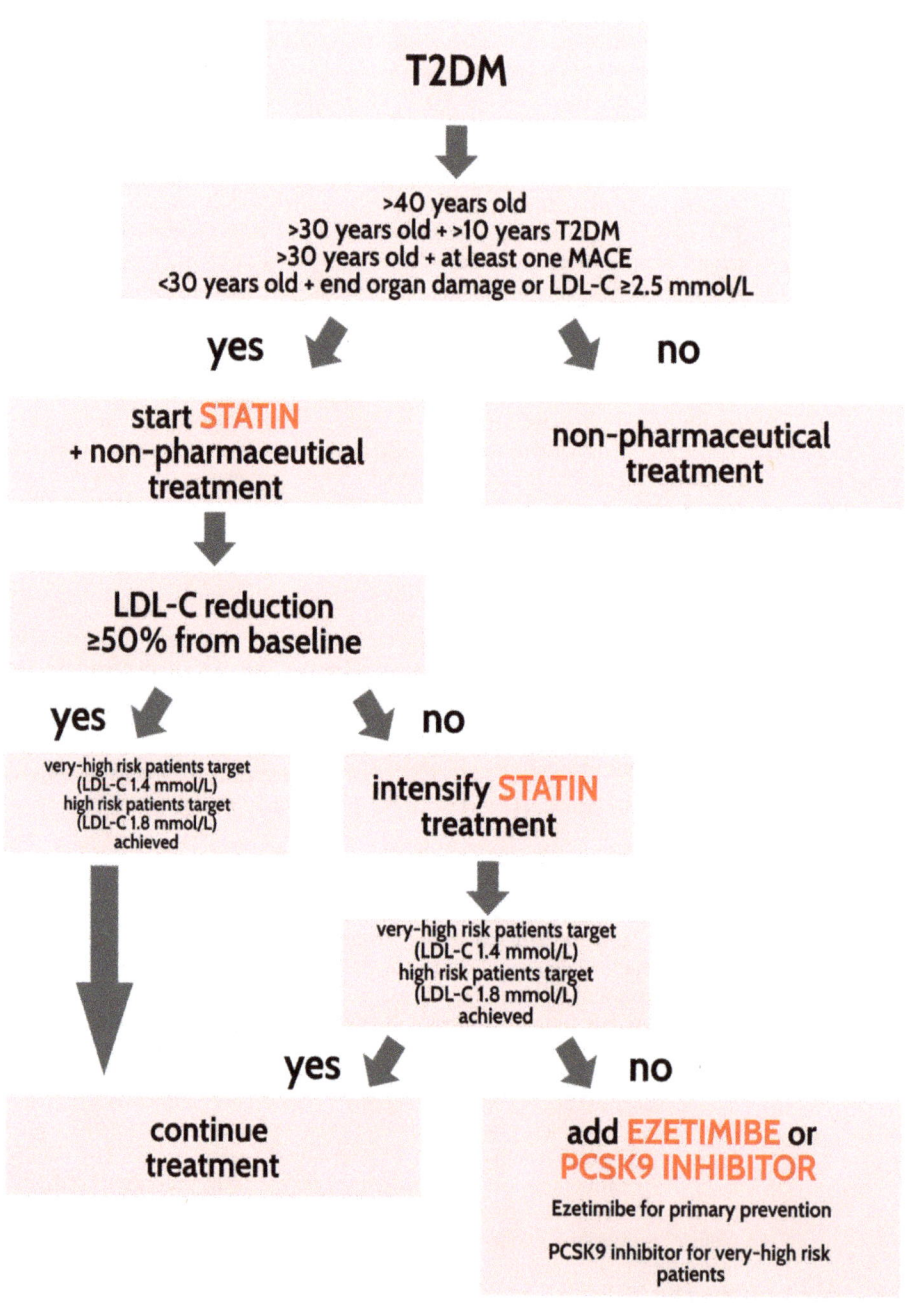

Figure 1. Recommendations for the treatment of dyslipidaemia in T2DM.

Table 2. Overview of the pharmacological approaches to dyslipidaemia in T2DM individuals.

Pharmacological Approach to Dyslipidaemia in T2DM Individuals				
Drug	Dosage	Mechanism of Action	Common Adverse Events	Monitoring (Except Lipid Profile)
Statins	10–80 mg Oral use/daily	HMG-3-CoA reductase antagonist	Statin-associated muscle disease	Serum aminotransferases
			Fatigue	Serum creatine-kinase
			Hepatic dysfunction	Regular blood count
Ezetimibe	10 mg Oral use/daily	NPC1L1 transporter inhibitor	Hepatic dysfunction	Serum aminotransferases
			Muscle-related effects	Serum creatine-kinase
Alirocumab Evolocumab	140 mg 75–300 mg Subcutaneous injections/2–4 weeks	PCSK9 inhibitors—monoclonal antibodies	Local injection reactions	-
Fibrates	145–215 mg Oral use/daily	PPARs activators	Hepatic dysfunction	Serum aminotransferases
			Muscle-related effects	Serum creatine-kinase
			Renal dysfunction	Serum renal function tests
				Regular blood count

5.3. PCSK9 Inhibitors

PCSK9 monoclonal antibodies such as evolocumab and alirocumab have attracted considerable attention due to their efficacy in lowering LDL-C levels, which is around 60% [33,34]. In the FOURIER study, the relative risk reduction for MACE was consistent in all patient groups with and without diabetes mellitus. However, the baseline risk profile of individuals with DM, characterised by an inherently higher cardiovascular risk, resulted in a more pronounced absolute risk reduction of 2.7% in MACE over 3 years [34]. These outstanding results are consistent with those of the ODYSSEY study, which demonstrated a consistent benefit of PCSK9 inhibitors, particularly in diabetic individuals after an acute coronary syndrome [35]. These studies highlight the potent LDL-C lowering effect of PCSK9 monoclonal antibody inhibitors and their potential to reduce the risk of MACE in both diabetics and non-diabetics [34,35]. A recent study that deepened our understanding of the effects of PCSK9 inhibitor therapy examined the effect of alirocumab in individuals of different glycaemic categories [34]. Importantly, alirocumab resulted in similar relative reductions in the incidence of primary cardiovascular endpoints in all glycaemic categories. However, in individuals with diabetes, there was a greater absolute reduction of 2.3% in the incidence of primary endpoints than in individuals with prediabetes (1.2%) or normoglycaemia (1.2%) [36]. Furthermore, in individuals without diabetes, the risk of new-onset diabetes was not increased by alirocumab therapy. These results highlight the safety profile of alirocumab with respect to new-onset diabetes [36,37]. Similar observations were made with evolocumab in a study that included individuals with and without diabetes. Evolocumab reduced cardiovascular outcomes in both patient groups [34,37]. These results suggest that the benefit of evolocumab is not dependent on diabetes status. Importantly, evolocumab did not increase the risk of new-onset diabetes in individuals without diabetes. In addition, haemoglobin A1c (HbA1c) and fasting plasma glucose (FPG) levels remained constant over time in all glycaemic categories between the evolocumab and placebo groups [38]. In addition, the frequency of adverse events was comparable between the evolocumab and placebo groups, further underscoring the safety profile of this PCSK9 inhibitor therapy regardless of diabetes status [34,35]. Overall, these comprehensive results highlight the robust efficacy and safety of monoclonal antibody PCSK9 inhibitors in both diabetic and non-diabetic individuals, supporting their role in controlling LDL-C levels and lowering MACE. However, the elephant in the room needs to be addressed, as the cost–benefit analysis of PCSK9 inhibitors is still ongoing. While some countries report further price reductions to increase cost-effectiveness, inclusion in T2DM treatment may justify their cost [39].

5.4. Fibrates

Fibrates are drugs used primarily to treat abnormal lipid profiles and conditions such as hypertriglyceridaemia and low levels of high-density lipoprotein cholesterol (HDL-C). These drugs work by activating peroxisome proliferator-activated receptors (PPARs), which regulate lipid metabolism [40]. The therapeutic efficacy of treating elevated triglyceride levels (TG) and low high-density lipoprotein cholesterol (HDL-C) levels, which are common in people with diabetes mellitus (DM), remains controversial. This debate arises from observations in studies such as FIELD and ACCORD, conducted in the context of T2DM cohorts, in which the effects of fenofibrate therapy on MACE did not yield positive results. In the FIELD study, fenofibrate showed a 27% reduction in CVD in individuals with elevated TG levels and elevated HDL-C levels [41]. Similarly, the ACCORD study confirmed that participants with both elevated TG and low HDL-C levels appeared to benefit from taking fenofibrate and statin at the same time [42]. The available evidence suggests that diabetics with dyslipidaemia may derive clinical benefits from TG -lowering therapy when administered concurrently with statin treatment.

5.5. Omega-3 Fatty Acids

Omega-3 fatty acids are essential polyunsaturated fats that provide a number of health benefits. These fats are abundant in certain fish such as salmon, mackerel, and sardines, as well as in flaxseeds, chia seeds, and walnuts [43]. They have the benefit of lowering triglyceride levels, improving blood vessel function and possibly reducing inflammation [44,45]. Omega-3 supplements are widely available in various forms such as fish oil capsules, krill oil, and algae-based supplements, so it is extremely difficult to regulate them and determine the exact dosage. There are limited data on the effects of adding omega-3 fatty acids to statin therapy in individuals with elevated plasma levels TG. The study REDUCE-IT sought to fill this gap by investigating the effects of icosapent ethyl at a dose of 2 grammes twice daily in high-risk HTG individuals taking statins concomitantly. The results showed a 25% reduction in the composite primary outcome, which includes cardiovascular death (CV), non-fatal myocardial infarction (MI), non-fatal stroke, coronary revascularisation, or unstable angina. This decrease corresponded to an absolute decrease of 4.8% [45]. Contrastingly, the ASCEND trial revealed that omega-3 fatty acids did not demonstrate a reduction in MACE [46] Although more research is needed, omega-3 fatty acids have an excellent safety profile. The most commonly reported adverse effects are gastrointestinal discomfort, increased risk of bleeding, and allergic reactions. While certain observations suggest the potential benefits of omega-3 fatty acids for individuals with T2DM, it is crucial to recognize that they cannot replace standard recommended treatments and are not in the guidelines for dyslipidaemia treatment. Both individuals and healthcare professionals should remain mindful of the potential impacts that supplements may have on patients [47].

5.6. Non-Pharmaceutical Treatment

A healthy lifestyle is a key element in the prevention of adverse cardiovascular events. A healthy lifestyle includes not only physical activity, but also improving dietary habits, reducing environmental risk factors, and maintaining mental health [48]. People who have type 2 diabetes mellitus have a higher risk of developing severe cardiovascular events. Expected lifestyle changes for these people therefore include improving dietary habits, increasing physical activity, and even taking medication to prevent further complications [49]. Added fats, sugars, or processed meats and sweetened beverages can significantly increase the risk of developing diabetes mellitus and cardiovascular disease. For example, drinking a single sweetened beverage per day can increase the risk of developing diabetes mellitus by up to 20% [50]. Physical activity and balanced dietary habits lead to weight loss in overweight individuals. Weight loss has a significant impact on lipid levels as well as on the treatment of type II diabetes mellitus, thus improving overall health. The effects of increased physical activity on lowering HbA1c levels have been known for several decades and point to the importance of a healthy lifestyle for blood glucose levels and cardiovascular-related morbidity and mortality in people with diabetes mellitus [51]. Exercise and increased physical activity have the greatest impact on HDL and triglyceride levels. In the study by Coillard and et al., participants were divided into four subgroups based on baseline HDL and triglyceride levels: The first consisted of people with normal levels (high HDL and low triglycerides), the second consisted of people with isolated low HDL and normal triglycerides, the third consisted of people with isolated high triglycerides and normal HDL levels, and the fourth subgroup included people with elevated triglycerides and low HDL. Among those with a combination of initially low HDL and elevated triglycerides, increased physical activity had the most significant effect, with a 4.9% increase in HDL levels, compared with a slight increase of 0.4% among those with isolated low HDL levels [52]. In addition, some studies suggest that not only physical activity but also its intensity has an impact on lipid management. In the STRRIDE study, changes in serum lipoproteins were monitored in participants with dyslipidaemia who took part in a range of physical activities. After eight months, HDL cholesterol levels and concentrations of large HDL particles were higher in those who engaged in intensive and vigorous physical activity than in the other groups. The STRIDDE-PD study included people with prediabetes, and global radiolabelled efflux capacity increased significantly (6.2%) in the high-volume/high-intensity group compared with all other STRRIDE-PD groups [53,54]. A combination of physical activity and healthy diet has shown a greater impact on lipid management. In a study of 22 obese men with metabolic syndrome, 3 weeks of physical activity combined with dietary changes resulted in an increase in platelet-activating factor acetylhydrolase activity [55]. Some diets tend to have a positive effect on the lipid profile of people with diabetes mellitus. For example, a ketogenic diet with 70% fat, 20% protein, and only 10% carbohydrate has been shown to reduce body mass, lower triglycerides and increase HDL levels in people with diabetes mellitus. In one study, no significant differences were found in the values for total cholesterol and LDL cholesterol. Another important outcome of the ketogenic diet is a reduction in waist circumference, which leads to a further reduction in the risk of complications of diabetes mellitus and the development of cardiovascular complications. In addition, in the same study, there is a significant improvement in blood glucose regulation due to a decrease in HbA1c [56]. Although there are studies that point to negative effects of the ketogenic diet on lipid levels, most studies report a reduction in weight and a resulting improvement in the lipid profile [57]. The Mediterranean diet, characterised by ingredients such as olive oil, seeds, whole grains, nuts, and fruits, is usually recommended as a golden model for the prevention of metabolic syndrome and its components. There are data indicating a significant impact of this diet on LDL cholesterol levels and triglyceride levels, especially in people suffering from type 2 diabetes mellitus. In a study by Elhayany and et al.

three different dietary approaches were compared during a one-year follow-up period. All participants had diabetes mellitus and were followed in a community-based setting. During this period, participants strictly followed the dietary recommendations for the low-carbohydrate Mediterranean diet, the classic Mediterranean diet, or the diet recommended by the American Diabetic Association in 2003. The low-carbohydrate Mediterranean diet has been shown to be particularly beneficial in lowering HbA1c and has been the only one associated with an increase in HDL cholesterol. The classic Mediterranean diet and the low-carbohydrate diet resulted in a greater reduction in triglyceride levels [58] (Figure 2). Olive oil, a major component of the Mediterranean diet, has shown positive effects on regulating lipid profiles, improving HDL functions such as cholesterol metabolism and cholesterol efflux capacity, and promoting an anti-inflammatory effect [59]. Consumption of phenol-containing olive oil increased HDL cholesterol and lowered total cholesterol and LDL cholesterol, resulting in a reduction in the ratio of total cholesterol/HDL cholesterol and LDL cholesterol/HDL cholesterol [60]. The CORDIOPREV (Coronary Diet Intervention with Olive Oil and Cardiovascular Prevention) trial showed that a 1.5-year intervention with a Mediterranean diet resulted in improved flow-mediated vasodilation and endothelial function and reduced overall cardiovascular risk in participants with diabetes mellitus and dyslipidaemia [61]. According to some studies, taking probiotics has also been shown to be beneficial. There is data to suggest that probiotics can lead to a reduction in total cholesterol and LDL cholesterol. The combination of probiotics and fermented dairy products can lead to an even greater reduction in LDL cholesterol than when probiotics are taken in capsule form [62]. Certain probiotic species such as Lactobacillus acidophilus and Lactobacillus plantarum have been shown to have more lipid-lowering effects and have been successful in lowering LDL cholesterol and total cholesterol [63]. The decrease in lipid levels varies from study to study and needs further investigation. On the other hand, in patients with dyslipidaemia and type 2 diabetes mellitus, synbiotics have shown an effect of significantly lowering fasting blood glucose levels and increasing HDL [64]. Probiotics have been shown to be beneficial in lowering liver enzymes and total cholesterol in patients with non-alcoholic fatty liver disease (NAFLD) [65]. In one study, NAFLD was induced in Iberian pigs fed a high-fat diet, as opposed to the control group, with or without probiotic supplementation. The high-fat diet caused inflammation and ectopic lipid accumulation in skeletal muscle, with no significant difference found between the groups with and without probiotic addition [66]. The full potential of probiotic supplementation in patients with metabolic syndrome and its components is often controversial, but it is certainly an interesting field waiting to be explored and used in the nonpharmacological treatment of patients. The microbiome diet, a new dietary trend, focuses on consuming less processed foods and increasing the intake of foods rich in prebiotics. Prebiotics are dietary fibres that promote beneficial gut bacteria. By promoting a healthier gut balance, this diet aims to improve metabolic function and reduce inflammation. Research has shown that a high-fat diet can disrupt the balance of the gut microbiome, leading to metabolic problems such as insulin resistance and inflammation. It is thought that by promoting a diverse and balanced gut microbiome community, the microbiome diet can positively influence conditions such as T2DM and dyslipidaemia [67]. The exact model of dietary habits and physical activity that will lead to adequate control of the risk of major cardiovascular events has yet to be found, but research to date may lead to a new answer to this dilemma.

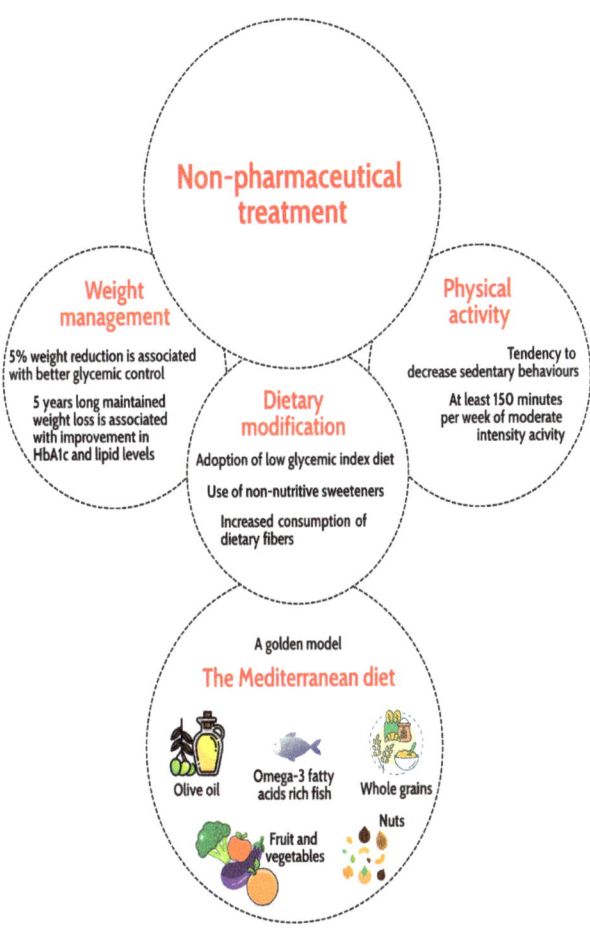

Figure 2. Overview of nonpharmaceutical treatment options in T2DM.

6. Conclusions

The treatment of dyslipidaemia in individuals with type 2 diabetes mellitus (T2DM) is of paramount importance because of the high risk of cardiovascular disease (CVD). T2DM is a complex metabolic disorder that not only affects glucose metabolism but also strongly influences lipid profiles, contributing to the development and progression of atherosclerosis—a key process underlying CVD. The pathophysiology of atherosclerosis in T2DM involves a complex interplay of metabolic abnormalities, inflammation, oxidative stress, and endothelial dysfunction. High glucose levels, a hallmark of T2DM, can damage blood vessels and lead to inflammation and oxidative stress that further increase CVD risk. Dyslipidaemia is common in T2DM. It is characterised by elevated triglycerides, reduced HDL cholesterol levels and the presence of small, dense low-density lipoprotein (LDL) particles. These lipid abnormalities contribute to the formation of atherosclerotic plaques. A comprehensive approach that includes pharmacological therapies, lifestyle modifications, and individualised treatment plans can significantly improve lipid profiles and reduce the risk of major cardiovascular events, ultimately improving the overall health and well-being of people with T2DM. While we have known therapeutical approaches to dyslipidaemia treatment in T2DM individuals, clear primary and secondary prevention protocols are still up for debate. However, treatment initiation at the earliest moment is of the utmost importance.

Author Contributions: Conceptualization, D.P., D.L. and D.S.; methodology, A.V.; software D.P., K.P., D.L. and D.S.; validation, D.P. and K.P.; formal analysis, A.V. and D.S.; investigation, I.P.; resources, I.P.; data curation, K.P. and D.L.; writing—original draft preparation, A.V.; writing—review and editing, D.S.; visualization, D.S.; supervision, I.M. and I.P.; project administration, I.M.; funding acquisition, I.M. and I.P. All authors have read and agreed to the published version of the manuscript.

Funding: This research received no external funding.

Data Availability Statement: The data presented in this study are openly available in PubMed database.

Conflicts of Interest: The authors declare no conflict of interest.

References

1. Khan, M.A.B.; Hashim, M.J.; King, J.K.; Govender, R.D.; Mustafa, H.; Al Kaabi, J. Epidemiology of Type 2 Diabetes—Global Burden of Disease and Forecasted Trends. *J. Epidemiol. Glob. Health* **2019**, *10*, 107. [CrossRef] [PubMed]
2. Andersson, E.; Persson, S.; Hallén, N.; Ericsson, Å.; Thielke, D.; Lindgren, P.; Steen Carlsson, K.; Jendle, J. Costs of diabetes complications: Hospital-based care and absence from work for 392,200 people with type 2 diabetes and matched control participants in Sweden. *Diabetologia* **2020**, *63*, 2582–2594. [CrossRef] [PubMed]
3. Poznyak, A.; Grechko, A.V.; Poggio, P.; Myasoedova, V.A.; Alfieri, V.; Orekhov, A.N. The Diabetes Mellitus–Atherosclerosis Connection: The Role of Lipid and Glucose Metabolism and Chronic Inflammation. *Int. J. Mol. Sci.* **2020**, *21*, 1835. [CrossRef] [PubMed]
4. Henning, R.J. Type-2 diabetes mellitus and cardiovascular disease. *Future Cardiol.* **2018**, *14*, 491–509. [CrossRef]
5. Gardner, D.G.; Shoback, D. *Greenspan's Basic & Clinical Endocrinology*, 10th ed.; McGrawHill: New York, NY, USA, 2018.
6. Low Wang, C.C.; Hess, C.N.; Hiatt, W.R.; Goldfine, A.B. Clinical Update: Cardiovascular Disease in Diabetes Mellitus: Atherosclerotic Cardiovascular Disease and Heart Failure in Type 2 Diabetes Mellitus—Mechanisms, Management, and Clinical Considerations. *Circulation* **2016**, *133*, 2459–2502. [CrossRef]
7. Faselis, C.; Katsimardou, A.; Imprialos, K.; Deligkaris, P.; Kallistratos, M.; Dimitriadis, K. Microvascular Complications of Type 2 Diabetes Mellitus. *Curr. Vasc. Pharmacol.* **2019**, *18*, 117–124. [CrossRef]
8. Kaur, R.; Kaur, M.; Singh, J. Endothelial dysfunction and platelet hyperactivity in type 2 diabetes mellitus: Molecular insights and therapeutic strategies. *Cardiovasc. Diabetol.* **2018**, *17*, 121. [CrossRef]
9. Vergès, B. Pathophysiology of diabetic dyslipidaemia: Where are we? *Diabetologia* **2015**, *58*, 886–899. [CrossRef]
10. Wang, J.; Stančáková, A.; Soininen, P.; Kangas, A.J.; Paananen, J.; Kuusisto, J.; Ala-Korpela, M.; Laakso, M. Lipoprotein Subclass Profiles in Individuals with Varying Degrees of Glucose Tolerance: A Population-Based Study of 9399 Finnish Men: Lipids and Glucose Tolerance. *J. Intern. Med.* **2012**, *272*, 562–572. [CrossRef]
11. Nogueira, J.P.; Maraninchi, M.; Béliard, S.; Padilla, N.; Duvillard, L.; Mancini, J.; Nicolay, A.; Xiao, C.; Vialettes, B.; Lewis, G.F.; et al. Absence of acute inhibitory effect of insulin on chylomicron production in type 2 diabetes. *Arterioscler. Thromb. Vasc. Biol.* **2012**, *32*, 1039–1044. [CrossRef]
12. Vergès, B. Intestinal lipid absorption and transport in type 2 diabetes. *Diabetologia* **2022**, *65*, 1587–1600. [CrossRef] [PubMed]
13. Taskinen, M.-R.; Nikkilä, E.A.; Kuusi, T.; Harno, K. Lipoprotein Lipase Activity and Serum Lipoproteins in Untreated Type 2 (Insulin-Independent) Diabetes Associated with Obesity. *Diabetologia* **1982**, *22*, 46–50. [CrossRef] [PubMed]
14. Adiels, M.; Taskinen, M.-R.; Packard, C.; Caslake, M.J.; Soro-Paavonen, A.; Westerbacka, J.; Vehkavaara, S.; Häkkinen, A.; Olofsson, S.-O.; Yki-Järvinen, H.; et al. Overproduction of Large VLDL Particles Is Driven by Increased Liver Fat Content in Man. *Diabetologia* **2006**, *49*, 755–765. [CrossRef] [PubMed]
15. Makita, T.; Tanaka, A.; Nakano, T.; Nakajima, K.; Numano, F. Importance of Glycation in the Acceleration of Low Density Lipoprotein (LDL) Uptake into Macrophages in Patients with Diabetes Mellitus. *Int. Angiol. J. Int. Union Angiol.* **1999**, *18*, 149–153.
16. Duvillard, L.; Pont, F.; Florentin, E.; Gambert, P.; Vergès, B. Inefficiency of Insulin Therapy to Correct Apolipoprotein A-I Metabolic Abnormalities in Non-Insulin-Dependent Diabetes Mellitus. *Atherosclerosis* **2000**, *152*, 229–237. [CrossRef] [PubMed]
17. Fisher, R. American Diabetes Association Releases 2023 Standards of Care in Diabetes to Guide Prevention, Diagnosis, and Treatment for People Living with Diabetes. *Diabetes Care* **2023**, *46*, 1715. [CrossRef]
18. Solano, M.P.; Goldberg, R.B. Lipid Management in Type 2 Diabetes. *Clin. Diabetes* **2006**, *24*, 27–33. [CrossRef]
19. Mach, F.; Baigent, C.; Catapano, A.L.; Koskinas, K.C.; Casula, M.; Badimon, L.; Chapman, M.J.; De Backer, G.G.; Delgado, V.; Ference, B.A.; et al. 2019 ESC/EAS Guidelines for the Management of Dyslipidaemias: Lipid Modification to Reduce Cardiovascular Risk. *Eur. Heart J.* **2020**, *41*, 111–188. [CrossRef]
20. Mancini, G.B.J.; Hegele, R.A.; Leiter, L.A. Dyslipidemia. *Can. J. Diabetes* **2018**, *42*, S178–S185. [CrossRef]
21. Cholesterol Treatment Trialists' (CTT) Collaborators. Efficacy of Cholesterol-Lowering Therapy in 18 686 People with Diabetes in 14 Randomised Trials of Statins: A Meta-Analysis. *Lancet* **2008**, *371*, 117–125. [CrossRef]

22. Colhoun, H.M.; Betteridge, D.J.; Durrington, P.N.; Hitman, G.A.; Neil, H.A.W.; Livingstone, S.J.; Thomason, M.J.; Mackness, M.I.; Charlton-Menys, V.; Fuller, J.H. Primary Prevention of Cardiovascular Disease with Atorvastatin in Type 2 Diabetes in the Collaborative Atorvastatin Diabetes Study (CARDS): Multicentre Randomised Placebo-Controlled Trial. *Lancet* **2004**, *364*, 685–696. [CrossRef] [PubMed]
23. Knopp, R.H.; d'Emden, M.; Smilde, J.G.; Pocock, S.J.; on behalf of the ASPEN Study Group. Efficacy and Safety of Atorvastatin in the Prevention of Cardiovascular End Points in Subjects with Type 2 Diabetes. *Diabetes Care* **2006**, *29*, 1478–1485. [CrossRef] [PubMed]
24. Ganda, O.P. Statin-Induced Diabetes: Incidence, Mechanisms, and Implications. *F1000Research* **2016**, *5*, 1499. [CrossRef] [PubMed]
25. Galicia-Garcia, U.; Jebari, S.; Larrea-Sebal, A.; Uribe, K.B.; Siddiqi, H.; Ostolaza, H.; Benito-Vicente, A.; Martín, C. Statin Treatment-Induced Development of Type 2 Diabetes: From Clinical Evidence to Mechanistic Insights. *Int. J. Mol. Sci.* **2020**, *21*, 4725. [CrossRef] [PubMed]
26. Abbasi, F.; Lamendola, C.; Harris, C.S.; Harris, V.; Tsai, M.-S.; Tripathi, P.; Abbas, F.; Reaven, G.M.; Reaven, P.D.; Snyder, M.P.; et al. Statins Are Associated with Increased Insulin Resistance and Secretion. *Arterioscler. Thromb. Vasc. Biol.* **2021**, *41*, 2786–2797. [CrossRef] [PubMed]
27. Davis, T.M.E.; Badshah, I.; Chubb, S.A.P.; Davis, W.A. Dose-Response Relationship between Statin Therapy and Glycaemia in Community-Based Patients with Type 2 Diabetes: The Fremantle Diabetes Study. *Diabetes Obes. Metab.* **2016**, *18*, 1143–1146. [CrossRef]
28. Merćep, I.; Strikić, D.; Slišković, A.M.; Reiner, Ž. New Therapeutic Approaches in Treatment of Dyslipidaemia—A Narrative Review. *Pharmaceuticals* **2022**, *15*, 839. [CrossRef]
29. Castellano, J.M.; Pocock, S.J.; Bhatt, D.L.; Quesada, A.J.; Owen, R.; Fernandez-Ortiz, A.; Sanchez, P.L.; Ortuño, F.M.; Rodriguez, J.M.V.; Domingo-Fernández, A.; et al. Polypill Strategy in Secondary Cardiovascular Prevention. *N. Engl. J. Med.* **2022**, *387*, 967–977. [CrossRef]
30. Pandor, A.; Ara, R.M.; Tumur, I.; Wilkinson, A.J.; Paisley, S.; Duenas, A.; Durrington, P.N.; Chilcott, J. Ezetimibe Monotherapy for Cholesterol Lowering in 2722 People: Systematic Review and Meta-Analysis of Randomized Controlled Trials. *J. Intern. Med.* **2009**, *265*, 568–580. [CrossRef]
31. Cannon, C.P.; Blazing, M.A.; Giugliano, R.P.; McCagg, A.; White, J.A.; Theroux, P.; Darius, H.; Lewis, B.S.; Ophuis, T.O.; Jukema, J.W.; et al. Ezetimibe Added to Statin Therapy after Acute Coronary Syndromes. *N. Engl. J. Med.* **2015**, *372*, 2387–2397. [CrossRef]
32. Giugliano, R.P.; Cannon, C.P.; Blazing, M.A.; Nicolau, J.C.; Corbalán, R.; Špinar, J.; Park, J.-G.; White, J.A.; Bohula, E.A.; Braunwald, E. Benefit of Adding Ezetimibe to Statin Therapy on Cardiovascular Outcomes and Safety in Patients with Versus without Diabetes Mellitus: Results from IMPROVE-IT (Improved Reduction of Outcomes: Vytorin Efficacy International Trial). *Circulation* **2018**, *137*, 1571–1582. [CrossRef] [PubMed]
33. Kosoglou, T.; Statkevich, P.; Johnson-Levonas, A.O.; Paolini, J.F.; Bergman, A.J.; Alton, K.B. Ezetimibe: A Review of Its Metabolism, Pharmacokinetics and Drug Interactions. *Clin. Pharmacokinet.* **2005**, *44*, 467–494. [CrossRef] [PubMed]
34. Sabatine, M.S.; Giugliano, R.P.; Keech, A.C.; Honarpour, N.; Wiviott, S.D.; Murphy, S.A.; Kuder, J.F.; Wang, H.; Liu, T.; Wasserman, S.M.; et al. Evolocumab and Clinical Outcomes in Patients with Cardiovascular Disease. *N. Engl. J. Med.* **2017**, *376*, 1713–1722. [CrossRef] [PubMed]
35. Ray, K.K.; Colhoun, H.M.; Szarek, M.; Baccara-Dinet, M.; Bhatt, D.L.; Bittner, V.A.; Budaj, A.J.; Diaz, R.; Goodman, S.G.; Hanotin, C.; et al. Effects of Alirocumab on Cardiovascular and Metabolic Outcomes after Acute Coronary Syndrome in Patients with or without Diabetes: A Prespecified Analysis of the ODYSSEY OUTCOMES Randomised Controlled Trial. *Lancet Diabetes Endocrinol.* **2019**, *7*, 618–628. [CrossRef] [PubMed]
36. Rana, K.; Reid, J.; Rosenwasser, J.N.; Lewis, T.; Sheikh-Ali, M.; Choksi, R.R.; Goldfaden, R.F. A Spotlight on Alirocumab in High Cardiovascular Risk Patients with Type 2 Diabetes and Mixed Dyslipidemia: A Review on the Emerging Data. *Diabetes Metab. Syndr. Obes. Targets Ther.* **2019**, *12*, 1897–1911. [CrossRef] [PubMed]
37. Carugo, S.; Sirtori, C.R.; Corsini, A.; Tokgozoglu, L.; Ruscica, M. PCSK9 Inhibition and Risk of Diabetes: Should We Worry? *Curr. Atheroscler. Rep.* **2022**, *24*, 995–1004. [CrossRef] [PubMed]
38. Memon, R.; Malek, R.; Munir, K.M. Doubling of Hemoglobin A1c on PCSK9 Inhibitor Therapy. *Am. J. Med.* **2019**, *132*, e17–e18. [CrossRef]
39. Civeira, F.; Pedro-Botet, J. Cost-Effectiveness Evaluation of the Use of PCSK9 Inhibitors. *Endocrinol. Diabetes Nutr. Engl. Ed.* **2021**, *68*, 369–371. [CrossRef]
40. Staels, B.; Dallongeville, J.; Auwerx, J.; Schoonjans, K.; Leitersdorf, E.; Fruchart, J.-C. Mechanism of Action of Fibrates on Lipid and Lipoprotein Metabolism. *Circulation* **1998**, *98*, 2088–2093. [CrossRef]
41. FIELD Study Investigators. Effects of Long-Term Fenofibrate Therapy on Cardiovascular Events in 9795 People with Type 2 Diabetes Mellitus (the FIELD Study): Randomised Controlled Trial. *Lancet* **2005**, *366*, 1849–1861. [CrossRef]
42. The ACCORD Study Group. Effects of Combination Lipid Therapy in Type 2 Diabetes Mellitus. *N. Engl. J. Med.* **2010**, *362*, 1563–1574. [CrossRef] [PubMed]
43. Willett, W.C. The Role of Dietary N-6 Fatty Acids in the Prevention of Cardiovascular Disease. *J. Cardiovasc. Med.* **2007**, *8* (Suppl. S1), S42–S45. [CrossRef] [PubMed]

44. Yokoyama, M.; Origasa, H.; Matsuzaki, M.; Matsuzawa, Y.; Saito, Y.; Ishikawa, Y.; Oikawa, S.; Sasaki, J.; Hishida, H.; Itakura, H.; et al. Effects of Eicosapentaenoic Acid on Major Coronary Events in Hypercholesterolaemic Patients (JELIS): A Randomised Open-Label, Blinded Endpoint Analysis. *Lancet* **2007**, *369*, 1090–1098. [CrossRef] [PubMed]
45. Bhatt, D.L.; Steg, P.G.; Miller, M.; Brinton, E.A.; Jacobson, T.A.; Ketchum, S.B.; Doyle, R.T., Jr.; Juliano, R.A.; Jiao, L.; Granowitz, C.; et al. Cardiovascular Risk Reduction with Icosapent Ethyl for Hypertriglyceridemia. *N. Engl. J. Med.* **2019**, *380*, 11–22. [CrossRef] [PubMed]
46. ASCEND Study Collaborative Group; Bowman, L.; Mafham, M.; Wallendszus, K.; Stevens, W.; Buck, G.; Barton, J.; Murphy, K.; Aung, T.; Haynes, R.; et al. Effects of Aspirin for Primary Prevention in Persons with Diabetes Mellitus. *N. Engl. J. Med.* **2018**, *379*, 1529–1539.
47. Backes, J.; Anzalone, D.; Hilleman, D.; Catini, J. The Clinical Relevance of Omega-3 Fatty Acids in the Management of Hypertriglyceridemia. *Lipids Health Dis.* **2016**, *15*, 118. [CrossRef]
48. Gonzalez, J.S.; Tanenbaum, M.L.; Commissariat, P.V. Psychosocial Factors in Medication Adherence and Diabetes Self-Management: Implications for Research and Practice. *Am. Psychol.* **2016**, *71*, 539–551. [CrossRef]
49. Arnett, D.K.; Blumenthal, R.S.; Albert, M.A.; Buroker, A.B.; Goldberger, Z.D.; Hahn, E.J.; Himmelfarb, C.D.; Khera, A.; Lloyd-Jones, D.; McEvoy, J.W.; et al. 2019 ACC/AHA Guideline on the Primary Prevention of Cardiovascular Disease. *J. Am. Coll. Cardiol.* **2019**, *74*, e177–e232. [CrossRef]
50. Löfvenborg, J.E.; Andersson, T.; Carlsson, P.-O.; Dorkhan, M.; Groop, L.; Martinell, M.; Tuomi, T.; Wolk, A.; Carlsson, S. Sweetened Beverage Intake and Risk of Latent Autoimmune Diabetes in Adults (LADA) and Type 2 Diabetes. *Eur. J. Endocrinol.* **2016**, *175*, 605–614. [CrossRef]
51. Boule, N.G.; Haddad, E.; Kenny, G.P.; Wells, G.A.; Sigal, R.J. Effects of Exercise on Glycemic Control and Body Mass in Type 2 Diabetes Mellitus: A Meta-Analysis of Controlled Clinical Trials: Sports Medicine Update. *Scand. J. Med. Sci. Sports* **2002**, *12*, 60–61. [CrossRef]
52. Couillard, C.; Després, J.-P.; Lamarche, B.; Bergeron, J.; Gagnon, J.; Leon, A.S.; Rao, D.C.; Skinner, J.S.; Wilmore, J.H.; Bouchard, C. Effects of Endurance Exercise Training on Plasma HDL Cholesterol Levels Depend on Levels of Triglycerides: Evidence From Men of the Health, Risk Factors, Exercise Training and Genetics (HERITAGE) Family Study. *Arterioscler. Thromb. Vasc. Biol.* **2001**, *21*, 1226–1232. [CrossRef] [PubMed]
53. Kraus, W.E.; Houmard, J.A.; Duscha, B.D.; Knetzger, K.J.; Wharton, M.B.; McCartney, J.S.; Bales, C.W.; Henes, S.; Samsa, G.P.; Otvos, J.D.; et al. Effects of the Amount and Intensity of Exercise on Plasma Lipoproteins. *N. Engl. J. Med.* **2002**, *347*, 1483–1492. [CrossRef] [PubMed]
54. Sarzynski, M.A.; Ruiz-Ramie, J.J.; Barber, J.L.; Slentz, C.A.; Apolzan, J.W.; McGarrah, R.W.; Harris, M.N.; Church, T.S.; Borja, M.S.; He, Y.; et al. Effects of Increasing Exercise Intensity and Dose on Multiple Measures of HDL (High-Density Lipoprotein) Function. *Arterioscler. Thromb. Vasc. Biol.* **2018**, *38*, 943–952. [CrossRef] [PubMed]
55. Roberts, C.K.; Ng, C.; Hama, S.; Eliseo, A.J.; Barnard, R.J. Effect of a Short-Term Diet and Exercise Intervention on Inflammatory/Anti-Inflammatory Properties of HDL in Overweight/Obese Men with Cardiovascular Risk Factors. *J. Appl. Physiol.* **2006**, *101*, 1727–1732. [CrossRef]
56. Zhou, C.; Wang, M.; Liang, J.; He, G.; Chen, N. Ketogenic Diet Benefits to Weight Loss, Glycemic Control, and Lipid Profiles in Overweight Patients with Type 2 Diabetes Mellitus: A Meta-Analysis of Randomized Controlled Trails. *Int. J. Environ. Res. Public. Health* **2022**, *19*, 10429. [CrossRef]
57. Leow, Z.Z.X.; Guelfi, K.J.; Davis, E.A.; Jones, T.W.; Fournier, P.A. The Glycaemic Benefits of a Very-Low-Carbohydrate Ketogenic Diet in Adults with Type 1 Diabetes Mellitus May Be Opposed by Increased Hypoglycaemia Risk and Dyslipidaemia. *Diabet. Med.* **2018**, *35*, 1258–1263. [CrossRef]
58. Elhayany, A.; Lustman, A.; Abel, R.; Attal-Singer, J.; Vinker, S. A Low Carbohydrate Mediterranean Diet Improves Cardiovascular Risk Factors and Diabetes Control among Overweight Patients with Type 2 Diabetes Mellitus: A 1-Year Prospective Randomized Intervention Study. *Diabetes Obes. Metab.* **2010**, *12*, 204–209. [CrossRef]
59. Mazzocchi, A.; Leone, L.; Agostoni, C.; Pali-Schöll, I. The Secrets of the Mediterranean Diet. Does [Only] Olive Oil Matter? *Nutrients* **2019**, *11*, 2941. [CrossRef]
60. Covas, M.-I.; Nyyssönen, K.; Poulsen, H.E.; Kaikkonen, J.; Zunft, H.-J.F.; Kiesewetter, H.; Gaddi, A.; de la Torre, R.; Mursu, J.; Bäumler, H.; et al. The Effect of Polyphenols in Olive Oil on Heart Disease Risk Factors. *Ann. Intern. Med.* **2006**, *145*, 333–341. [CrossRef]
61. Torres-Peña, J.D.; Garcia-Rios, A.; Delgado-Casado, N.; Gomez-Luna, P.; Alcala-Diaz, J.F.; Yubero-Serrano, E.M.; Gomez-Delgado, F.; Leon-Acuña, A.; Lopez-Moreno, J.; Camargo, A.; et al. Mediterranean Diet Improves Endothelial Function in Patients with Diabetes and Prediabetes: A Report from the CORDIOPREV Study. *Atherosclerosis* **2018**, *269*, 50–56. [CrossRef]
62. Companys, J.; Pla-Pagà, L.; Calderón-Pérez, L.; Llauradó, E.; Solà, R.; Pedret, A.; Valls, R.M. Fermented Dairy Products, Probiotic Supplementation, and Cardiometabolic Diseases: A Systematic Review and Meta-analysis. *Adv. Nutr.* **2020**, *11*, 834–863. [CrossRef] [PubMed]
63. Cho, Y.A.; Kim, J. Effect of Probiotics on Blood Lipid Concentrations: A Meta-Analysis of Randomized Controlled Trials. *Medicine* **2015**, *94*, e1714. [CrossRef] [PubMed]

64. Moroti, C.; Souza Magri, L.F.; de Rezende Costa, M.; Cavallini, D.C.; Sivieri, K. Effect of the consumption of a new symbiotic shake on glycemia and cholesterol levels in elderly people with type 2 diabetes mellitus. *Lipids Health Dis.* **2012**, *11*, 29. [CrossRef] [PubMed]
65. Yang, R.; Shang, J.; Zhou, Y.; Liu, W.; Tian, Y.; Shang, H. Effects of probiotics on nonalcoholic fatty liver disease: A systematic review and meta-analysis. *Expert. Rev. Gastroenterol. Hepatol.* **2021**, *15*, 1401–1409. [CrossRef]
66. Spooner, H.C.; Derrick, S.A.; Maj, M.; Manjarín, R.; Hernandez, G.V.; Tailor, D.S.; Bastani, P.S.; Fanter, R.K.; Fiorotto, M.L.; Burrin, D.G.; et al. High-Fructose, High-Fat Diet Alters Muscle Composition and Fuel Utilization in a Juvenile Iberian Pig Model of Non-Alcoholic Fatty Liver Disease. *Nutrients* **2021**, *13*, 4195. [CrossRef]
67. Sikalidis, A.K.; Maykish, A. The Gut Microbiome and Type 2 Diabetes Mellitus: Discussing a Complex Relationship. *Biomedicines* **2020**, *8*, 8. [CrossRef]

Disclaimer/Publisher's Note: The statements, opinions and data contained in all publications are solely those of the individual author(s) and contributor(s) and not of MDPI and/or the editor(s). MDPI and/or the editor(s) disclaim responsibility for any injury to people or property resulting from any ideas, methods, instructions or products referred to in the content.

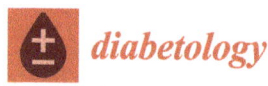

Review

Prevention of Type 2 Diabetes: The Role of Intermittent Fasting

Bright Test and Jay H. Shubrook *

Department of Clinical Sciences and Community Health, College of Osteopathic Medicine, Touro University California, Vallejo, CA 94592, USA; btest@student.touro.edu
* Correspondence: jshubroo@touro.edu

Abstract: Despite the progress in treatment options and improved understanding of pathophysiology, type 2 diabetes remains one of the costliest and most harmful global chronic diseases. The current guidelines encourage physicians to fight an uphill battle and react to an incubated disease state that has been propelled forward by clinical inertia. The authors completed a literature search of PubMed, ScienceDirect, and NIH, searching with the terms intermittent fasting, type 2 diabetes, and prediabetes, and excluded studies related to religion-based fasting. There is emerging evidence that intermittent fasting could be an option to aid in weight loss, reduce hepatic steatosis, and lower the level of biomarkers such as fasting glucose while improving insulin resistance. If incorporated into the lives of patients with risk factors for type 2 diabetes, intermittent fasting could prove to be a cost-effective and efficient tool for preventing this insidious disease. This clinical review examines current evidence supporting the implementation of this lifestyle to prevent the onset or exacerbation of type 2 diabetes and the hurdles that must still be overcome for physicians to confidently prescribe this to their patients.

Keywords: diabetes; intermittent fasting; prevention

Citation: Test, B.; Shubrook, J.H. Prevention of Type 2 Diabetes: The Role of Intermittent Fasting. *Diabetology* **2023**, *4*, 507–518. https://doi.org/10.3390/diabetology4040044

Academic Editors: Andrej Belančić, Sanja Klobučar and Dario Rahelić

Received: 26 September 2023
Revised: 12 October 2023
Accepted: 1 November 2023
Published: 13 November 2023

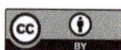

Copyright: © 2023 by the authors. Licensee MDPI, Basel, Switzerland. This article is an open access article distributed under the terms and conditions of the Creative Commons Attribution (CC BY) license (https://creativecommons.org/licenses/by/4.0/).

1. Introduction

1.1. Intermittent Fasting

Intermittent fasting (IF) is a popular dieting strategy that has been implemented by many to lose weight, but uncertainty remains as to whether this lifestyle change could be beneficial in the prevention of multiple metabolic disorders, including type 2 diabetes mellitus (T2DM). It is well understood that human evolution, on a biological level, lags behind rapid sociological and technological advancement. In other words, the same physical bodies our hunter–gatherer ancestors used to survive prolonged periods of fasting have not evolved to accommodate a lifestyle of working sedentary desk jobs 8 h a day with all kinds of processed foods readily available for snacking. The theory of IF is rooted in this evolutionary science and is reinforced by the biochemical processes in our bodies. When fasting, glycogenolysis activates in the short term to mobilize the glycogen stores from meals prior. After about 12 h, the stores are depleted, and the body finds energy through other metabolic pathways such as gluconeogenesis, lipolysis, and beta-oxidation (β-oxidation). As the fat stores are burned for fuel, there is a subsequent loss of weight and a decreased percentage of body fat. Alternating periods of fasting with periods of eating prevents total starvation and allows the body to function properly while still taking advantage of the above benefits. This aesthetic benefit has been one of the main incentives for people to adopt IF into their lives, but there are many more benefits to following this lifestyle than meets the eye.

Intermittent Fasting Schedules

There are different intermittent fasting schedules (Table 1). The most common one is the daily time-restricted variant (16:8), which involves fasting for about 16 h in a 24 h period [1]. During the 8 h feeding window, an individual can eat ad libitum with or without whatever restrictions they deem fit with help from their doctor. This plan allows for much flexibility but may require a motivated attitude for long-term adherence. Due to the inherent flexibility and multitude of variables involved with this regimen, there is significant variation in its results and outcomes. The nutritional quality of the food consumed during the feasting window most likely also affects the outcomes.

Table 1. Description of common IF schedules. The varying schedules of IF may be modified based on the individual's needs and capabilities.

Schedule	Description	Possible Modifications
Daily (16:8)	All days of the week involve a 16 h fasting period of zero calories, followed by an 8 h window of ad libitum eating.	Certain dietary restrictions can be added to modify results, or the fasting period may be increased to 18 h.
Alternate-day (4:3)	Fasting is carried out every other day for a 24 h period and alternates with days of ad libitum eating.	The fasting days typically involve a 25% caloric intake compared to normal, but this can be decreased to complete zero-calorie fasting.
Whole-day (5:2)	Zero-calorie fasting is completed for two days out of the week, usually in between a few days of ad libitum eating.	While zero-calorie fasting is the standard, a modified decrease in caloric intake, such as 25% of normal, may be implemented based on individual capabilities.

IF versus other dietary plans.

Other notable intermittent fasting schedules include the alternate-day (4:3) and whole-day (5:2) schedules. The 4:3 schedule involves 4 days of ad libitum eating with 3 days of complete zero-calorie fasting or a modified 25% typical caloric intake fasting interwoven weekly. The 5:2 schedule consists of 5 days of ad libitum eating with 2 days of complete, zero-calorie, intermittently paced fasting throughout the week. In a systematic review, these two schedules were compared for improving body composition and clinical markers for disease. Alternate-day fasting trials of 3 to 12 weeks in duration appear to be effective at reducing body weight, body fat, total cholesterol, and triglycerides in normal-weight, overweight, and obese humans as compared to whole-day fasting trials lasting 12 to 24 weeks, which also reduce body weight and body fat and favorably improve blood lipids [2].

Intermittent fasting has been compared to continuous energy restriction (CER) for weight loss and related benefits. While intermittent fasting appears to produce similar effects to continuous energy restriction in reducing body weight, fat mass, fat-free mass and appetite and improving glucose homeostasis, it does not appear to improve weight loss efficiency [3]. However, a systematic review analyzing 11 comparative studies concluded that there was a significant difference in the change in body weight that favored IF over continuous caloric restriction [4]. A different 12-month trial examining insulin-resistant individuals compared the effects of modified 4:3 IF with 25% caloric intake versus daily 75% caloric intake (CR) compared to a control [5]. The research found that in this population, the weight loss was not different between the IF ($-8\% \pm 2\%$) and CR ($-6\% \pm 1\%$) groups by month 12 relative to the controls ($p < 0.0001$), and the fat mass and BMI decreased ($p < 0.05$) similarly for the IF and CR. However, IF produced greater decreases ($p < 0.05$) in fasting insulin ($-52\% \pm 9\%$) and insulin resistance ($-53\% \pm 9\%$) compared with CR ($-14\% \pm 9\%$; $-17\% \pm 11\%$) and the controls by month 12 [5]. Research has shown that IF boosts verbal memory, improves blood pressure and resting heart rate, and can help obese adults lose weight [1]. As for patients with T2DM, most of the available research shows that IF can help people lose body weight and decrease their levels of fasting glucose, insulin, and leptin, all while reducing insulin resistance and increasing levels of adiponectin [1,6,7].

1.2. Fasting for the Future

There have been studies showing the benefits of IF on animal models. In animal models, intermittent feeding improves insulin sensitivity, counters obesity caused by a high-fat diet, and ameliorates diabetic retinopathy [8].

Metabolic syndrome (MS) has been strongly linked to diabetes. Rodent studies have shown the potential for MS reversal when subjects followed a 4:3 IF schedule. Subjects experienced reductions in abdominal fat, inflammation, and blood pressure as well as an increase in insulin sensitivity and improvement in cardiovascular system functionality [9,10]. Some medications, such as metformin, show similar benefits in animal models from alternate-day IF by challenging the metabolism to switch. However, the available data from animal models suggest that the safety and efficacy of such pharmacological approaches are likely to be inferior to naturally induced metabolism switching caused by intermittent fasting [6]. In a study where mice were kept on the 4:3 IF schedule vs. ad libitum feeding, the IF group on average had significantly lower serum glucose concentrations and insulin levels compared to the control group [11].

The mice on the IF diet also exhibited a two-fold increase in the fasting serum concentration of β-hydroxybutyrate compared with mice fed ad libitum, which aligns with the knowledge that fasting raises the concentration of ketone bodies in the blood due to lipolysis. This increase in blood ketones could offer some neuroprotection as well as the added benefit of resistance to epileptic seizures [12–14]. Further, there are multiple studies examining the effects of IF on the aging process of rodents, with some showing increased lifespans by as much as 80% compared to ad libitum feeding [15–18]. The evidence for the effects of time-restricted daily 16:8 IF in human models remains relatively scarce. This narrative review will delve into the available literature and attempt to illuminate the usefulness of implementing IF alongside established drug and surgical therapies for the prevention of T2DM.

1.3. At the Core of Prediabetes and Type 2 Diabetes

1.3.1. Visceral Fat

Ongoing research has elucidated the complex pathophysiology of T2DM, from the Triumvirate to the Ominous Octet [19] to the Egregious Eleven [20]. What seems to be of the greatest clinical interest currently is the relationship between visceral fat buildup and the progression of T2DM. In patients with established type 2 diabetes, visceral fat accumulation has a significant negative effect on glycemic control through a decrease in peripheral insulin sensitivity and an enhancement of gluconeogenesis [21]. The exact mechanism of this was not investigated in this study, but correlations were seen: insulin-mediated glucose clearance was inversely related to visceral fat levels in a nonlinear fashion, and this relationship remained weakly significant after adjusting for BMI (partial $r = 0.33$; $p = 0.01$) [21]. To examine whether visceral fat contributed to enhanced gluconeogenesis, the percent gluconeogenesis was regressed against visceral fat levels, first purely and then after adjustment for confounders. In both models, the association between percent gluconeogenesis and visceral fat was positive ($r = 0.28$; $p < 0.03$ and partial $r = 0.30$; $p = 0.04$, respectively). When gluconeogenesis fluxes were calculated, they were more strongly associated with visceral fat in a direct fashion (partial $r = 0.45$; $p = 0.003$) [21]. Screening for visceral fat levels while implementing feasible exercise regimens and healthier eating habits early could be the key in keeping T2DM at bay.

1.3.2. Hepatic Steatosis

Hepatic steatosis has also been linked to the progression of prediabetes (higher likelihood of impaired fasting glucose (IFG) and impaired glucose tolerance (IGT) or both) [22]. It has been established that a fatty liver has increased hepatic glucose production due to impaired insulin signaling [23]. In this study, the adjusted liver fat metric was significantly correlated with prediabetes progression since, most notably, insulin sensitivity was inversely correlated (r = −0.44, p < 0.0001) and sensitivity decreased from the normal glucose tolerance (NGT) group to the IFG+IGT group [22]. Individuals with IGT or IFG + IGT more often had a fatty liver than individuals with NGT or isolated IFG [22]. Screening for levels of hepatic steatosis could be another useful tool for patients who have a risk of developing T2DM.

Intermittent fasting has demonstrated beneficial effects on hepatic steatosis. Using MRI technology and the 5:2 IF schedule, a small study was conducted with participants with prediabetes evaluating probiotics during a 12-week IF program. The results showed that, after 12 weeks of intermittent fasting, subcutaneous fat (%) changed from 35.9 ± 3.1 to 34.4 ± 3.2, visceral fat (%) changed from 15.8 ± 1.3 to 14.8 ± 1.2, liver fat (%) changed from 8.7 ± 0.8 to 7.5 ± 0.7, and pancreatic fat (%) changed from 7.7 ± 0.5 to 6.5 ± 0.5 (all p < 0.001) [24]. In mice, despite being fed a high-fat or a high-fructose diet for 8 weeks, alternate-day IF for 4 weeks was effective in decreasing hepatic lipogenesis and increasing β-oxidation markers, resulting in a reduction in hepatic steatosis and inflammation [25]. In a proteomic analysis involving rats undergoing a modified daily IF schedule of 18:6 (time-restricted feeding between 1600 and 2200) for 15 weeks, the results showed that, compared with the comparison group that consumed a 60% high-fat diet ad libitum, the expression of *PPARα* (a transcription factor that is the primary regulator of liver β-oxidation) in the 6 h IF group on the same diet was significantly increased, and the lipid synthesis gene *FAS* was decreased [26]. This means that these IF rats experienced more breakdown of liver fat and stored less liver fat compared to the ad libitum group. In a human study, adults with obesity and non-alcoholic fatty liver disease (NAFLD) were randomized between four groups for 3 months: 4:3 IF with 25% caloric intake only (fasting group), 4:3 IF with 60 min of aerobic exercise five times a week (combo group), exercise-only group, and no-intervention control group [27]. This randomized controlled trial found that by month 3, the intrahepatic triglyceride content was significantly reduced in the combo group (−5.48%; 95% CI, −7.77% to −3.18%) compared with the exercise group (−1.30%; 95% CI, −3.80% to 1.20%; p = 0.02) and the control group (−0.17%; 95% CI, −2.17% to 1.83%; p < 0.01) but was not significantly different compared to the fasting group (−2.25%; 95% CI, −4.46% to −0.04%; p = 0.05) [27]. Also, body weight, fat mass, waist circumference, and alanine transaminase levels significantly decreased, while insulin sensitivity significantly increased in the combination group compared with the control group [27]. These studies alone highlight the importance of lifestyle changes in combating hepatic steatosis and allude to the effectiveness of intermittent fasting as an option.

Preventing visceral adiposity and liver fat accumulation could slow or prevent the onset of T2DM, relieving both the health burden as well as a significant economic burden. In the U.S. healthcare system, one out every four dollars is spent on caring for people with diabetes. And 48% to 64% of lifetime medical costs for a person with diabetes are for disease-related complications [28]. By the time someone is diagnosed with T2DM and intervention is initiated, it is already very difficult to effectively treat the disease. Maintaining a healthy and non-sedentary lifestyle proves to be the best deterrent and can be reinforced with proper patient education [29].

2. The Role of Intermittent Fasting in Combating Type 2 Diabetes Mellitus

2.1. What Is at Stake?

Diabetes has become a non-communicable pandemic. An estimated total of 37.3 million people (11.3%) in the United States have diabetes [30]. There are 96 million people (38%) who live with prediabetes at an estimated rate of progression of 1.5 million people per year [30]. The costs associated with treating this disease through classical methods are enough to prioritize treatment and prevention through affordable and straightforward interventions such as IF. According to the American Diabetes Association (ADA), the total estimated cost of diagnosed diabetes in 2017 was USD 327 billion, including USD 237 billion in direct medical costs and USD 90 billion in reduced productivity at work [31]. Understanding and effectively implementing IF into the lifestyles of at-risk patients for diabetes may prove to be beneficial before medication and insulin interventions become involved.

2.2. The Effects of Intermittent Fasting on HbA1c Levels

The INTERFAST-2 trial demonstrated safety and efficacy in reducing the total daily insulin dose and body weight in insulin-treated people with T2DM [32]. Forty-six participants were randomly assigned between a 4:3 schedule IF group and a control group for 12 weeks. The IF group spent significantly less time on average above the blood glucose range compared to the control group, significantly more time on average within this range, and a similar amount of time on average below this range as compared to the control group. There was also a significant difference between the groups for the endpoint measurements set by the trial investigators. An HbA1c reduction ≥ 3 mmol/mol was seen in 60% of the IF group compared to 25% in the control group ($p < 0.05$). An insulin dose reduction $\geq 10\%$ was seen in 75% of the IF group compared to 0% in the control group ($p < 0.001$). A weight reduction $\geq 2\%$ was seen in 80% of the IF group compared to 4% in the control group ($p < 0.001$). And all three endpoints combined were achieved by 40% of the IF group versus 0% in the control group ($p < 0.001$) [32]. While this study observed the treatment of people with T2DM, the positive benefits may be extrapolated to diabetes prevention as well. Lifestyle modification with an intermittent fasting protocol and proper diet help lower blood glucose levels, maintain body mass index, and reduce inflammation, which is the main cause of chronic diseases among the general population [33].

Intermittent fasting using a 16:8 schedule with a 25% energy restriction has shown similar results in lowering fasting glucose, insulin, and HbA1c compared to a 25% continuous energy restriction [34]. In a trial of patients with T2DM and an average HbA1c of 7.3%, a modified 5:2 IF schedule with two fasting days having a 25% calorie intake was not significantly different from CER [35]. The IF group lowered their mean HbA1c by 0.3%, while the CER group's mean was lower by 0.5% [35]. Obesity is widely known to be the most significant modifiable risk factor for developing T2DM. Calorie-restrictive regiments such as IF have been shown time and time again to help decrease weight and BMI fat mass. In an observational analysis of participants in the Look AHEAD trial, those who lost 5–10% of their body weight had 3.5:1 increased odds of decreasing HbA1c levels by 0.5% as well as seeing beneficial reductions in other metabolic markers [36]. Due to the scarcity of randomized human trials and variations in fasting schedules, there remains ambiguity about the true relationship between IF and levels of HbA1c; however, there does seem to be a positive correlation that must be explored more with long-term studies.

2.3. From Healthy to Prediabetes to Type 2 Diabetes Mellitus

Preventing the crossover from healthy to prediabetes to T2DM is difficult for many reasons, one of which is the need for consistent and accurate monitoring. This may be difficult to achieve. When should one begin monitoring for metabolic changes? When should one implement an IF schedule if they are concerned about developing T2DM? The exact beginning of elevated biomarkers is difficult to trace and varies greatly, as illuminated by the variable data from studies. As many as 183 million people globally are unaware that they have T2DM [37], and it can be present for up to 12 years in some cases before being diagnosed [38]. If a patient has a relevant family history, it is important to educate and empower them as early as possible since T2DM has a strong genetic component [39]. Despite this, genetic testing is still not clinically useful due to reasons such as the low discriminative ability of genetic testing and the non-significant added value of observable clinical risk factors [40]. The sooner the individual is made aware of these risk factors, the sooner they can begin adopting important lifestyle modifications such as IF to prevent progression from prediabetes to type 2 diabetes.

Both IFG and IGT can be used to measure and predict progression from prediabetes to T2DM. However, because IGT is more prevalent than IFG in most populations, consistently conducting 2 h oral glucose tolerance tests (OGTT) to identify those with IGT often yields a greater proportion of people at risk for developing T2DM than simply looking at fasting plasma glucose (FPG) [41]. This is not a common first-line screening tool due to its cost and inconvenience compared to other initial analyses [42]. Prediabetes and T2DM have insidious onsets that begin to develop many years before they are diagnosed in a clinic. The exact onset varies across individuals and populations. A large retrospective analysis concluded that significantly elevated FPG can be seen 10 years ahead of a diagnosis with T2DM, and glucose dysregulation could precede a diagnosis by 20 years [43]. This inherent variability between individuals makes timely assessment and response difficult. Hopefully, though, these challenges will be resolved in the future with the development of new medical technologies in this sphere.

2.4. Current Alternative Therapies for the Prevention of Type 2 Diabetes Mellitus

It is now common knowledge that moderate weight loss, an active exercise routine, and a healthy whole food diet are all positive lifestyle changes that can aid in the prevention of T2DM [44]. There are also pharmacological interventions available for high-risk populations, such as those with IFG and IGT, that can be used in conjunction with lifestyle modifications. Metformin is the most commonly used medication in the treatment of T2DM, but it may prove useful as a method of prevention too. In the Diabetes Prevention Program (DPP) trial, 1073 participants with IGT were administered 850 mg of metformin twice a day, and 1082 participants were administered a placebo. Both groups were followed up for a median period of 2.8 years, which showed in the end that metformin reduced the incidence of T2DM by 31% compared with a placebo [45]. Some of the active participants followed up 10 years later when it was determined that T2DM incidence was still reduced more with metformin (18% compared to the placebo) [46]. The relative risk reduction (RRR) and number needed to treat (NNT) are compared to other studies examining lifestyle interventions (Table 2). In a Finnish study, 523 overweight subjects received seven sessions of nutritional and activity guidance, followed by visits every three months thereafter to help in reducing weight [47]. Weight loss and blood glucose levels were significantly improved in the intervention group and were maintained during a 3-year median follow-up period [47,48]. In a Da Qing study, 577 participants were distributed into a control group and three different intervention groups: diet, exercise, or combined [49]. Compared with the control group, those in the combined lifestyle intervention groups had a 51% lower incidence of diabetes (95% CI 0.33–0.73) during the active intervention period and a 43% lower incidence (0.41–0.81) over the 20-year period after the follow-up in 2006, controlled for age and clustering [49].

Table 2. Randomized controlled trials for lifestyle interventions for the prevention of type 2 diabetes.

Study	Country	N	Baseline BMI (kg/m^2)	Intervention Period (Years)	RRR (%)	NNT
Diabetes Prevention Program [45]	USA	3234	34.0	2.8	58	21
Diabetes Prevention Study [47,48]	Finland	523	31.0	4	39	22
Da Qing [49]	China	577	25.8	6	51	30

References. DPP Research Group. N Engl J Med. 2002, 346, 393–403 [44]. Eriksson, J.; et al. Diabetologia. 1999, 42, 793–801 [45]. Lindstrom, J.; et al. Lancet. 2006, 368, 1673–1679 [46]. Li, G.; et al. Lancet. 2008, 371, 1783–1789 [47].

Other pharmacologic agents, such as alpha glucosidase inhibitors and thiazolidinediones, have also proven to be effective in the delay of or prevention of T2DM. The STOP-NIDDM trial randomly assigned individuals with IGT to thrice daily 100 mg acarbose for a mean period of 3.3 years and demonstrated a 35.8% relative reduction in T2DM when compared to a placebo [50]. Treatment with troglitazone in the TRIPOD study delayed or prevented the onset of T2DM, wherein the protective effect was associated with the preservation of pancreatic beta-cell function [51]. The DREAM trial recruited 5269 patients with IFG, IGT, or both. The results revealed that rosiglitazone was very effective in lowering the incidence of T2DM, (60% compared to the placebo) [52]. A later study included 207 patients with IGT who received a combination of 2 mg rosiglitazone and 500 mg metformin twice daily for a median period of 3.9 years. This low-dose combination therapy was highly effective in the prevention of T2DM, with a low incidence of clinically relevant adverse effects [53].

There are many options currently available for the prevention and treatment of T2DM. The lipase inhibitor orlistat was utilized in a randomized study. When compared to lifestyle changes alone, orlistat plus these changes resulted in a 37.3% reduction in the risk of developing T2DM in patients with obesity over the course of four years [54]. The bile acid sequestrant colesevelam has been shown to improve insulin sensitivity and β-cell function similarly in subjects with IFG and T2DM, which led to a follow-up study illustrating the positive effects of this drug in patients with prediabetes by significantly reducing A1c levels and normalizing FPG compared to a placebo [55,56].

DPP-4 inhibitors and GLP-1 receptor agonists are versatile medications implemented to combat diabetes but could also be used in prediabetes stages. Vidagliptin was compared to a placebo in 179 subjects with IGT, and the participants saw a 32% reduction in postprandial glucose [57]. There are strong studies with GLP-1RA that could be added to this discussion. Human studies using exenatide or liraglutide have demonstrated significantly substantial weight loss and glucose tolerance improvement in patients with IFG or IGT, with benefits very apparent by about 20 weeks and, in the case of liraglutide, lasting for as long as 2 years [58,59].

Although it is not a common first-line method of prevention or treatment, metabolic surgery is another tool used to prevent type 2 diabetes among those at risk. Metabolic (bariatric) surgery is an effective and cost-effective therapy for people with T2DM and obesity. With an acceptable safety profile, it provides an appropriate treatment for people who struggle with achieving treatment goals through medication and lifestyle modifications alone [60]. Patients who undergo bariatric surgery tend to see significant improvements in A1c levels and a reduction in the number of their medications and insulin doses [61]. These findings could possibly extend to those with obesity and prediabetes. Compared to standard typical care, metabolic surgery reduces the long-term incidence of T2DM by 78% in obese individuals and by 87% in individuals with IFG [62]. This intervention is usually reserved for individuals struggling with morbid obesity, and it is unclear if the benefits seen from this surgery are merely due to the weight loss accompanied by it. Regardless, this modality is the least likely to be used in the prevention of T2DM, mainly due to the cost and risks associated with surgical procedures.

3. The Challenges to Overcome

3.1. Catching It Early

As mentioned previously, T2DM is a disease with an insidious onset, which makes early detection and intervention tremendously important. It is better to prevent the onset of a disease than to treat an ongoing one, especially when the excess lifetime medical expense is roughly USD 124,600 per person diagnosed with T2DM at the age of 40 [63]. The American Diabetes Association recommends beginning screening for diabetes in adults aged 45 years or older and then following up once every 3 years if the results are normal, with screening beginning earlier in overweight adults with one or more risk factors [64]. Compared with the ADA recommendations, the USPSTF recommendation is broader because it sets a minimum age of 35 years for screening and does not require any additional risk factors other than an elevated BMI [65]. There is a case to be made for beginning screening earlier as a US-population-based analysis found that screening for type 2 diabetes is cost-effective when started between the ages of 30 years and 45 years, with screening repeated every 3–5 years [66]. There are no established criteria for screening in healthy adults without risk factors, although visceral adiposity and hepatic steatosis could already be building up inside unaware individuals. This is where lifestyle modification, education on self-management, and patient empowerment become so crucial [67].

There are many biochemical tests conducted to monitor disease progression and diagnose T2DM. The "gold standard" is the 2 h OGTT, but it requires an 8 h fasting period beforehand and a time commitment from nursing staff that is not readily convenient, along with other limitations [68]. It is an accurate test for measuring 2 h post-prandial glucose (2hPG) and IGT, which may be a better predictor of outcomes than FPG or HbA1c. A multicenter study demonstrated that 2hPG is an independent predictor of diabetes and a novel risk assessment for cardiovascular disease, and mortality was better in this case than with FPG and HbA1c [69]. Developing a more streamlined version of the OGTT with fewer limitations could allow it to become a more common first-line monitoring tool in clinics. Combining FPG and HbA1c testing may be an optimal approach to identifying prediabetes and T2DM in clinics, but it is not used very often this way. Using both simultaneously could be more effective than choosing one over the other for initial screening. A community-based study showcased support for the clinical utility of using a combination of FPG and HbA1c levels from a single blood sample to identify undiagnosed T2DM in a population, as a high positive predictive value was seen for subsequent diagnoses of diabetes [70].

3.2. Implementing and Adhering to Intermittent Fasting

Implementing consistent and long-term lifestyle changes is a difficult task, and intermittent fasting is no exception. Helping patients go through these changes through strong motivation and support is one of the intrinsic responsibilities of a clinician. The authors provide some best practice suggestions for helping patients with therapeutic lifestyle changes (Figure 1). It is already evident that adherence to calorie-restriction diets tends to decline over time, perhaps because patients lose motivation or feel like they have reached a good point to stop [71]. A study examining the effects of four popular diets showed that, regardless of diet, about 25% of the participants adhered to a self-reported level of six out of ten by the end of the 1-year period, with adherence levels declining steadily over the 12 months [72]. On average, weight regain post-diet initiation begins about 6–9 months into the program, reflecting temporal decreases in adherence to the relevant prescribed regimen [73]. Key factors that promote adherence to IF include, but are not limited to, improvements in physical health, positive psychological impacts, and strong social support [74]. Some barriers to adherence include feelings of hunger and sluggishness, difficulties with self-monitoring, and social situations that discourage fasting schedules [74]. Most studies specifically target populations that struggle with obesity in observation of the weight-loss benefits, but other populations may see benefits as well. Although patients with certain health conditions should avoid IF, it has been linked to improving other metabolic ailments, such as dyslipidemia and hypertension [75]. Regardless, the data on the long-term effects of intermittent fasting remain very limited.

The absence of large long-term studies on the direct relationship between IF and its effects for people with T2DM is also a challenge to overcome. Most currently available published research articles, systematic reviews excluded, do not contain sample sizes in the thousands. It would be helpful to have larger sample sizes in future studies to draw more robust conclusions. Although there is a large study in progress at this time of writing known as DRIFT [71], more randomized human trials are needed.

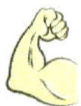

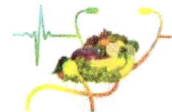

Celebrate and Reinforce Positive Behavior
Key facilitators as to why individuals adhere to IF include but are not limited to; improvements in physical health, positive psychological impacts, and strong social support.

Support Patient During Struggles
Some barriers to adherence include; feelings of hunger and sluggishness, difficulties with self-monitoring, and social situations that discourage the fasting schedule.

Adjust Meds and Lifestyle Changes Accordingly
Being flexible with medication dosing and fasting schedules as well as working together with the patient's needs and goals can help achieve long-term success with results that reduce overall cost and improve patient wellbeing.

Figure 1. An example of implementing IF into the lives of patients. This represents a generalized strategy that may be modified to fit the situation.

4. Conclusions

Intermittent fasting is a popular lifestyle dietary plan that may prove to be a useful and cost-effective tool in preventing T2DM. Currently, the most pronounced results of integrating IF occur in the population of people struggling with obesity. While IF is generally a safe plan to follow, it should be avoided by individuals who require a higher caloric diet, such as children and women who are pregnant or breastfeeding, and by those who are susceptible to eating disorders like bulimia nervosa. People with type 1 diabetes who require insulin should also avoid IF, as prolonged episodes of hypoglycemia may occur. Although animal models and short-term human trials have demonstrated the positive effects of IF, more research involving long-term multi-year timelines must be conducted to examine the chronic metabolic changes associated with IF. With more established and long-term evidence, physicians can gain confidence and may be more likely to recommend IF to their patients. IF is easily assessable and affordable compared to other interventions. Since T2DM is a chronic condition, it requires a chronic prophylactic and cure, and future studies involving IF might demonstrate it to practically and effectively function as both.

Author Contributions: Conceptualization, B.T. and J.H.S.; methodology, B.T. and J.H.S.; software, B.T. and J.H.S.; validation, B.T. and J.H.S.; formal analysis, B.T. and J.H.S.; investigation, B.T. and J.H.S.; resources, B.T. and J.H.S.; data curation, B.T. and J.H.S.; writing—original draft preparation, B.T.; writing—review and editing, J.H.S.; visualization, B.T.; supervision, J.H.S.; project administration, J.H.S. All authors have read and agreed to the published version of the manuscript.

Funding: This research received no external funding.

Data Availability Statement: Not applicable.

Conflicts of Interest: The authors declare no conflict of interest.

References

1. Intermittent Fasting: What Is It, and How Does It Work? Available online: https://www.hopkinsmedicine.org/health/wellness-and-prevention/intermittent-fasting-what-is-it-and-how-does-it-work (accessed on 14 June 2023).
2. Tinsley, G.M.; La Bounty, P.M. Effects of Intermittent Fasting on Body Composition and Clinical Health Markers in Humans. *Nutr. Rev.* **2015**, *73*, 661–674. [CrossRef] [PubMed]
3. Seimon, R.V.; Roekenes, J.A.; Zibellini, J.; Zhu, B.; Gibson, A.A.; Hills, A.P.; Wood, R.E.; King, N.A.; Byrne, N.M.; Sainsbury, A. Do Intermittent Diets Provide Physiological Benefits over Continuous Diets for Weight Loss? A Systematic Review of Clinical Trials. *Mol. Cell. Endocrinol.* **2015**, *418*, 153–172. [CrossRef] [PubMed]

4. Zhang, Q.; Zhang, C.; Wang, H.; Ma, Z.; Liu, D.; Guan, X.; Liu, Y.; Fu, Y.; Cui, M.; Dong, J. Intermittent Fasting versus Continuous Calorie Restriction: Which Is Better for Weight Loss? *Nutrients* **2022**, *14*, 1781. [CrossRef] [PubMed]
5. Gabel, K.; Kroeger, C.M.; Trepanowski, J.F.; Hoddy, K.K.; Cienfuegos, S.; Kalam, F.; Varady, K.A. Differential Effects of Alternate-Day Fasting Versus Daily Calorie Restriction on Insulin Resistance. *Obesity* **2019**, *27*, 1443–1450. [CrossRef]
6. De Cabo, R.; Mattson, M.P. Effects of Intermittent Fasting on Health, Aging, and Disease. *N. Engl. J. Med.* **2019**, *381*, 2541–2551. [CrossRef]
7. Redman, L.M.; Smith, S.R.; Burton, J.H.; Martin, C.K.; Il'yasova, D.; Ravussin, E. Metabolic Slowing and Reduced Oxidative Damage with Sustained Caloric Restriction Support the Rate of Living and Oxidative Damage Theories of Aging. *Cell Metab.* **2018**, *27*, 805–815.e4. [CrossRef]
8. Wan, R.; Camandola, S.; Mattson, M.P. Intermittent Food Deprivation Improves Cardiovascular and Neuroendocrine Responses to Stress in Rats. *J. Nutr.* **2003**, *133*, 1921–1929. [CrossRef]
9. Castello, L.; Froio, T.; Maina, M.; Cavallini, G.; Biasi, F.; Leonarduzzi, G.; Donati, A.; Bergamini, E.; Poli, G.; Chiarpotto, E. Alternate-Day Fasting Protects the Rat Heart against Age-Induced Inflammation and Fibrosis by Inhibiting Oxidative Damage and NF-κB Activation. *Free Radic. Biol. Med.* **2010**, *48*, 47–54. [CrossRef]
10. Wan, R.; Camandola, S.; Mattson, M.P. Intermittent Fasting and Dietary Supplementation with 2-Deoxy-D-Glucose Improve Functional and Metabolic Cardiovascular Risk Factors in Rats. *FASEB J.* **2003**, *17*, 1133–1134. [CrossRef]
11. Anson, R.M.; Guo, Z.; de Cabo, R.; Iyun, T.; Rios, M.; Hagepanos, A.; Ingram, D.K.; Lane, M.A.; Mattson, M.P. Intermittent Fasting Dissociates Beneficial Effects of Dietary Restriction on Glucose Metabolism and Neuronal Resistance to Injury from Calorie Intake. *Proc. Natl. Acad. Sci. USA* **2003**, *100*, 6216–6220. [CrossRef]
12. Bough, K.J.; Valiyil, R.; Han, F.T.; Eagles, D.A. Seizure Resistance Is Dependent upon Age and Calorie Restriction in Rats Fed a Ketogenic Diet. *Epilepsy Res.* **1999**, *35*, 21–28. [CrossRef] [PubMed]
13. Gilbert, D.L.; Pyzik, P.L.; Freeman, J.M. The Ketogenic Diet: Seizure Control Correlates Better with Serum Beta-Hydroxybutyrate than with Urine Ketones. *J. Child Neurol.* **2000**, *15*, 787–790. [CrossRef] [PubMed]
14. Kashiwaya, Y.; Takeshima, T.; Mori, N.; Nakashima, K.; Clarke, K.; Veech, R.L. D-Beta-Hydroxybutyrate Protects Neurons in Models of Alzheimer's and Parkinson's Disease. *Proc. Natl. Acad. Sci. USA* **2000**, *97*, 5440–5444. [CrossRef]
15. Varady, K.A.; Hellerstein, M.K. Alternate-Day Fasting and Chronic Disease Prevention: A Review of Human and Animal Trials. *Am. J. Clin. Nutr.* **2007**, *86*, 7–13. [CrossRef]
16. Arum, O.; Bonkowski, M.S.; Rocha, J.S.; Bartke, A. The Growth Hormone Receptor Gene-Disrupted Mouse Fails to Respond to an Intermittent Fasting Diet. *Aging Cell* **2009**, *8*, 756–760. [CrossRef] [PubMed]
17. Kendrick, D.C. The Effects of Infantile Stimulation and Intermittent Fasting and Feeding on Life Span in the Black-Hooded Rat. *Dev. Psychobiol.* **1973**, *6*, 225–234. [CrossRef]
18. Goodrick, C.L.; Ingram, D.K.; Reynolds, M.A.; Freeman, J.R.; Cider, N. Effects of Intermittent Feeding upon Body Weight and Lifespan in Inbred Mice: Interaction of Genotype and Age. *Mech. Ageing Dev.* **1990**, *55*, 69–87. [CrossRef]
19. DeFronzo, R.A. From the Triumvirate to the Ominous Octet: A New Paradigm for the Treatment of Type 2 Diabetes Mellitus. *Diabetes* **2009**, *58*, 773–795. [CrossRef]
20. Schwartz, S.S.; Epstein, S.; Corkey, B.E.; Grant, S.F.A.; Gavin, J.R.; Aguilar, R.B. The Time Is Right for a New Classification System for Diabetes: Rationale and Implications of the β-Cell-Centric Classification Schema. *Diabetes Care* **2016**, *39*, 179–186. [CrossRef]
21. Gastaldelli, A.; Miyazaki, Y.; Pettiti, M.; Matsuda, M.; Mahankali, S.; Santini, E.; DeFronzo, R.A.; Ferrannini, E. Metabolic Effects of Visceral Fat Accumulation in Type 2 Diabetes. *J. Clin. Endocrinol. Metab.* **2002**, *87*, 5098–5103. [CrossRef]
22. Kantartzis, K.; Machann, J.; Schick, F.; Fritsche, A.; Häring, H.-U.; Stefan, N. The Impact of Liver Fat vs. Visceral Fat in Determining Categories of Prediabetes. *Diabetologia* **2010**, *53*, 882–889. [CrossRef] [PubMed]
23. Samuel, V.T.; Liu, Z.-X.; Qu, X.; Elder, B.D.; Bilz, S.; Befroy, D.; Romanelli, A.J.; Shulman, G.I. Mechanism of Hepatic Insulin Resistance in Non-Alcoholic Fatty Liver Disease. *J. Biol. Chem.* **2004**, *279*, 32345–32353. [CrossRef] [PubMed]
24. Dokpuang, D.; Zhiyong Yang, J.; Nemati, H.; He, K.; Plank, L.D.; Murphy, R.; Lu, J. Magnetic Resonance Study of Visceral, Subcutaneous, Liver and Pancreas Fat Changes after 12 Weeks Intermittent Fasting in Obese Participants with Prediabetes. *Diabetes Res. Clin. Pract.* **2023**, *202*, 110775. [CrossRef] [PubMed]
25. de Souza Marinho, T.; Ornellas, F.; Barbosa-da-Silva, S.; Mandarim-de-Lacerda, C.A.; Aguila, M.B. Beneficial Effects of Intermittent Fasting on Steatosis and Inflammation of the Liver in Mice Fed a High-Fat or a High-Fructose Diet. *Nutrition* **2019**, *65*, 103–112. [CrossRef] [PubMed]
26. Deng, J.; Feng, D.; Jia, X.; Zhai, S.; Liu, Y.; Gao, N.; Zhang, X.; Li, M.; Lu, M.; Liu, C.; et al. Efficacy and Mechanism of Intermittent Fasting in Metabolic Associated Fatty Liver Disease Based on Ultraperformance Liquid Chromatography-Tandem Mass Spectrometry. *Front. Nutr.* **2022**, *9*, 838091. [CrossRef]
27. Ezpeleta, M.; Gabel, K.; Cienfuegos, S.; Kalam, F.; Lin, S.; Pavlou, V.; Song, Z.; Haus, J.M.; Koppe, S.; Alexandria, S.J.; et al. Effect of Alternate Day Fasting Combined with Aerobic Exercise on Non-Alcoholic Fatty Liver Disease: A Randomized Controlled Trial. *Cell Metab.* **2023**, *35*, 56–70.e3. [CrossRef]
28. Health and Economic Benefits of Diabetes Interventions | Power of Prevention. Available online: https://www.cdc.gov/chronicdisease/programs-impact/pop/diabetes.htm (accessed on 1 July 2023).
29. Galaviz, K.I.; Narayan, K.M.V.; Lobelo, F.; Weber, M.B. Lifestyle and the Prevention of Type 2 Diabetes: A Status Report. *Am. J. Lifestyle Med.* **2015**, *12*, 4–20. [CrossRef]

30. National Diabetes Statistics Report | Diabetes | CDC. Available online: https://www.cdc.gov/diabetes/data/statistics-report/index.html (accessed on 14 June 2023).
31. American Diabetes Association. Economic Costs of Diabetes in the U.S. in 2017. *Diabetes Care* **2018**, *41*, 917–928. [CrossRef]
32. Obermayer, A.; Tripolt, N.J.; Pferschy, P.N.; Kojzar, H.; Aziz, F.; Müller, A.; Schauer, M.; Oulhaj, A.; Aberer, F.; Sourij, C.; et al. Efficacy and Safety of Intermittent Fasting in People With Insulin-Treated Type 2 Diabetes (INTERFAST-2)-A Randomized Controlled Trial. *Diabetes Care* **2023**, *46*, 463–468. [CrossRef]
33. Tagde, P.; Tagde, S.; Bhattacharya, T.; Tagde, P.; Akter, R.; Rahman, M.H. Multifaceted Effects of Intermittent Fasting on the Treatment and Prevention of Diabetes, Cancer, Obesity or Other Chronic Diseases. *Curr. Diabetes Rev.* **2022**, *18*, e131221198789. [CrossRef]
34. Kunduraci, Y.E.; Ozbek, H. Does the Energy Restriction Intermittent Fasting Diet Alleviate Metabolic Syndrome Biomarkers? A Randomized Controlled Trial. *Nutrients* **2020**, *12*, 3213. [CrossRef] [PubMed]
35. Carter, S.; Clifton, P.M.; Keogh, J.B. Effect of Intermittent Compared With Continuous Energy Restricted Diet on Glycemic Control in Patients With Type 2 Diabetes: A Randomized Noninferiority Trial. *JAMA Netw. Open* **2018**, *1*, e180756. [CrossRef] [PubMed]
36. Wing, R.R.; Lang, W.; Wadden, T.A.; Safford, M.; Knowler, W.C.; Bertoni, A.G.; Hill, J.O.; Brancati, F.L.; Peters, A.; Wagenknecht, L. Benefits of Modest Weight Loss in Improving Cardiovascular Risk Factors in Overweight and Obese Individuals with Type 2 Diabetes. *Diabetes Care* **2011**, *34*, 1481–1486. [CrossRef] [PubMed]
37. Guariguata, L.; Whiting, D.; Weil, C.; Unwin, N. The International Diabetes Federation Diabetes Atlas Methodology for Estimating Global and National Prevalence of Diabetes in Adults. *Diabetes Res. Clin. Pract.* **2011**, *94*, 322–332. [CrossRef]
38. Harris, M.I.; Klein, R.; Welborn, T.A.; Knuiman, M.W. Onset of NIDDM Occurs at Least 4–7 Yr before Clinical Diagnosis. *Diabetes Care* **1992**, *15*, 815–819. [CrossRef]
39. Ali, O. Genetics of Type 2 Diabetes. *World J. Diabetes* **2013**, *4*, 114–123. [CrossRef]
40. Lyssenko, V.; Laakso, M. Genetic Screening for the Risk of Type 2 Diabetes. *Diabetes Care* **2013**, *36*, S120–S126. [CrossRef]
41. Shaw, J. Diagnosis of Prediabetes. *Med. Clin. N. Am.* **2011**, *95*, 341–352. [CrossRef]
42. Stern, M.P.; Williams, K.; Haffner, S.M. Identification of Persons at High Risk for Type 2 Diabetes Mellitus: Do We Need the Oral Glucose Tolerance Test? *Ann. Intern. Med.* **2002**, *136*, 575–581. [CrossRef]
43. Sagesaka, H.; Sato, Y.; Someya, Y.; Tamura, Y.; Shimodaira, M.; Miyakoshi, T.; Hirabayashi, K.; Koike, H.; Yamashita, K.; Watada, H.; et al. Type 2 Diabetes: When Does It Start? *J. Endocr. Soc.* **2018**, *2*, 476–484. [CrossRef]
44. Uusitupa, M.; Khan, T.A.; Viguiliouk, E.; Kahleova, H.; Rivellese, A.A.; Hermansen, K.; Pfeiffer, A.; Thanopoulou, A.; Salas-Salvadó, J.; Schwab, U.; et al. Prevention of Type 2 Diabetes by Lifestyle Changes: A Systematic Review and Meta-Analysis. *Nutrients* **2019**, *11*, 2611. [CrossRef]
45. Knowler, W.C.; Barrett-Connor, E.; Fowler, S.E.; Hamman, R.F.; Lachin, J.M.; Walker, E.A.; Nathan, D.M. Diabetes Prevention Program Research Group Reduction in the Incidence of Type 2 Diabetes with Lifestyle Intervention or Metformin. *N. Engl. J. Med.* **2002**, *346*, 393–403. [CrossRef] [PubMed]
46. Diabetes Prevention Program Research Group; Knowler, W.C.; Fowler, S.E.; Hamman, R.F.; Christophi, C.A.; Hoffman, H.J.; Brenneman, A.T.; Brown-Friday, J.O.; Goldberg, R.; Venditti, E.; et al. 10-Year Follow-up of Diabetes Incidence and Weight Loss in the Diabetes Prevention Program Outcomes Study. *Lancet* **2009**, *374*, 1677–1686. [CrossRef] [PubMed]
47. Eriksson, J.; Lindström, J.; Valle, T.; Aunola, S.; Hämäläinen, H.; Ilanne-Parikka, P.; Keinänen-Kiukaanniemi, S.; Laakso, M.; Lauhkonen, M.; Lehto, P.; et al. Prevention of Type II Diabetes in Subjects with Impaired Glucose Tolerance: The Diabetes Prevention Study (DPS) in Finland. Study Design and 1-Year Interim Report on the Feasibility of the Lifestyle Intervention Programme. *Diabetologia* **1999**, *42*, 793–801. [CrossRef] [PubMed]
48. Lindström, J.; Ilanne-Parikka, P.; Peltonen, M.; Aunola, S.; Eriksson, J.G.; Hemiö, K.; Hämäläinen, H.; Härkönen, P.; Keinänen-Kiukaanniemi, S.; Laakso, M.; et al. Sustained Reduction in the Incidence of Type 2 Diabetes by Lifestyle Intervention: Follow-up of the Finnish Diabetes Prevention Study. *Lancet* **2006**, *368*, 1673–1679. [CrossRef] [PubMed]
49. Li, G.; Zhang, P.; Wang, J.; Gregg, E.W.; Yang, W.; Gong, Q.; Li, H.; Li, H.; Jiang, Y.; An, Y.; et al. The Long-Term Effect of Lifestyle Interventions to Prevent Diabetes in the China Da Qing Diabetes Prevention Study: A 20-Year Follow-up Study. *Lancet* **2008**, *371*, 1783–1789. [CrossRef]
50. Chiasson, J.-L.; Josse, R.G.; Gomis, R.; Hanefeld, M.; Karasik, A.; Laakso, M. STOP-NIDDM Trail Research Group Acarbose for Prevention of Type 2 Diabetes Mellitus: The STOP-NIDDM Randomised Trial. *Lancet* **2002**, *359*, 2072–2077. [CrossRef]
51. Buchanan, T.A.; Xiang, A.H.; Peters, R.K.; Kjos, S.L.; Marroquin, A.; Goico, J.; Ochoa, C.; Tan, S.; Berkowitz, K.; Hodis, H.N.; et al. Preservation of Pancreatic Beta-Cell Function and Prevention of Type 2 Diabetes by Pharmacological Treatment of Insulin Resistance in High-Risk Hispanic Women. *Diabetes* **2002**, *51*, 2796–2803. [CrossRef]
52. DREAM (Diabetes REduction Assessment with ramipril and rosiglitazone Medication) Trial Investigators; Gerstein, H.C.; Yusuf, S.; Bosch, J.; Pogue, J.; Sheridan, P.; Dinccag, N.; Hanefeld, M.; Hoogwerf, B.; Laakso, M.; et al. Effect of Rosiglitazone on the Frequency of Diabetes in Patients with Impaired Glucose Tolerance or Impaired Fasting Glucose: A Randomised Controlled Trial. *Lancet* **2006**, *368*, 1096–1105. [CrossRef]
53. Zinman, B.; Harris, S.B.; Neuman, J.; Gerstein, H.C.; Retnakaran, R.R.; Raboud, J.; Qi, Y.; Hanley, A.J.G. Low-Dose Combination Therapy with Rosiglitazone and Metformin to Prevent Type 2 Diabetes Mellitus (CANOE Trial): A Double-Blind Randomised Controlled Study. *Lancet* **2010**, *376*, 103–111. [CrossRef]

54. Torgerson, J.S.; Hauptman, J.; Boldrin, M.N.; Sjöström, L. XENical in the Prevention of Diabetes in Obese Subjects (XENDOS) Study: A Randomized Study of Orlistat as an Adjunct to Lifestyle Changes for the Prevention of Type 2 Diabetes in Obese Patients. *Diabetes Care* **2004**, *27*, 155–161. [CrossRef] [PubMed]
55. Marina, A.L.; Utzschneider, K.M.; Wright, L.A.; Montgomery, B.K.; Marcovina, S.M.; Kahn, S.E. Colesevelam Improves Oral but Not Intravenous Glucose Tolerance by a Mechanism Independent of Insulin Sensitivity and β-Cell Function. *Diabetes Care* **2012**, *35*, 1119–1125. [CrossRef] [PubMed]
56. Handelsman, Y.; Goldberg, R.B.; Garvey, W.T.; Fonseca, V.A.; Rosenstock, J.; Jones, M.R.; Lai, Y.-L.; Jin, X.; Misir, S.; Nagendran, S.; et al. Colesevelam Hydrochloride to Treat Hypercholesterolemia and Improve Glycemia in Prediabetes: A Randomized, Prospective Study. *Endocr. Pract.* **2010**, *16*, 617–628. [CrossRef]
57. Rosenstock, J.; Foley, J.E.; Rendell, M.; Landin-Olsson, M.; Holst, J.J.; Deacon, C.F.; Rochotte, E.; Baron, M.A. Effects of the Dipeptidyl Peptidase-IV Inhibitor Vildagliptin on Incretin Hormones, Islet Function, and Postprandial Glycemia in Subjects with Impaired Glucose Tolerance. *Diabetes Care* **2008**, *31*, 30–35. [CrossRef]
58. Rosenstock, J.; Klaff, L.J.; Schwartz, S.; Northrup, J.; Holcombe, J.H.; Wilhelm, K.; Trautmann, M. Effects of Exenatide and Lifestyle Modification on Body Weight and Glucose Tolerance in Obese Subjects with and without Pre-Diabetes. *Diabetes Care* **2010**, *33*, 1173–1175. [CrossRef] [PubMed]
59. Astrup, A.; Carraro, R.; Finer, N.; Harper, A.; Kunesova, M.; Lean, M.E.J.; Niskanen, L.; Rasmussen, M.F.; Rissanen, A.; Rössner, S.; et al. Safety, Tolerability and Sustained Weight Loss over 2 Years with the Once-Daily Human GLP-1 Analog, Liraglutide. *Int. J. Obes.* **2012**, *36*, 843–854. [CrossRef]
60. Dixon, J.B.; Zimmet, P.; Alberti, K.G.; Rubino, F. Bariatric Surgery: An IDF Statement for Obese Type 2 Diabetes. *Diabet. Med.* **2011**, *28*, 628–642. [CrossRef]
61. de la Cruz-Muñoz, N.; Messiah, S.E.; Arheart, K.L.; Lopez-Mitnik, G.; Lipshultz, S.E.; Livingstone, A. Bariatric Surgery Significantly Decreases the Prevalence of Type 2 Diabetes Mellitus and Pre-Diabetes among Morbidly Obese Multiethnic Adults: Long-Term Results. *J. Am. Coll. Surg.* **2011**, *212*, 505–511; discussion 512–513. [CrossRef]
62. Carlsson, L.M.S.; Peltonen, M.; Ahlin, S.; Anveden, Å.; Bouchard, C.; Carlsson, B.; Jacobson, P.; Lönroth, H.; Maglio, C.; Näslund, I.; et al. Bariatric Surgery and Prevention of Type 2 Diabetes in Swedish Obese Subjects. *N. Engl. J. Med.* **2012**, *367*, 695–704. [CrossRef]
63. Zhuo, X.; Zhang, P.; Barker, L.; Albright, A.; Thompson, T.J.; Gregg, E. The Lifetime Cost of Diabetes and Its Implications for Diabetes Prevention. *Diabetes Care* **2014**, *37*, 2557–2564. [CrossRef]
64. Vasavada, A.; Taub, L.F.M. Diabetes Mellitus Screening. In *StatPearls*; StatPearls Publishing: Treasure Island, FL, USA, 2023.
65. US Preventive Services Task Force. Screening for Prediabetes and Type 2 Diabetes: US Preventive Services Task Force Recommendation Statement. *JAMA* **2021**, *326*, 736–743. [CrossRef] [PubMed]
66. Kahn, R.; Alperin, P.; Eddy, D.; Borch-Johnsen, K.; Buse, J.; Feigelman, J.; Gregg, E.; Holman, R.R.; Kirkman, M.S.; Stern, M.; et al. Age at Initiation and Frequency of Screening to Detect Type 2 Diabetes: A Cost-Effectiveness Analysis. *Lancet* **2010**, *375*, 1365–1374. [CrossRef] [PubMed]
67. Lambrinou, E.; Hansen, T.B.; Beulens, J.W. Lifestyle Factors, Self-Management and Patient Empowerment in Diabetes Care. *Eur. J. Prev. Cardiol.* **2019**, *26*, 55–63. [CrossRef] [PubMed]
68. Bartoli, E.; Fra, G.P.; Carnevale Schianca, G.P. The Oral Glucose Tolerance Test (OGTT) Revisited. *Eur. J. Intern. Med.* **2011**, *22*, 8–12. [CrossRef]
69. Lu, J.; He, J.; Li, M.; Tang, X.; Hu, R.; Shi, L.; Su, Q.; Peng, K.; Xu, M.; Xu, Y.; et al. Predictive Value of Fasting Glucose, Postload Glucose, and Hemoglobin A1c on Risk of Diabetes and Complications in Chinese Adults. *Diabetes Care* **2019**, *42*, 1539–1548. [CrossRef]
70. Selvin, E.; Wang, D.; Matsushita, K.; Grams, M.E.; Coresh, J. Prognostic Implications of Single-Sample Confirmatory Testing for Undiagnosed Diabetes: A Prospective Cohort Study. *Ann. Intern. Med.* **2018**, *169*, 156–164. [CrossRef]
71. Ostendorf, D.M.; Caldwell, A.E.; Zaman, A.; Pan, Z.; Bing, K.; Wayland, L.T.; Creasy, S.A.; Bessesen, D.H.; MacLean, P.; Melanson, E.L.; et al. Comparison of Weight Loss Induced by Daily Caloric Restriction versus Intermittent Fasting (DRIFT) in Individuals with Obesity: Study Protocol for a 52-Week Randomized Clinical Trial. *Trials* **2022**, *23*, 718. [CrossRef]
72. Dansinger, M.L.; Gleason, J.A.; Griffith, J.L.; Selker, H.P.; Schaefer, E.J. Comparison of the Atkins, Ornish, Weight Watchers, and Zone Diets for Weight Loss and Heart Disease Risk ReductionA Randomized Trial. *JAMA* **2005**, *293*, 43–53. [CrossRef]
73. MacLean, P.S.; Wing, R.R.; Davidson, T.; Epstein, L.; Goodpaster, B.; Hall, K.D.; Levin, B.E.; Perri, M.G.; Rolls, B.J.; Rosenbaum, M.; et al. NIH Working Group Report: Innovative Research to Improve Maintenance of Weight Loss. *Obesity* **2015**, *23*, 7–15. [CrossRef]
74. O'Connor, S.G.; Boyd, P.; Bailey, C.P.; Nebeling, L.; Reedy, J.; Czajkowski, S.M.; Shams-White, M.M. A Qualitative Exploration of Facilitators and Barriers of Adherence to Time-Restricted Eating. *Appetite* **2022**, *178*, 106266. [CrossRef]
75. Vasim, I.; Majeed, C.N.; DeBoer, M.D. Intermittent Fasting and Metabolic Health. *Nutrients* **2022**, *14*, 631. [CrossRef] [PubMed]

Disclaimer/Publisher's Note: The statements, opinions and data contained in all publications are solely those of the individual author(s) and contributor(s) and not of MDPI and/or the editor(s). MDPI and/or the editor(s) disclaim responsibility for any injury to people or property resulting from any ideas, methods, instructions or products referred to in the content.

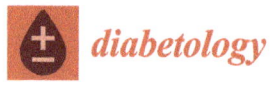

Review

Recent Advances in Psychotherapeutic Treatment and Understanding of Alexithymia in Patients with Obesity and Diabetes Mellitus Type 2

Filip Mustač [1,*], Tin Galijašević [2], Eva Podolski [2], Andrej Belančić [3,4], Martina Matovinović [5,*] and Darko Marčinko [1,2]

1. Department of Psychiatry and Psychological Medicine, University Hospital Centre Zagreb, 10000 Zagreb, Croatia; niarveda@gmail.com
2. School of Medicine, University of Zagreb, 10000 Zagreb, Croatia; kopaka@oems.hr (T.G.); eva.podolski3@gmail.com (E.P.)
3. Department of Clinical Pharmacology, Clinical Hospital Centre Rijeka, Krešimirova 42, 51000 Rijeka, Croatia; a.belancic93@gmail.com
4. Department of Basic and Clinical Pharmacology with Toxicology, Faculty of Medicine, University of Rijeka, Braće Branchetta 20, 51000 Rijeka, Croatia
5. Department of Internal Medicine, Division of Endocrinology, Croatian Obesity Treatment Referral Centre, University Hospital Centre Zagreb, 10000 Zagreb, Croatia
* Correspondence: filip.mustac@gmail.com (F.M.); martina_10000@yahoo.com (M.M.)

Abstract: Alexithymia is the inability to describe one's own feelings and is being increasingly researched. According to contemporary psychodynamic theories, negative emotions cannot be adequately named and externalized, but remain trapped in the body. Recent research shows the connection of alexithymia with numerous somatic diseases. Diabetes mellitus type 2 and obesity represent great challenges in treatment, and the psychological profiles in these diseases are being studied more and more often. Therefore, alexithymia enters the focus of some research as a factor that could play a significant role in these diseases, namely as the one that makes a difference. The aim of this paper is a review of the literature with the purpose of understanding the current knowledge about the interconnection between alexithymia, obesity and type 2 diabetes mellitus.

Keywords: alexithymia; obesity; diabetes mellitus type 2; psychodynamic psychotherapy

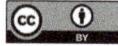

1. Introduction

Alexithymia is a psychological term used to describe a personality trait or psychological construct characterized by difficulties in identifying, describing, and expressing one's emotions. People with alexithymia have trouble understanding and verbalizing their own emotional experiences and recognizing emotions in others. The term was first coined in 1970s [1], meaning "no words for emotions". It is characterized by restricted imaginal processes, difficulties in recognizing and identifying subjective feelings and describing them to others. Another key feature is an externally orientated cognitive style which causes individuals to rely on external stimuli or behaviors to regulate their emotions rather than internally processing and understanding their emotional experiences. In addition to this, emotional apathy is often present, causing alexithymic individuals to appear emotionally distant or indifferent to others because of their difficulties in understanding and expressing emotions. It is considered a stable personality factor, that varies in intensity among individuals. It is important to highlight that having alexithymia does not mean that a person lacks emotions altogether; instead, they experience emotions differently and find it challenging to articulate and understand them in a typical way. Although it is not classified as a mental disorder itself, it is often associated with other psychological conditions and medical conditions, such as depression, anxiety, and eating disorders, making it an important treatment target as it is related to poorer treatment outcomes [1]. Obesity, a medical condition characterized by excessive body fat accumulation and defined as Body Mass Index (BMI) ≥ 30 kg/m^2, is not strictly considered an eating disorder, yet some studies have found a positive correlation between obesity and alexithymia [2]. Apart from alexithymia as a psychological factor, obesity is also characterized by genetic, biological, social, cultural, and environmental factors, making it one of the biggest public health concerns nowadays, due to its multidimensionality and growing prevalence [2]. As such, it significantly affects the latter development of cardiovascular diseases and diabetes. In this paper, we explore the current literature on the impact of alexithymia as an independent factor in the development and outcome prediction of obesity and DM type 2.

2. Materials and Methods

Our primary focus in writing this paper was to find the correlation between type 2 diabetes mellitus and alexithymia and how they are interconnected. We conducted our research by analyzing the literature on PubMed, concentrating on studies which spoke about our topics of interest. Our inclusion criteria were following. We searched only articles that are in English language. There was no strict time limit for the papers that are included, but mainly we focused on recent studies. On the other hand, we have not rejected all the older studies, so we included all the studies that three authors (FM, TG, EP) found relevant. The process of that deciding was through in-person and telephone meetings and discussing the literature that we found. What was considered relevant was based on our research experience and looking into research methodology and the number of participants. Searching the literature, we found that phenomena like emotional eating and binge eating disorders in most cases link diabetic and alexithymic patients. We also included a summary table (Table 1) in our paper that presents findings from different study groups regarding the relationship between alexithymia and obesity. The table provides insights from various studies, showcasing the diverse results observed in different research contexts. Moreover, in Table 2 the varied relationships between alexithymia and T2DM are presented and summarized, including the findings of the studies which we observed.

3. The Complex Relationship between Alexithymia and Obesity

The underlying mechanisms connecting alexithymia and obesity are complex and not fully understood, but several factors may contribute to this relationship. One of the most important ones is emotional eating. Alexithymic individuals may struggle to recognize and cope with their emotions, leading them to use food as a way to manage their feelings. Emotional eating can lead to overeating and contribute to weight gain and obesity. This finding is in perfect accordance with the addiction theory developed by McDougal, which explains the function of acting, in this case eating, as a way of avoiding psychic work—which in alexithymic individuals includes processing emotions [3]. Some studies have suggested that alexithymia may be linked to impulsive behaviors, including impulsive eating patterns. This impulsivity can lead to a lack of self-control and overeating, contributing to weight gain. Stress plays another significant role in the relationship between these conditions, especially as it is becoming deep-rooted phenomenon in people's lives. As alexithymia is associated with difficulties in managing stress and negative emotions, individuals with this trait may be more prone to experiencing chronic stress, which can lead to unhealthy eating habits and significant weight gain over time. Another possibility upon which has been argued is the fact that alexithymic individuals may have a limited awareness of their physical and emotional states, including hunger and fullness cues. This lack of self-awareness can lead to overeating and difficulties in maintaining a healthy weight. Finally, since alexithymic individuals present with significantly reduced motivation for weight loss and thus difficulty in engaging in weight loss efforts, the entire process of weight reduction therapy is more challenging for them. It is important to note that not all individuals with alexithymia will experience obesity, and not all obese individuals will have alexithymia. The relationship between these factors is, as already mentioned, still an area of ongoing research, and individual differences play a significant role in how these traits manifest. Many studies on this topic conclude that alexithymia only exists in people with obesity, with other psychological characteristics (e.g., eating disorders), but rarely in patients with no mental health issues. Different hypotheses may explain the strong correlation between alexithymia and mental illness. The first one considers alexithymia to be a primary personality psychological factor, thus highly correlated to mental health problems, in particular depression, anxiety and binge eating. In that context, alexithymia, through a facilitating role in endangering mental health, results in emotional eating, which is involved in weight gain and inadequate weight loss in obese subjects. On the other hand, alexithymia could be a "secondary trait", in this manner presenting itself with the difficulty to identify and describe feelings in a response to a certain event where, e.g., depression or anxiety is a primary condition [4]. These findings collectively suggest that there may be a complex relationship between alexithymia and obesity. While some studies found positive correlations between alexithymia and body weight, others found associations with emotional eating, depression, and different facets of emotional processing (Table 1).

Table 1. This table offers an overview of different study groups and their findings regarding the relationship between alexithymia and obesity.

Study Group	Results
Troisi et al. (2001) [5]	No significant association between BMI and TAS total score was found.
Pinaqui et al. (2003) [3]	Alexithymia was the predictor of emotional eating in population of obese women suffering from BED.
Zak-Golab et al. (2013) [6]	Higher BMI was associated with severe depression symptoms, but not alexithymia.
Pinna et al. (2011) [4]	Alexithymia was significantly more frequent among obese patients compared to controls with normal BMI, with this group of obese subjects achieving higher mean scores on TAS. BED was associated with a significantly higher frequency of alexithymic traits and higher TAS scores.
Fernandes et al. (2017) [7]	Meta-analyses of 31 studies comparing emotional processing in individuals with obesity demonstrated that obese individuals had higher scores of alexithymia, difficulty in identifying feelings, and externally oriented thinking style, when compared with control groups.
C. Di Monte et al. (2020) [2]	A significant positive correlation between alexithymia level, measured with TSIA scale, and body weight was found.

TSIA—Toronto Structured Interview for Alexithymia; BED—binge eating disorder; BMI—Body Mass Index, TAS—Toronto Alexithymia Scale.

It is important to note that the relationship between these factors may vary among different populations and individuals. Further research may be needed to better understand the mechanisms and implications of this relationship.

4. The Importance of an Adequate Assessment Tool for Alexithymia

It is worth noting that in all these studies, alexithymia was assessed using a self-report instrument, the 20-item Toronto Alexithymia Scale (TAS-20), the most widely used instrument to assess alexithymia. The TAS-20, as a self-report test, shows some limitations. One of them is the fact that some individuals may not be able to properly rate their deficits in emotional awareness through the form of a self-report measure. Moreover, reduced fantasy and imaginal thinking, which are both distinctive features of the alexithymia construct, are not taken into consideration in TAS-20. To beat these limitations, a new instrument for alexithymia assessment, the Toronto Structured Interview for Alexithymia (TSIA) was developed. It consists of four subscales which correlate with four predominant aspects of alexithymia construct: difficulty in identifying feelings, difficulty in describing feelings, externally orientated thinking, and imaginal processes. This assessment proved to be better because it is the interviewer who applies a score to each of these aspects, thus avoiding self-evaluation bias. Furthermore, a complete set of prompts and probes is asked in each question, leading to more precise comprehension of the meaning of the given responses. Therefore, TSIA presents as a more sensitive assessment tool for alexithymia, and many researchers advocate for the implementation of TSIA in everyday practice, underlining the importance of a multimethod assessment for the evaluation of alexithymia [2].

5. How Alexithymia Influences Coping with Diabetes Mellitus Type 2

Alexithymia further represents a complex construct that goes beyond the basic definition of the mere inability to describe one's own emotions, but rather predicts how an individual experience himself and his emotions, as well as the world around him, and speaks of a lack of the possibility of symbolism, which will mean that these patients tend to focus on concrete topics [8,9]. If these patients are inclined to a concrete, non-phantasmatic interpretation of internal and external reality and then we may consider alexithymia to be very pronounced [8,10]. Diabetes mellitus type 2 represents a very demanding and difficult diagnosis regarding the importance of discipline not only when taking medication, but also maintaining a healthy lifestyle. Thus, a person with diabetes mellitus type 2 must pay attention to the therapy regimen, caloric intake, and qualitative food intake, if on insulin therapy, have the necessary equipment in every situation, pay attention to foot care, etc. [11,12]. Eating represents a very essential and important sociocultural role, and such a level of engagement with one's own illness certainly makes an individual tired and frustrated after a while and can lead to some mental health problems [13,14]. Also, things like continuous glucose monitor implants facilitate disease control and comfort, which is still relatively challenging in Croatia [15]. However, CGM implants still change the external appearance and the patient may feel different, ashamed or stigmatized, which can also be a problem for a certain number of patients. A person with diabetes mellitus can thus find her/himself in a rather unfavorable position. It should be noted that for some people, food represents a certain type of escape from reality and comfort. It can also be present with symptoms associated with atypical depression [9,16], but for some people, food also represents a small joy during the day, such as eating something sweet (a cake or the like). A person with diabetes mellitus type 2 must also pay attention to this. This alone brings us to the very important concept of one's own awareness and reaction to the disease and the recognition of one's own emotions and conditions related to the reaction to a disease such as diabetes mellitus. Alexithymia in patients with diabetes mellitus has been investigated for some time, but the results and conclusions are still sometimes contradictory and the discussion about the exact connection and causal effect is still being investigated. Melin et al., 2017, in a study comparing patients with DM type 1 and 2, reported that depression is strongly associated with alexithymia in patients with DM type 2 and that this is attributable to features of atypical depression since other results indicated no association with anxiety and elevated levels secretion of cortisol. Furthermore, their results indicate that people with DM type 2 and depressive symptoms also have a high prevalence of obesity [9]. Friedman et al. found that alexithymia is associated with depression in type 1 DM patients as well [17]. In 2021, Dincer et al. published a paper in which during 2020 (the pandemic period) they studied the connection between alexithymia, depressive symptoms, and changes in sexual behavior in patients with DM type 2, and their results show that after diabetes, 83.3% of patients had impaired sexual functioning, which could be associated with high levels of depressive and anxiety symptoms, especially during a pandemic, and alexithymia stands out as a possible connection [12]. Our team's research from 2021 revealed that approximately one third of obese patients have sexual dysfunction and that this association is more pronounced in female obese patients, as well as those who have more pronounced anxiety and depressive symptoms [18]. All of the above indicates that difficulties in sexual functioning could be related to depressive symptoms in patients with DM type 2 and obesity, where alexithymia could play a significant role, which is still insufficiently defined. The connection between cognition and alexithymia is increasingly being investigated, including in patients with DM type 2. Hintistan et al., 2013, in patients with DM type 2 older than 60 years without a psychiatric diagnosis, found the presence of alexithymia in 75.8% of patients, and the association was not related to professional status or level of education. Furthermore, other studies also question whether alexithymia is only a consequence of a certain cognitive deficit, especially in patients with obesity and DM type 2 [11,19,20]. Martino et al. note in their review that the prevalence of alexithymia in patients with DM type 2 ranges from 25 to 50% which is noteworthy as they found that alexithymia is a predictor of poor glycemic control. They hypothesize that poor awareness of bodily sensations in alexithymic patents negatively impacts coping strategies in the management of DM type 2 in both self-care and disease knowledge. They also highlight how patients with alexithymia may be less prone to recognize their illness and seriously follow their doctors' instructions. On the other hand, they explain that poor glycemic control might negatively impact cognitive and emotional processing, resulting in greater alexithymia levels overall, which might explain the increased hospitalization rates some studies found in patients, with those studies finding a correlation between alexithymia and diabetes. Martino et al. also note the correlation of alexithymia with depression and anxiety which might prevent the patient making sense of the illness without adequate psychotherapeutic intervention [14]. Lemche et al. conducted a study exploring the connection between alexithymic symptoms in patients with metabolic syndrome and those patients developing DM type 2. They found that alexithymia severity is a predictor of DM type 2 in patients with metabolic syndrome as well as that alexithymia statistically significantly predicts other indicators of obesity like BMI and waist girth and risk factors like dyslipidemia, hypertension, and microalbuminuria, all relevant biomarkers in long-term outcomes in metabolic syndrome patients [21]. These findings collectively highlight the potential relationship between alexithymia and T2DM, as well as their impact on glycemic control and emotional well-being. However, it is important to note that research in this area may vary in terms of study populations and methodologies, and more research may be needed to further understand the complex interactions between alexithymia, T2DM, and related factors. (Table 2).

Table 2. This table summarizes findings from various studies regarding the relationship between alexithymia and type 2 diabetes mellitus (T2DM), as well as their potential impact on glycemic control and related factors.

Study	Results
Melin et al. (2017) [9]	Depression was associated with alexithymia in T2DM patients
Luca et al. (2014) [13]	Alexithymic patients presented higher HBA1c levels compared to non-alexithymic ones
Martino et al. (2020) [14]	Patients with T2DM reflected greater values of alexithymia
Avci et al. (2016) [16]	Alexithymia was 2.09 times higher among T2DM patients who had HbA1c $\geq 7\%$
Friedman et al. (2003) [17]	Alexithymia is not correlated with glycemic control
Lemche et al. (2014) [21]	Alexithymia is a substantial indicator of T2DM and cardiovascular risks in patients with metabolic syndrome
Celik et al. (2022) [22]	The majority of T2DM patients showed signs of alexithymia and positive relationship between HBA1c and alexithymia score was found

T2DM—type 2 diabetes mellitus.

A cross-sectional study by Avci and Kelleci, which enrolled 326 DM2 patients (37.3% determined to have alexithymia), reported that alexithymia was 2.09 times higher among those who had worse glycaemia control (HbA1c $\geq$ 7.0% vs. <7.0% group), as well as 3.77 and 2.57 times higher for those in whom anxiety ($\geq$11 vs. $\leq$10) and depression ($\geq$8 vs. $\leq$7) were more expressed, respectively. The latter is obviously an interesting finding; however, the obtained results should be interpreted accordingly bearing in mind the study methodology [16]. What is more, as per Luca et al. data, alexithymia more than depression influenced glycemic control, and HbA1c was only significantly associated (logistic regression), with alexithymia and insulin therapy, which clearly highlights the importance of this topic [13]. To deduce, a well-summarized body of the literature within the Martino et al. systematic review revealed a strong correlation between alexithymia, HbA1c and fasting blood glucose levels: 0.75 and 0.77 (for TAS-20 total scores), respectively. Also, significantly higher levels of HbA1c and blood glucose were present among alexithymic (25–50% of DM2 population in general) compared to the non-alexithymic participants [14]. To the best of our knowledge, there are no RCT designs yet, so we can only talk on association, but not on causality. However, we can speculate that improving glycemic control, and decreasing anxiety and depression levels, might result in better alexithymia control, and vice versa. All things considered, it is evident that management of patients living with DM2 should be arranged to include psychopathological alterations screening and mental health care services for those at risk in order to improve both DM2 control as well as quality of life [14,23]. On the other hand, well-management of alexithymia is a cornerstone for improving the psychiatric treatment outcomes in general also [24,25]; thus, it can be seen as a strong 'knot' within the DM2–psychiatry vicious circle. To clarify, alexithymia is implicated in a wide variety of psychological problems (depression and schizophrenia), emotional deficits in autism spectrum disorder, suicidality, increased psychosomatic complaints, and elevated mortality rates; thus, achieving optimal/rational and personalized antidepressant, antipsychotic, mood stabilizer, and anxiolytic prescribing (alongside cognitive-behavioral therapy and psychodynamic therapy) is a hard, but indispensable task for clinicians working with patients in such a setting [26]. Simultaneously, it is of utmost importance to choose an optimal antihyperglycemic therapeutic approach (always, but especially in alexithymic patients), bearing in mind the efficacy/effectiveness, safety profile, comorbidity profile (both potential benefits and harms), as well as medication adherence rates, and costs [27]. A recent meta-analysis by Pei et al. 2022 [28] aimed to explore the prevalence of alexithymia in T2DM patients and its implications. The analysis found a high prevalence of alexithymia in T2DM patients, with 43.0% of individuals affected, which was much higher than the general population (12.8%), which suggests that a significant proportion of T2DM patients are at risk of developing alexithymic traits. It should be noted that most studies excluded individuals with pre-existing psychiatric disorders. The analysis highlighted the potential impact of alexithymia on glycemic control, as patients with alexithymia may struggle to recognize bodily sensations, leading to poorer disease management. Conversely, poor glycemic control may exacerbate alexithymia due to vascular and neural effects of T2DM. The study noted differences in alexithymia prevalence between China and non-China populations which was likely influenced by cultural, religious, and socio-demographic factors, and it should be noted that the majority of studies originated from China, which means more research on this topic may further elaborate this phenomenon. The authors highlight the importance of screening T2DM patients for alexithymia and raising awareness of the condition among healthcare professionals. The study also notes that most studies use self-report questionnaires for alexithymia assessment, which may limit the accuracy of current research.

6. Ways to Fight Alexithymia and Diabetes Mellitus Type 2

When we discuss the therapeutic options for patients with pronounced alexithymia, it is important to think about how we will consider alexithymia. This points us to the fact that alexithymia is probably not an entity in itself, but a phenomenon that most likely occurs either as a symptom or even more likely as some kind of personality trait [24,29,30]. However, it is clearly present in a large proportion of patients, as our review of the literature shows. Managing obesity and type 2 diabetes mellitus (T2DM) through psychotherapy can be a valuable component of a comprehensive treatment plan. Psychotherapy can address various psychological and emotional factors that contribute to these conditions, helping individuals make sustainable lifestyle changes, manage stress, and improve overall well-being. There are various types of psychotherapy which have been shown to be helpful in coping with obesity and TD2M. Psychodynamic psychotherapy stands out as a therapeutic option. Modern psychodynamic therapy primary concentrates on enhancing self-awareness, through which an individual can achieve a higher level of self-control, leading to improved decision making regarding diet and exercise. It aims to call into the preconscious and conscious an unconscious part of the self that is inhibited by the outer armor, that is, the part from which the inner world of the psyche defends itself, mainly through various defense mechanisms. However, with psychodynamic psychotherapy, it is possible to change the personality level and thus empower the person to abandon the alexithymic pattern [24,29,31]. Furthermore, group psychotherapy, as well as supportive therapy in general, also shows positive therapeutic effects [30], although in general, alexithymia is associated with a minor recovery of psychological symptoms [32]. It is sometimes stated that difficulties in expressing emotions and verbalizing them are the most resistant and least responsive symptom, but that other domains respond better to psychodynamic psychotherapy [29,32]. It was also shown that group therapy or family therapy provides social support, reducing feelings of isolation and increasing motivation. Motivational interviewing techniques also proved effective in finding internal motivation for adopting healthier behaviors. Another therapy worth mentioning is mindfulness-based therapy which through mindful eating techniques promotes awareness of eating habits, making individuals more conscious of portion sizes and food choices. In addition to this, mindfulness meditation can reduce stress, which is beneficial for both weight management and glycemic control. Creative therapies such as drama, music, and art could also be taken in consideration when discussing treatment options of alexithymic patients. Engaging in creative activities can help individuals express emotions indirectly. Creative therapies provide non-verbal outlets for emotional expression, making it easier for some individuals to explore their feelings and therefore fight alexithymia. Cognitive-behavioral therapy (CBT) can be helpful in management of both stress and cravings management as it teaches stress reduction techniques, reducing the likelihood of stress-induced eating. Moreover, it can influence changes in behavioral patterns and therefore help individuals identify and change behaviors related to overeating, emotional eating and sedentary lifestyle. When we talk about patients with DM type 2 and the pharmacological therapy to which they have been exposed, the studies available to date have not determined a difference in the alexithymic status with regard to the exposed therapy (in the sense of a difference depending on whether the patient is on insulin therapy, oral antidiabetic drugs, or diet) [13,14,16]. What is considered important is certainly to be aware of the severity of diseases such as DM type 2 and obesity, and to be aware of one's own reaction to the disease and to act accordingly, accepting one's own weakness and vulnerability, since the acceptance of any disease is also a process, especially when it is a disease that requires a lot of commitment and lifestyle control, which DM type 2 and obesity certainly are.

7. Conclusions

The spread of obesity and diabetes mellitus type 2 today is very high and worrisome, and since these are diseases that, in addition to pharmacological treatment methods, also require lifestyle changes, the study of psychological factors certainly contributes to a better knowledge of the entities themselves and the creation of an environment that would be supportive for people with the mentioned diseases. Studying alexithymia as a factor that makes a difference in these diseases can significantly explain some of the mentioned phenomena. Further well-designed studies that would explain the role of alexithymia in patients with obesity and type 2 diabetes mellitus in more detail are definitely needed.

Author Contributions: Conceptualization and design of article: F.M.; literature search, writing—original draft preparation: F.M., T.G., E.P. and A.B.; supervision: M.M. and D.M.; writing—review and editing: all authors. All authors have read and agreed to the published version of the manuscript.

Funding: This research received no external funding.

Institutional Review Board Statement: Not applicable.

Informed Consent Statement: Not applicable.

Data Availability Statement: Not applicable.

Conflicts of Interest: The authors declare no conflict of interest.

References

1. Westwood, H.; Kerr-Gaffney, J.; Stahl, D.; Tchanturia, K. Alexithymia in Eating Disorders: Systematic Review and Meta-Analyses of Studies Using the Toronto Alexithymia Scale. *J. Psychosom. Res.* **2017**, *99*, 66–81. [CrossRef] [PubMed]
2. Di Monte, C.; Renzi, A.; Paone, E.; Silecchia, G.; Solano, L.; Di Trani, M. Alexithymia and Obesity: Controversial Findings from a Multimethod Assessment. *Eur. Rev. Med. Pharmacol. Sci.* **2020**, *24*, 831–836. [CrossRef] [PubMed]
3. Pinaquy, S.; Chabrol, H.; Simon, C.; Louvet, J.-P.; Barbe, P. Emotional Eating, Alexithymia, and Binge-Eating Disorder in Obese Women. *Obes. Res.* **2003**, *11*, 195–201. [CrossRef] [PubMed]
4. Pinna, F.; Lai, L.; Pirarba, S.; Orrù, W.; Velluzzi, F.; Loviselli, A.; Carpiniello, B. Obesity, Alexithymia and Psychopathology: A Case-Control Study. *Eat. Weight Disord. EWD* **2011**, *16*, e164–e170. [CrossRef]
5. Troisi, A.; Scucchi, S.; San Martino, L.; Montera, P.; d'Amore, A.; Moles, A. Age Specificity of the Relationship between Serum Cholesterol and Mood in Obese Women. *Physiol. Behav.* **2001**, *72*, 409–413. [CrossRef]
6. Zak-Gołąb, A.; Olszanecka-Glinianowicz, M.; Kocełak, P.; Chudek, J. [The role of gut microbiota in the pathogenesis of obesity]. *Postep. Hig. Med. Dosw. Online* **2014**, *68*, 84–90. [CrossRef]
7. Fernandes, J.; Ferreira-Santos, F.; Miller, K.; Torres, S. Emotional Processing in Obesity: A Systematic Review and Exploratory Meta-Analysis. *Obes. Rev.* **2018**, *19*, 111–120. [CrossRef]
8. Marchini, F.; Caputo, A.; Napoli, A.; Balonan, J.; Martino, G.; Nannini, V.; Langher, V. Chronic Illness as Loss of Good Self: Underlying Mechanisms Affecting Diabetes Adaptation. *Mediterr. J. Clin. Psychol.* **2019**, *6*. [CrossRef]
9. Melin, E.O.; Thunander, M.; Landin-Olsson, M.; Hillman, M.; Thulesius, H.O. Depression Differed by Midnight Cortisol Secretion, Alexithymia and Anxiety between Diabetes Types: A Cross Sectional Comparison. *BMC Psychiatry* **2017**, *17*, 335. [CrossRef]
10. Luminet, O.; de Timary, P.; Buysschaert, M.; Luts, A. The Role of Alexithymia Factors in Glucose Control of Persons with Type 1 Diabetes: A Pilot Study. *Diabetes Metab.* **2006**, *32*, 417–424. [CrossRef]
11. Hintistan, S.; Cilingir, D.; Birinci, N. Alexithymia among Elderly Patients with Diabetes. *Pak. J. Med. Sci.* **2013**, *29*, 1344–1348. [CrossRef] [PubMed]
12. Dincer, B.; Yıldırım Ayaz, E.; Oğuz, A. Changes in Sexual Functions and Alexithymia Levels of Patients with Type 2 Diabetes During the COVID-19 Pandemic. *Sex. Disabil.* **2021**, *39*, 461–478. [CrossRef] [PubMed]
13. Luca, A.; Luca, M.; Di Mauro, M.; Palermo, F.; Rampulla, F.; Calandra, C. Alexithymia, More than Depression, Influences Glycaemic Control of Type 2 Diabetic Patients. *J. Endocrinol. Investig.* **2015**, *38*, 653–660. [CrossRef] [PubMed]
14. Martino, G.; Caputo, A.; Vicario, C.M.; Catalano, A.; Schwarz, P.; Quattropani, M.C. The Relationship between Alexithymia and Type 2 Diabetes: A Systematic Review. *Front. Psychol.* **2020**, *11*, 2026. [CrossRef] [PubMed]
15. Belančić, A.; Klobučar, S.; Rahelić, D. Current Obstacles (With Solutions) in Type 2 Diabetes Management, Alongside Future Directions. *Diabetology* **2023**, *4*, 31. [CrossRef]
16. Avci, D.; Kelleci, M. Alexithymia in Patients with Type 2 Diabetes Mellitus: The Role of Anxiety, Depression, and Glycemic Control. *Patient Prefer. Adherence* **2016**, *10*, 1271–1277. [CrossRef]
17. Friedman, S.; Vila, G.; Even, C.; Timsit, J.; Boitard, C.; Dardennes, R.; Guelfi, J.D.; Mouren-Simeoni, M.C. Alexithymia in Insulin-Dependent Diabetes Mellitus Is Related to Depression and Not to Somatic Variables or Compliance. *J. Psychosom. Res.* **2003**, *55*, 285–287. [CrossRef]
18. Matovinović, M.; IvanaTudor, K.; Mustač, F.; MarioTudor, D.; Kovačević, A.; Bilić, E. Sexual dysfunction in croatian patients with obesity. *Psychiatr. Danub.* **2021**, *33*, 191.
19. Reynolds, R.M.; Strachan, M.W.J.; Labad, J.; Lee, A.J.; Frier, B.M.; Fowkes, F.G.; Mitchell, R.; Seckl, J.R.; Deary, I.J.; Walker, B.R.; et al. Morning Cortisol Levels and Cognitive Abilities in People with Type 2 Diabetes: The Edinburgh Type 2 Diabetes Study. *Diabetes Care* **2010**, *33*, 714–720. [CrossRef]
20. Cukierman, T.; Gerstein, H.C.; Williamson, J.D. Cognitive Decline and Dementia in Diabetes–Systematic Overview of Prospective Observational Studies. *Diabetologia* **2005**, *48*, 2460–2469. [CrossRef]
21. Lemche, A.V.; Chaban, O.S.; Lemche, E. Alexithymia as a Risk Factor for Type 2 Diabetes Mellitus in the Metabolic Syndrome: A Cross-Sectional Study. *Psychiatry Res.* **2014**, *215*, 438–443. [CrossRef] [PubMed]
22. Celik, S.; Taskin Yilmaz, F.; Yurtsever Celik, S.; Anataca, G.; Bulbul, E. Alexithymia in Diabetes Patients: Its Relationship with Perceived Social Support and Glycaemic Control. *J. Clin. Nurs.* **2022**, *31*, 2612–2620. [CrossRef] [PubMed]

23. Marcovecchio, M.L.; Chiarelli, F. The Effects of Acute and Chronic Stress on Diabetes Control. *Sci. Signal.* **2012**, *5*, pt10. [CrossRef]
24. Pinna, F.; Manchia, M.; Paribello, P.; Carpiniello, B. The Impact of Alexithymia on Treatment Response in Psychiatric Disorders: A Systematic Review. *Front. Psychiatry* **2020**, *11*, 311. [CrossRef] [PubMed]
25. Lane, R.D. Alexithymia 3.0: Reimagining Alexithymia from a Medical Perspective. *Biopsychosoc. Med.* **2020**, *14*, 21. [CrossRef]
26. Samur, D.; Tops, M.; Schlinkert, C.; Quirin, M.; Cuijpers, P.; Koole, S.L. Four Decades of Research on Alexithymia: Moving toward Clinical Applications. *Front. Psychol.* **2013**, *4*, 861. [CrossRef]
27. Davies, M.J.; Aroda, V.R.; Collins, B.S.; Gabbay, R.A.; Green, J.; Maruthur, N.M.; Rosas, S.E.; Del Prato, S.; Mathieu, C.; Mingrone, G.; et al. Management of Hyperglycemia in Type 2 Diabetes, 2022. A Consensus Report by the American Diabetes Association (ADA) and the European Association for the Study of Diabetes (EASD). *Diabetes Care* **2022**, *45*, 2753–2786. [CrossRef]
28. Pei, J.-H.; Wei, Y.-T.; Tao, H.-X.; Yang, Q.-X.; Zhang, G.-L.; Guo, X.-J.; Guo, J.-L.; Yan, F.-H.; HanPhD, L. The Prevalence and Characteristics of Alexithymia in Patients with Type 2 Diabetes Mellitus: A Systematic Review and Meta-Analysis. *J. Psychosom. Res.* **2022**, *162*, 111018. [CrossRef]
29. Stingl, M.; Bausch, S.; Walter, B.; Kagerer, S.; Leichsenring, F.; Leweke, F. Effects of Inpatient Psychotherapy on the Stability of Alexithymia Characteristics. *J. Psychosom. Res.* **2008**, *65*, 173–180. [CrossRef]
30. Ogrodniczuk, J.S.; Piper, W.E.; Joyce, A.S. Effect of Alexithymia on the Process and Outcome of Psychotherapy: A Programmatic Review. *Psychiatry Res.* **2011**, *190*, 43–48. [CrossRef]
31. Cameron, K.; Ogrodniczuk, J.; Hadjipavlou, G. Changes in Alexithymia Following Psychological Intervention: A Review. *Harv. Rev. Psychiatry* **2014**, *22*, 162–178. [CrossRef] [PubMed]
32. Leweke, F.; Bausch, S.; Leichsenring, F.; Walter, B.; Stingl, M. Alexithymia as a Predictor of Outcome of Psychodynamically Oriented Inpatient Treatment. *Psychother. Res. J. Soc. Psychother. Res.* **2009**, *19*, 323–331. [CrossRef] [PubMed]

Disclaimer/Publisher's Note: The statements, opinions and data contained in all publications are solely those of the individual author(s) and contributor(s) and not of MDPI and/or the editor(s). MDPI and/or the editor(s) disclaim responsibility for any injury to people or property resulting from any ideas, methods, instructions or products referred to in the content.

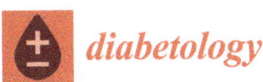

Review

Diabetes Mellitus—Digital Solutions to Improve Medication Adherence: Scoping Review

Nikol Georgieva *, Viktor Tenev, Maria Kamusheva and Guenka Petrova

Department of Organization and Economics of Pharmacy, Faculty of Pharmacy, Medical University of Sofia, 1000 Sofia, Bulgaria; viktortenev@abv.bg (V.T.); mkamusheva@pharmfac.mu-sofia.bg (M.K.); gpetrova@pharmfac.mu-sofia.bg (G.P.)
* Correspondence: nikol.georgieva25@yahoo.com

Abstract: Medication adherence (MA) is a major problem. On average 50% of chronic disease management medications are not taken as prescribed While digital healthcare tools like mobile apps offer benefits such as informative messages and prescription management, they must be personalized and offer support across all medication phases to effectively address individual patient factors and optimize adherence, with room for further improvements. This scoping review examined the impact of digital health technologies on MA in adults with diabetes as well as their benefits and barriers. Using PubMed and Scopus databases, 11 out of 385 studies (2.86%) from January 2017 to August 2023 met the criteria for digital health interventions in diabetes MA, assessed through the Chronic Care Model. The Chronic Care Model (CCM) is a patient-centered, evidence-based framework designed to improve the care and outcomes for chronic illness patients, consisting of six core elements and enhanced by eHealth tools that facilitate self-management and support through digital innovations. The results demonstrate the effectiveness of digital health technology in improving medication adherence among adults with diabetes. Specific digital interventions, including mobile apps like Gather and Medisafe, SMS text messaging, telemonitoring, and tailored care management have demonstrated effectiveness in enhancing MA. These interventions have shown positive outcomes, including enhanced glycemic control and increased patient engagement. Some of the limitations, which these technologies face, are the poor usability, digital illiteracy among the patients, low rates of sustainability and low accessibility among the elderly population. Digital health technology shows promise in enhancing medication adherence among adults with diabetes, as revealed in this scoping review. However, ongoing research is necessary to fine-tune these interventions for improved outcomes and the overall well-being of individuals with diabetes. Additional improvement of the technologies and adaptation to the diverse population might be a good field for exploration.

Keywords: digital health; diabetes; medication adherence

Citation: Georgieva, N.; Tenev, V.; Kamusheva, M.; Petrova, G. Diabetes Mellitus—Digital Solutions to Improve Medication Adherence: Scoping Review. *Diabetology* **2023**, *4*, 465–480. https://doi.org/10.3390/diabetology4040040

Academic Editors: Andrej Belančić, Sanja Klobučar and Dario Rahelić

Received: 9 September 2023
Revised: 4 October 2023
Accepted: 7 October 2023
Published: 19 October 2023

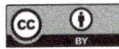

Copyright: © 2023 by the authors. Licensee MDPI, Basel, Switzerland. This article is an open access article distributed under the terms and conditions of the Creative Commons Attribution (CC BY) license (https:// creativecommons.org/licenses/by/ 4.0/).

1. Introduction

Chronic diseases are the epidemic of twenty-first century. They are common, costly and some of them could be prevented. Primary care providers are looking for new and innovative approaches to prevent chronic diseases. The MedTech industry has been working intensively during the recent years to benefit healthcare with advanced technological solutions. Electronic solutions help patients and physicians in many areas, by controlling physiological indicators, monitoring patient status, improving dosage, enhancing adherence. Self-management, as an important part of chronic illness prevention and management has to include different techniques as this occurs outside the primary healthcare provider. Creating tools to help the individual develop life skills to support self-management will lead to improving the patient outcomes [1].

The Ascertaining Barriers to Compliance (ABC) taxonomy was developed with the aim of systematizing definitions and operationalizations of medication adherence [2].

Medication adherence is the procedure through which patients follow their prescribed medication regimens. It can be broken down into three measurable phases as follows: "Initiation", "Implementation", and "Discontinuation" [3]. Medication adherence refers to patients following the prescribed medication's timing, dosage, and frequency, which hinges on their understanding of their health condition and collaboration with healthcare providers [4]. The significance of adhering to medication has been acknowledged for a while, yet it was only about 50 years ago that it started receiving proper attention in clinical settings. Originally referred to as "compliance with therapeutic regimen," the concept evolved to "adherence to medication" to emphasize the patient's more active role [5]. Over time, it was realized that non-adherence stems from intentional and unintentional factors [6]. Implementing the medication adherence concept is delicate; identifying and addressing non-adherence is crucial for enhancing treatment. However, labeling patients as non-adherent doesn't effectively improve adherence rates [4].

Lack of medication adherence (MA) is a common problem, which endangers the effectiveness of healthcare systems. The collaboration of the patients in taking the prescribed medications is highly important for reaching the desired clinical outcomes. While most healthcare systems are able to provide accessible and efficacy medications, the non-compliance remains high [6].

In the International Diabetes Federation (IDF) diabetes Atlas states that 537 million adults (20–79 years) are living with diabetes (1 in 10 persons) and that it is expected to rise to 643 million by 2030 and 783 million by 2045. In Europe 61 million adults are living with diabetes (1 in 11 persons) with the expectation that this number will rise to 67 million by 2030 and 69 million by 2045 [7].

The percentage of diabetic patients who adhere accurately to prescribed oral hypoglycemic therapy varies significantly. Depending on factors like the studied population, treatment plan, and measurement method, the high adherence group can range from 38.5% to 93.1% of patients [8]. Several factors influence how well patients with T2DM stick to their medication regimen. The most consistent obstacles to treatment adherence for this condition involve the patient (such as depression and understanding of the disease and treatment), the treatment itself (including experiencing adverse reactions and the complexity of therapy), and the healthcare system (like difficulties in access and high medication costs) [9].

In cases of type 2 diabetes mellitus (T2DM), not taking medication regularly or following the correct schedule harms patients' health. It also raises healthcare costs due to poor control, more medical visits, higher expenses, and increased mortality. Ultimately, it leads to higher outpatient, ER, and hospitalization costs for T2D complications [10–13].

A systematic review conducted by Cheen and colleagues [14] showed a pooled primary medication non-adherence (PMN) rate of 10% for diabetes mellitus patients, and 12% and 14% for depression and asthma, respectively, which are the lowest compared to 25–43% for newly diagnosed patients with osteoporosis. The lower non-adherence of these patients is a result of the symptoms that are visible after non-compliance to the medication regimen [14]. In a study tracking over 11,000 veterans with T2D for at least 5 years, poor medication adherence (with medication possession ratio <80%) was significantly associated with inadequate glycemic control [15]. According to the National Health and Wellness Survey involving 1198 patients with T2D, each 1-point decrease in self-reported medication adherence (using the Morisky Medication Adherence Scale) correlated with a 0.21% increase in HbA1c, and increases of 4.6%, 20.4%, and 20.9% in physician visits, ER visits, and hospitalizations respectively [16].

Significantly, poor medication adherence in type 2 diabetes (T2D) has also been tied to higher mortality rates [13]. Similarly, Ho et al. found a significant connection between poor medication adherence in T2D and all-cause mortality over time [17].

Simple changes in the lifestyle of individuals could prevent type 2 diabetes. Early diagnosis and prevention could improve the results of the pre-diabetic population. Letting individuals have control over their health and support the self-management of the health with new technologies, would lead not only to the prevention of diabetes but also improve the quality of life [5].

The purpose of this narrative review is to search for evidence for the benefits of the digital health technologies used to improve medication adherence in adults with diabetes. The following questions were asked to guide the review:

1. Is there evidence that digital health technologies improve medication adherence in adults with diabetes?
2. What are the benefits and barriers of the digital health technology for medication adherence when used by adult patients with diabetes?

2. Materials and Methods

This scoping review follows five stages: (1) problem identification, (2) literature search, (3) data evaluation, (4) data analysis, and (5) presentation [18]. A literature search was conducted to find relevant studies published from January 2017 to August 2023.

One researcher conducted the search using: PubMed and Scopus. A combination of keywords was used, including "digital", "technology", "health", "diabetes", "medication", and "adherence".

For inclusion in this review, studies were required to explore a digital health technology intervention for medication adherence among patients with diabetes mellitus. The inclusion criteria encompassed the following: (1) randomized controlled trials (RCTs) that were peer-reviewed and conducted in English language, employing quasi-experimental, observational, or qualitative designs; (2) studies that involved digital health interventions aimed at enhancing adherence to prescribed medications among individuals aged 18 years or older; and (3) studies that specifically concentrated on diabetes type 1 and T2D.

On the other hand, studies were excluded if they met the following criteria: (1) lack of data regarding medication adherence; or (2) were classified as pilot studies. The process involved evaluating titles and abstracts to determine their relevance. Then, the selected studies were reviewed as full text publications.

In this scoping review, the Chronic Care Model (CCM) was employed to assess the utilization of digital health technology for enhancing medication adherence in diabetes. The MA interventions were categorized according to the CCM. We categorized the various MA interventions based on the components of the CCM. This aligned each intervention with the relevant CCM elements.

The Chronic Care Model (CCM) (Table 1) is a well-established framework focused on compassionate care for chronic illness patients. It emphasizes improving functionality and clinical outcomes. This patient-centered, evidence-based framework aims to reshape outpatient care and enhance healthcare results for those with chronic conditions [19–23].

Table 1. Chronic Care Model components and descriptions.

Chronic Care Model Components	Description
Self-management support	To empower patients to manage their health and cope with their condition.
Decision support	To promote clinical care that is consistent with scientific evidence and patient preferences.
Clinical information systems	To organize patient and population data to facilitate efficient and effective care.
Delivery system design	To ensure that care is coordinated, proactive, and patient-centered.
Community support	To mobilize community resources to meet the needs of patients.
Health systems	To create a culture and organization that promote high-quality care.

The Chronic Care Model consists of six core elements: health system or organization (HSHO), clinical information systems (CIS), decision support (DS), delivery system design (DSD), self-management support (SMS), and community resources for patients (CORP) [20,21,24].

The eHealth-enhanced CCM (eCCM) integrates digital health tools into chronic condition self-management. It assesses digital health innovations, extending beyond the traditional CCM by including eHealth tools and a broader definition of eCommunity, which covers various digital health support and education. The CCM and eCCM are interconnected, emphasizing the importance of eHealth [19].

Each digital technology for MA used in patients with diabetes was analyzed from the perspective of the CCM.

3. Results

3.1. Overview

Of the 385 abstracts, 11 articles (2.86%) that used a digital health intervention to promote medication adherence to prescribed medications for diabetes were selected in full text (Appendix A) and evaluated with the Chronic Care Model (see Table 2). Studies included eight RCTs, and three observational studies. Two studies were conducted in the USA, two in India, two in Spain, one in the United Kingdom, one in China, one in Singapore, one in Saudi Arabia, one in the United Arab Emirates. Medication adherence findings for the intervention and data extraction categories, including the study objective, design, sample, intervention length, and participant age, are included in Appendix A.

Strategies used to improve medication adherence included three primary approaches: SMS text messaging, telemonitoring and/or tailored care management, and web-based software. The subheadings in this section under "Utilization of the Chronic Care Model" consist of progressively interdependent components of the Chronic Care Model that influence patient-centered, evidence-based care and are designed to improve health outcomes by changing the routine delivery of care (ie, self-management support, decision support, clinical information systems, delivery system design, community support, and health systems) [25].

The examined research papers are shown in Appendix A, aiming to classify results according to components of the CCM, facilitating an evaluation of digital health interventions' impact on medication adherence. A summary of CCM elements used in each study is outlined in Table 2 [26–36].

Table 2. Chronic Care Model applied to studies.

Study Author, Year	Self-Management	Decision Support	Clinical Information Systems	Delivery System Design	Community Support
Kleinman, N.J. et al., 2017 [26]	X		X		
Huang, Z. et al., 2019 [27]	X				
Xu, R. et al., 2020 [28]				X	
Omar, M.A. et al., 2020 [29]					X
Almer, A. et al., 2020 [30]	X				
Shamanna, P. et al., 2020 [31]		X			
Katz, L.B. et al., 2022 [32]	X				
Lee, E.Y. et al., 2022 [33]	X				
Orozco-Beltrán, D., Morales, C. et al., 2022 [34]	X	X			
Al-Mutairi, A.M. et al., 2023 [35]			X		
Heald, A.H. et al., 2023 [36]	X				

3.2. Utilization of the Chronic Care Model

3.2.1. Self-Management

The objective of self-management support is to educate patients and families, providing training and health-related guidance to encourage self-care [25]. Additionally, the electronic Chronic Care Model (eCCM) introduces 24/7 accessibility, convenience, reminders, and notifications [19]. In a study conducted by Kleinman and colleagues [26], a m-Health app—Gather was found to improve medication adherence (39.0% vs. 12.8%;) and increase frequency of blood glucose (BG) self-testing (39.0% vs. 10.3%). The Gather m-Health platform offers a solution for individuals with diabetes, aiding in self-management and results in enhanced diabetes self-management [26]. In study by Huang and colleagues [27], the Medisafe app was evaluated and showed that the reduced obstacles to medication adherence in the intervention group. Although no improvement in HbA1c levels was observed, the app facilitated self-management and support in medication management, and it is likely to result in short-term enhancements in medication adherence [27]. In a study conducted by Alamer and colleagues [30], one-way automated SMS (OASMS) was assessed to study the effects of diabetes self-care messages delivered through non-tailored one-way automated SMS (OASMS) on managing blood sugar levels in type 2 diabetes). The study results revealed that the baseline HbA1c values were 10.2% in the intervention group vs. 9.9% in the control group. When adjusting for baseline HbA1c levels and age using an ANCOVA model, it was estimated that there was a reduction in HbA1c of −0.97% in favor of the intervention group. The study demonstrated the feasibility of using SMS for self-care messages in managing blood sugar levels, which again showed short-term improvement [29]. Similarly, RCT conducted by Katz and colleagues [32], aimed to showcase the effectiveness of the OneTouch (OT) Verio Flex glucose meter when used along with a Spanish-language version of the OT Reveal mobile app. The goal was to enhance diabetes care and enhance blood sugar control within an underserved Hispanic population dealing with type 2 diabetes. Over a period of 12 weeks, the individuals in the test group experienced a notable average decrease in A1C levels of 1.0%, which was considerably larger than the reduction seen in the control group). This improvement in A1C persisted during the following 12 weeks as well. Even those who switched to using the meter and mobile app showed significant enhancements in A1C. The intervention enhanced diabetes care, blood sugar control, and self-management within an underserved Hispanic population [32]. Another study conducted by Lee and colleagues [33] evaluated the impact of a mobile application that is integrated with an electronic medical record system, designed for personalized diabetes self-management. The focus of the assessment was on how this app affected glycemic control in individuals with type 2 diabetes mellitus, specifically in terms of self-monitoring of blood glucose levels and making lifestyle adjustments. The main measure of interest was the alteration in HbA1c levels after 26 weeks. Furthermore, the study also examined self-confidence in managing diabetes, engagement in self-care practices, and user satisfaction with the iCareD system after the intervention. The average reduction in HbA1c levels showed a significant decrease in HbA1c levels post-intervention. Furthermore, there was a substantial reduction in average blood glucose levels without an increase in hypoglycemic events The app supported self-monitoring of blood glucose levels and lifestyle adjustments, empowering individuals with type 2 diabetes [33]. Another study, an ambispective study (retrospective and prospective) was conducted by Orozco-Beltrán and colleagues [34] to examine how a home-based digital tool for patient empowerment and communication, known as the DeMpower App, impacts metabolic control of individuals with inadequately controlled type 2 diabetes mellitus (T2DM) over a 54-week period. The DeMpower app group showed a noticeable trend towards a higher proportion of patients reaching the study's glycemic target (46% vs. 18%). This trend became statistically significant when considering the target of HbA1c $\leq 7.5\%$ (64% vs. 24%) or HbA1c $\leq 8\%$ (85% vs. 53%). Additionally, improvements in other cardiovascular risk factors, medication adherence, and satisfaction were observed as well. The app empowered individuals with inadequately controlled type 2 diabetes for better self-management [34]. Finally, Heald and colleagues [36] conducted a RCT to assess how the Haelum app improved health outcomes and patient quality of life among patients with T2D over a 6-month period as well as if the app improved the patient's engagement levels [36]. Over 6 months, the treatment group's average HbA1c dropped by −7.4%, while the control group only saw a 1.8% decrease. Similarly, the treatment group's average BMI decreased by −0.7%, whereas the control group's average BMI reduction was −0.2%. A greater percentage of the active treatment group achieved reductions in both HbA1c and BMI compared to the control group. In terms of HbA1c, 72.4% of the active treatment group lowered their levels, while only 41.5% of the control group did Patients in the active treatment group also experienced an improvement in self-measured quality of life (QoL), as indicated by an average increase of 0.0464 in their EQ-5D-5L rating from pre-trial to post-trial. These results highlight that offering personalized care plans, along with support and education through a mobile app, can lead to reductions in HbA1c and BMI among individuals with T2D. The utilization of a patient management app, coupled with tailored care plans, also contributed to an enhancement in patient-reported quality of life (QoL) and engagement [36]. These studies emphasize the contribution of using digital technologies to medication adherence and self-management, key aspects of the Chronic Care Model in diabetes.

3.2.2. Decision Support

Decision support focuses on enhancing medical decision-making for healthcare providers and patients, with the aim of granting access to up-to-date care guidelines based on evidence [25]. Furthermore, eCCM covers topics like prompts and informational cues [19]. A study conducted by Shamanna and colleagues [31], examined the difference in hemoglobin A1c (HbA1c) in 64 patients with diabetes type 2 over a 3-month period using the Twin Precision Nutrition (TPN) program. The TPN machine learning algorithm utilized data from daily continuous glucose monitors (CGM) and food intake to offer personalized recommendations. These guidelines aimed to help patients steer clear of foods that led to spikes in blood glucose, suggesting alternatives that didn't cause spikes. In the 90-day follow-up, the program resulted in significant improvements in decision-making and glycemic control. HbA1c levels decreased from 8.8% to 6.9%, weight decreased, and fasting blood glucose levels improved. Physicians used the CGM data to make informed medication adjustments [31]. The ambispective study by Orozco-Beltrán and colleagues [34] for the DeMpower app implies that utilizing home digital tools for patient empowerment could have a meaningful impact on metabolic control. This app served as a home-based digital tool for patient empowerment, offering decision support for individuals with inadequately controlled type 2 diabetes. It helped patients make informed choices about their diabetes management. The study suggested that using home digital tools, like the DeMpower app, had a significant impact on metabolic control. This type of decision support is particularly valuable during situations like the COVID-19 pandemic and within the context of digital health advancements [34].

3.2.3. Clinical Information Systems

Clinical information systems serve the purpose of gathering, managing, and applying healthcare-related information, including patient registries and electronic medical records [18]. Furthermore, eCCM highlights the creation of patient portals, utilization of the Internet, mHealth, mobile phones, wearable devices, and patient health records [19]. Digital health technology enables potential integration of secure messaging, virtual appointments, remote monitoring with feedback, health risk assessment with feedback, prescription refills, personalized interventions, and connections to community initiatives [37]. The RCT conducted by Kleinman and colleagues [26], investigated the Gather app (m-Health diabetes platform) and the impact on the clinical outcomes, patient-reported outcomes, patient and provider satisfaction, and app usage. From the clinical information systems perspective of the Chronic Care Model, the Gather app serves as a tool that enhances information flow and communication between patients and providers. It offers the potential to improve access to high-quality care and empower patients to actively manage their condition. The study's positive outcomes suggest that such clinical information systems can contribute significantly to effective chronic disease management. [26]. A retrospective study in Saudi Arabia by Al-Mutari and colleagues [35] examined the impact of telemedicine on glycemic control (measured by HbA1c levels) in patients with type 2 diabetes during a specific period, particularly the COVID-19 lockdown. Telemedicine, as a component of clinical information systems, played a critical role in maintaining patient care during challenging times like the lockdown. It facilitated remote monitoring and communication between patients and healthcare providers, enabling the assessment of glycemic control. While the average HbA1c levels increased slightly, the study highlighted that a significant proportion of patients (63.1%) maintained or improved their glycemic control through telemedicine. The gender-based differences in outcomes also suggested that tailoring telemedicine interventions based on patient characteristics can be important. However, persistent elevated HbA1c levels in some patients may indicate the influence of other factors beyond telemedicine, such as lifestyle and comorbidities [35]. Both studies demonstrate the value of clinical information systems, including mobile apps and telemedicine, in supporting chronic care management. These systems enhance information exchange, patient-provider interactions, and monitoring, aligning with the Chronic Care Model's emphasis on proactive, well-informed, and collaborative care for chronic diseases like diabetes.

3.2.4. Delivery System Design

Delivery system design encompasses the significance of interdisciplinary clinical teams and the cooperation between patients and multiple healthcare providers [25]. Bluetooth-enabled devices and the utilization of chat, voice, and video communication enable the healthcare team to offer many aspects similar to a conventional in-person appointment. The incorporation of advanced technology offers an affordable and adaptable way to complement formal healthcare practices [37]. Ran and colleagues [28], conducted a study to evaluate the effectiveness of the EpxDiabetes automated phone calls or text messages as an intervention for patients with type 2 diabetes. The study assessed patient engagement and changes in HbA1c levels between the intervention group and the control group. The study demonstrated that the EpxDiabetes intervention led to increased patient engagement, with 58% of the intervention group actively responding to $\geq 25\%$ of texts or calls over 4 weeks. This high level of engagement indicates that the delivery system design effectively reached and involved patients in their diabetes management. The intervention group showed an absolute reduction of 0.69% in HbA1c levels, particularly among patients with a baseline HbA1c level greater than 8%, where there was a significant decrease of 1.17%. In contrast, the control group had minimal HbA1c reductions. These findings highlight the effectiveness of the EpxDiabetes intervention in improving clinical outcomes, especially for patients with uncontrolled diabetes. The EpxDiabetes intervention's success in reducing HbA1c levels suggests that it promotes effective communication between patients and healthcare providers. This aligns with the delivery system design aspect of the Chronic Care Model, emphasizing the importance of well-organized, coordinated care delivery to achieve positive outcomes. Overall, Ran and colleagues' study showcases the value of a delivery system designed to facilitate automated communication with patients. It not only enhances patient engagement but also leads to significant improvements in clinical outcomes, particularly for those with uncontrolled diabetes. This approach aligns well with the Chronic Care Model's emphasis on organized, proactive care delivery to effectively manage chronic conditions [28].

3.2.5. Community Support

Community support connects patients to nearby resources and offers a chance for organizational leaders to forge new connections and broaden their reach. Within the eCCM framework, eHealth education is integrated as part of the eCommunity element, covering message training, health education, technology instruction, numeracy, literacy, usability, and security [19]. In the randomized two-arm parallel interventional study conducted by Omar and colleagues [29] over a 6-month period, a self-management education through social media network application (i.e., WhatsApp) was assessed. The study aimed to evaluate how a patient-centered diabetes education program, delivered via WhatsApp, influenced glycosylated hemoglobin (HbA1c) levels. Additionally, the research aimed to examine whether there was a correlation between health literacy, numeracy, and the outcomes of the intervention. This study aligns with the community support aspect of the Chronic Care Model by leveraging a social media network application (WhatsApp) to deliver diabetes self-management education. WhatsApp serves as a digital platform that can foster community-like interactions among participants. The use of WhatsApp for self-management education had a beneficial impact on glycemic control, as evidenced by a 0.7% reduction in HbA1c levels on average. This suggests that the intervention provided valuable support to individuals with diabetes in managing their condition. One noteworthy aspect is that the positive influence of social media on HbA1c levels remained consistent across patients with varying levels of health literacy and numeracy skills. This implies that the intervention was accessible and inclusive, addressing the needs of a diverse patient population. Overall, Omar et al.'s study demonstrates the potential of leveraging digital platforms like WhatsApp to provide community support for diabetes self-management. The positive impact on glycemic control, regardless of patients' literacy and numeracy skills, emphasizes the value of such interventions within the Chronic Care Model's community support framework [29].

3.2.6. Health Systems

The healthcare system establishes a context where organizational initiatives enhance patient care [25]. No studies were found that addressed the organization of healthcare and health systems.

3.3. Benefits and Barriers of Medication Adherence by Digital Health Technology 2

The second aim of this review was to determine the benefits and barriers of MA technology studied in adults with diabetes. Overall, the strongest benefit of digital health technologies to measure medication adherence involves patient engagement in diabetes and hypertension self-management through either one-way or two-way interactive reminders or educational information. Barriers to digital health technology for medication adherence in diabetes encompass limited smartphone access, staffing requirements, user engagement challenges, HbA1c level improvements, holiday season disruptions, digital literacy gaps, complex relationships between response rates and glucose levels, patient perceptions, message burden, scalability issues, time-limited interventions, age-related differences, one-way reminders, dietary maintenance difficulties, high costs, language and cultural barriers, legal concerns, patient experience, information access, low literacy (especially in the elderly), and training needs. The benefits and barriers are listed in Table 3.

Table 3. Benefits and barriers of digital health technology for medication adherence.

Study Author, Year	Digital Health Technology	Benefits	Barriers
Kleinman, N.J. et al., 2017 [26]	Gather app (m-Health diabetes platform)	• Improved medication adherence and blood glucose testing • Participants have high satisfaction for all aspects of the application	• The usage of smartphones is not among all the population • There should be an additional staff member, whose responsibilities will be to run the system in the hospitals • Users may become bored to using the application within the course of their treatment

Table 3. Cont.

Study Author, Year	Digital Health Technology	Benefits	Barriers
Huang, Z. et al., 2019 [27]	Medisafe app	• Improved medication adherence • Physician advocacy • Digital data collection	• No improvement in HbA1c levels • Holiday seasons impact • Digital literacy and usability
Xu, R. et al., 2020 [28]	EpxDiabetes	• Increased feeling of connection between patient-healthcare provider, which leads to better adherence to the therapy	• Complex relationship between response rate and fasting blood glucose • Patients' perception of benefit • Initial message burden before the adjustments • Scalability and physician feedback
Omar, M.A. et al., 2020 [29]	Self-management education through WhatsApp	• Improved glycemic control • Convenient access to Information • Effective communication • Inclusivity (regardless of literacy) • Higher engagement among younger • Cost-effective • Enhanced patient satisfaction	• Limited duration (6 months) • Age-related differences in response
Almer, A. et al., 2020 [30]	One-way automated short message service (OASMS)	• Reduction in HbA1c levels • Simplicity in messaging strategy • Potential impact on diabetes self-care • Enhanced patient satisfaction	• One-way reminders
Shamanna, P. et al., 2020 [31]	Digital Twin Technology-Enabled Precision Nutrition (TPN program)	• Personalized patient treatment • Precision nutrition guidance	• Patient experience difficulties in maintaining the low-calorie diet and the improvements cannot be maintained in the long-term
Katz, L.B. et al., 2022 [32]	OneTouch OT Verio Flex glucose meter	• The application is well tolerated within the underserved, low-numeracy, low-literacy population • Real time access of the patient data from the health care providers • The platform gives the opportunity of the health-care providers to make quick conclusions and decisions	• High expenses • Language and cultural barriers

Table 3. Cont.

Study Author, Year	Digital Health Technology	Benefits	Barriers
Lee, E.Y. et al., 2022 [33]	iCareD system	• High satisfaction of the participants from the iCareD program, which improves their self-care skills	• Age is a barrier to digital healthcare adoption
Orozco-Beltrán, D., Morales, C. et al., 2022 [34]	DeMpower app	• Improved metabolic control • Positive impact on HbA1c levels • Improved medication adherence	• Legal and logistical concerns • Patient experience and satisfaction • Information access
Al-Mutairi, A.M. et al., 2023 [35]	Telemedicine—virtual clinics	• Improvement in treatment satisfaction and glycemic control • Cost-effective solution	• Low literacy levels (elderly population)
Heald, A.H. et al., 2023 [36]	Healum Collaborative Care Planning Software and App	• Improved HbA1c levels • Improved patient self-reported QoL	• Digital literacy • Access to smartphones • Training and support needs

4. Discussion

4.1. Improvement of Medication Adherence Using Digital Health Technology

The results of this scoping review provide substantial evidence supporting the notion that digital health technology can significantly improve medication adherence among adults with diabetes. Several studies [26–28,30,32–36] demonstrated positive outcomes in terms of medication adherence through the use of various digital interventions. These interventions included mobile applications (e.g., Gather app, Medisafe app, iCareD system), SMS text messaging, telemonitoring, and tailored care management.

For instance, the Gather app [26] resulted in a substantial improvement in medication adherence, with a 39.0% adherence rate compared to 12.8% in the control group. Similarly, the EpxDiabetes intervention [28] led to increased patient engagement, with 58% of the intervention group actively responding to ≥25% of texts or calls over 4 weeks, and a significant reduction in HbA1c levels. The OneTouch OT Verio Flex glucose meter [32] demonstrated the effectiveness of the Spanish-language version of the OT Reveal mobile app in enhancing medication adherence and blood sugar control within an underserved Hispanic population.

The DeMpower app [34] showcased a noticeable trend toward improved metabolic control and medication adherence, with significant reductions in HbA1c levels. Furthermore, the Healdum Collaborative Care Planning Software and App [36] demonstrated improvements in HbA1c levels and patient-reported quality of life (QoL), highlighting the positive impact of digital interventions on medication adherence and overall well-being.

These findings collectively indicate that digital health technology can play a pivotal role in enhancing medication adherence among adults with diabetes, offering tailored solutions that range from reminders to self-monitoring tools, personalized care plans, and access to health information.

4.2. Other Similar Studies

In comparison to similar research studies, our scoping review contributes to the growing body of evidence supporting the use of digital health technology to improve medication adherence in diabetes patients. While previous reviews [38,39] have explored digital interventions' impact on medication adherence, our review utilizes the Chronic Care Model (CCM) framework to categorize and assess these interventions comprehensively. CCM-based interventions, even without digital tools, effectively enhance clinical, behavioral, psychological, and diabetic knowledge outcomes, including medication adherence in diabetes patients [40]. Malaysia has successfully implemented the CCM, leading to improved patient outcomes and enhanced practice-centered care delivery [41].

As digital health advances, technology has integrated medication adherence strategies for chronic conditions like diabetes [40,42–44]. The CCM has been applied to various chronic conditions such as asthma, bipolar disorder, breast cancer, diabetes, hypertension, and obesity [19–25,40–45].

This is a continuation of the integrative review performed by Conway et al. [37] which covered studies published in the period between January 2006 and October 2016. This review examined various digital health technologies aimed at improving medication adherence in adults aged 18 and older with diabetes type 1 and type 2. These technologies included IVR, SMS text messaging, telehealth, and web-based software. In some cases, interventions involved one-way communication to the patient or two-way communication between patients and healthcare providers, often involving the timely reporting of monitored results like blood glucose and blood pressure. The study found that digital health technologies were diverse, and the populations studied varied in size, ethnicity, and age range. There is considerable potential for further improving patient-provider communication through emerging mobile and electronic media, particularly in populations accustomed to mobile phones, tablets, and similar devices.

Overall, our review corroborates and expands upon existing research by categorizing digital interventions within the CCM framework, offering a structured perspective on how these interventions align with established models of chronic care and improve medication adherence in diabetes patients.

4.3. Limitations and Strengths of This Research

This research paper has several limitations that warrant consideration. Firstly, the inclusion criteria limited studies to those published in English between January 2017 and August 2023 which is the period after the research conducted by Conway et al. [37] which covered studies published in the period between January 2006 and October 2016. Consequently, relevant studies in other languages or published before this timeframe may have been omitted, potentially introducing language and publication bias.

Additionally, while efforts were made to identify studies focused on diabetes, the exclusion of pilot studies and those lacking data on medication adherence rates could have excluded valuable insights. Furthermore, the heterogeneity of interventions and outcome measures across the selected studies may limit the ability to make direct comparisons between interventions.

On the positive side, this research paper adhered to a structured scoping review methodology based on the CCM framework, providing a comprehensive overview of digital interventions for medication adherence in diabetes. By categorizing interventions within the CCM, this research paper offers a novel perspective on how digital solutions align with established models of chronic care.

The selected studies collectively contribute to the evidence base supporting the efficacy of digital health technology in improving medication adherence among adults with diabetes. The positive outcomes reported in terms of medication adherence, glycemic control, and patient satisfaction highlight the strengths of these interventions in enhancing diabetes care.

4.4. Future Research Directions

Future research directions in the field of digital health interventions for medication adherence for patients with diabetes encompass several key areas to enhance their effectiveness and accessibility. Diverse populations: Future research should explore the impact of digital health interventions on medication adherence in diverse populations, including those with varying levels of health literacy, numeracy, and cultural backgrounds. This will help ensure that interventions are accessible and effective for all segments of the population.

Long-term effects: Investigating the long-term effects of digital interventions on medication adherence and clinical outcomes is essential. Studies with extended follow-up periods can provide insights into the sustainability of improvements and potential challenges over time.

Integration with healthcare system: Future research should explore strategies for the seamless integration of digital health interventions into existing healthcare systems. This includes addressing issues related to scalability, healthcare provider feedback, and the coordination of care.

Comparative studies: Comparative studies that directly compare different types of digital interventions (e.g., mobile apps, SMS, telemonitoring) can help identify which approaches are most effective for improving medication adherence in specific patient populations.

Cost-effectiveness: Evaluating the cost-effectiveness of digital interventions is crucial for healthcare decision-makers. Future research should include economic analyses to assess the value of these interventions in relation to their impact on medication adherence and health outcomes.

Patient-centered research: Engaging patients in the design and evaluation of digital interventions is essential. Future studies should prioritize patient-centered research approaches to ensure that interventions align with patient preferences and needs.

5. Conclusions

In conclusion, digital health technology holds great promise for improving medication adherence in adults with diabetes. While this scoping review provides valuable insights into the effectiveness of these interventions, continued research is needed to further refine and optimize digital solutions to enhance medication adherence and, ultimately, the overall health and well-being of individuals living with diabetes.

Author Contributions: Conceptualization, N.G. and M.K.; formal analysis, N.G. and V.T.; writing—original draft, N.G.; writing—review and editing, M.K. and G.P.; supervision, M.K. and G.P.; project administration, N.G. and V.T.; funding acquisition, M.K. All authors have read and agreed to the published version of the manuscript.

Funding: This research was funded by financed by the European Union-NextGenerationEU, through the National Recovery and Resilience Plan of the Republic of Bulgaria, project № BG-RRP2.004-0004-C01.

Data Availability Statement: No new data were created or analyzed in this study. Data sharing is not applicable to this article.

Conflicts of Interest: The authors declare no conflict of interest.

Appendix A

Table A1. Diabetes Mellitus—Digital Solutions to Improve Medication Adherence: Integrative Review.

Autor, Year, (Country)	Sample, Intervention Length, Age and Study Purpose	Intervention	Medication Adherence Finding
Kleinman NJ et al., 2017 [26] (India) link	91 patients aged 18–65; 6 months. To assess the impact of an m-Health diabetes platform on clinical outcomes, patient-reported outcomes, patient and provider satisfaction, and app usage. RCT	Gather app (m-Health diabetes platform)	In the intervention group, more participants improved medication adherence (39.0% vs. 12.8%; $p = 0.03$) and increased blood glucose self-testing (39.0% vs. 10.3%) at 6 months. No other significant differences were observed.

Table A1. *Cont.*

Autor, Year, (Country)	Sample, Intervention Length, Age and Study Purpose	Intervention	Medication Adherence Finding
Huang Z et al., 2019 [27] (Singapore) Link	51 nonadherent and digitally literate patients with type 2 diabetes between the ages of 21 and 75 years, 12 weeks follow up. To determine the feasibility, acceptability, and clinical outcomes of using a smartphone app to improve medication adherence in a multiethnic Asian population with type 2 diabetes. RCT	Medisafe app	The intervention group had a lower post-study ASK-12 score. Medication adherence ranged from 38.3% to 100%, and most participants found the app easy to use.
Xu R et al., 2020 [28] (USA) link	65 patients, 6 months. To determine reduction of HbA1c and fasting blood glucose (FBG) among patients with type 2 diabetes mellitus (T2DM). RCT	EpxDiabetes	Intervention group saw a significant HbA1c reduction of 0.69%, especially for those with baseline HbA1c >8%. FBG decreased by 21.6 mg/dL in the intervention group. Engagement was 58% for the intervention and 48% for the control.
Alamer A et al., 2020 [30] (USA) Link	69 patients, ≥18 years; To evaluate the impact of diabetes self-care promoting messages via non-tailored one-way automated SMS (OASMS) on glycemic control in type 2 diabetes (T2DM). Observational	One-way automated short message service (OASMS)	ANCOVA model favored the intervention, showing an estimated HbA1c reduction difference of −0.97%. This suggests improved glycemic control in poorly controlled T2DM.
Shamanna P et al., 2020 [31] (India) link	64 patients, ≥18 years, 3 months follow up. To examine changes in hemoglobin A1c (HbA1c), anti-diabetic medication use, insulin resistance, and other ambulatory glucose profile metrics. Observational	Digital twin technology-enabled precision nutrition (TPN program)	Achieving a 1.9% HbA1c decrease, 6.1% weight loss, 56.9% reduction in HOMA-IR, reduced glucose time below range, and less diabetes medication use.
Omar MA et al., 2020 [29] (United Arab Emirates) link	218 patients (intervention and controlled group 109 each), aged ≥ 18, 6 months, To assess the effects on MA of self-management education through social media network application (i.e., WhatsApp). RCT	Self-management education through social media network application (i.e., WhatsApp)	After six months, HbA1c dropped significantly in the intervention group (7.7) compared to the control (8.4;). The intervention had a clinically significant reduction of 0.6%.
Laurence B Katz et al., 2022 [32] (Spain) link	81 subjects, aged ≥18, 6 months. To demonstrate the clinical value of OneTouch (OT) Verio Flex glucose meter used in combination with a Spanish-language version of the OT Reveal mobile application (app) to support diabetes care and improve glycemic control in an underserved Hispanic population with type 2 diabetes., RCT	OneTouch OT Verio Flex glucose meter	A significant 1.0% reduction in A1C was observed after 12 weeks, indicating improved glycemic control with the OT meter and app.

Table A1. Cont.

Autor, Year, (Country)	Sample, Intervention Length, Age and Study Purpose	Intervention	Medication Adherence Finding
Lee EY et al., 2022 [33] (China) Link	234 patients, ≥18 years, 6 months, to assess the effect of an electronic medical record-integrated mobile app for personalized diabetes self-care, focusing on the self-monitoring of blood glucose and lifestyle modifications, on glycemic control, RCT	iCareD system	At 12 weeks, HbA1c levels differed significantly among groups. HbA1c levels showed a statistically significant decrease after the intervention (UC vs. MC vs. MPC: −0.49% vs. −0.86% vs. −1.04%;).
Orozco-Beltrán D, Morales C et al., 2022 [34] (Spain) Link	50 patients, aged ≥ 18 and ≤80 years, observational: 52 weeks of follow-up and interventional: 52 weeks of follow-up, to analyze the effect of a home digital patient empowerment and communication tool (DeMpower App) on metabolic control in people with inadequately controlled T2DM, Observational	DeMpower app	The DeMpower app group showed a significant trend toward achieving glycemic targets, particularly HbA1c ≤ 7.5% and HbA1c ≤ 8%. Mean HbA1c was significantly reduced at week 24.
Al-Mutairi AM et al., 2023 [35] (Saudi Arabia) Link	4266 patients, aged ≥ 18, 3 months, to investigate the impact telemedicine had during this period on glycemic control (HbA1c) in patients with T2DM, RCT	Telemedicine—virtual clinics	In 24.9% of the patients HbA1c decreased by ≥0.5%, 36.9% of the patients whose HbA1c increased by ≥0.5% and 38.2% whose HbA1c changed by <0.5% in either direction. More males had significant improvements in glycemia compared to females (28.1% vs. 22.8%), as were individuals below the age of 60 years (28.1% vs. 22.5%). Hypertensive individuals were less likely than non-hypertensive to have glycemic improvement (23.7% vs. 27.9%). More patients on sulfonylureas had improvements in HbA1c (42.3% vs. 37.9%, whereas patients on insulin had higher HbA1c (62.7% vs. 56.2%). Patient groups exhibited varying changes in HbA1c, with notable gender and age differences. Hypertensive patients were less likely to have glycemic improvement, while medication types played a role.
Heald AH et al., 2023, [36] (UK) link	197 patients, aged ≥ 18, 6 months, to evaluate whether personalized care planning software and a patient-facing mobile app could improve health outcomes amongst patients with T2D through the delivery of personalized plans of care, support and education to allow patients to self-manage their diabetes more effectively, all accessible on a mobile device, RCT	Healum Collaborative Care Planning Software and App	The active treatment group had significant reductions in HbA1c (− 7.4%) and BMI (− 0.7%) compared to the control group (−0.2%). A higher percentage of the active treatment group improved their HbA1c and BMI, and quality of life also improved by an average of 0.0464.

References

1. Merck, S.F. Chronic Disease and Mobile Technology: An Innovative Tool for Clinicians. *Nurs. Forum.* **2017**, *52*, 298–305. [CrossRef]
2. Bernardo, C.; Tosin, M.H.S.; Almada, M.; Sampaio, R.; Oliveira, B.G.R.B.; Costa, E.; Vrijens, B.; Alves da Costa, F. Translation and cross-cultural adaptation of the ABC taxonomy for medication adherence into Portuguese—Updating patients into people. *Res. Soc. Adm. Pharm.* **2023**, *19*, 653–659. [CrossRef]
3. Haag, M.; Lehmann, A.; Hersberger, K.E.; Schneider, M.P.; Gauchet, A.; Vrijens, B.; Arnet, I.; Allenet, B. The ABC taxonomy for medication adherence translated into French and German. *Br. J. Clin. Pharmacol.* **2020**, *86*, 734–744. [CrossRef] [PubMed]
4. Vrijens, B.; De Geest, S.; Hughes, D.A.; Przemyslaw, K.; Demonceau, J.; Ruppar, T.; Dobbels, F.; Fargher, E.; Morrison, V.; Lewek, P.; et al. ABC Project Team A new taxonomy for describing and defining adherence to medications. *Br. J. Clin. Pharmacol.* **2012**, *73*, 691–705. [CrossRef] [PubMed]
5. Osterberg, L.; Blaschke, T. Adherence to medication. *N. Engl. J. Med.* **2005**, *353*, 487–497. [CrossRef]
6. Lehane, E.; McCarthy, G. Intentional and unintentional medication non-adherence: A comprehensive framework for clinical research and practice? A discussion paper. *Int. J. Nurs. Stud.* **2007**, *44*, 1468–1477. [CrossRef]
7. IDF Diabetes Atlas. Available online: https://diabetesatlas.org/ (accessed on 23 August 2023).
8. Krass, I.; Schieback, P.; Dhippayom, T. Adherence to diabetes medication: A systematic review. *Diabet. Med.* **2015**, *32*, 725–737. [CrossRef] [PubMed]
9. Jaam, M.; Awaisu, A.; Ibrahim, M.I.; Kheir, N. Synthesizing and Appraising the Quality of the Evidence on Factors Associated with Medication Adherence in Diabetes: A Systematic Review of Systematic Reviews. *Value Health Reg. Issues* **2017**, *13*, 82–91. [CrossRef]
10. Khunti, K.; Seidu, S.; Kunutsor, S.; Davies, M. Association Between Adherence to Pharmacotherapy and Outcomes in Type 2 Diabetes: A Meta-analysis. *Diabetes Care* **2017**, *40*, 1588–1596. [CrossRef]
11. Egede, L.E.; Gebregziabher, M.; Dismuke, C.E.; Lynch, C.P.; Axon, R.N.; Zhao, Y.; Mauldin, P.D. Medication Nonadherence in Diabetes: Longitudinal effects on costs and potential cost savings from improvement. *Diabetes Care* **2012**, *35*, 2533–2539. [CrossRef]
12. Polonsky, W.H.; Henry, R.R. Poor medication adherence in type 2 diabetes: Recognizing the scope of the problem and its key contributors. *Patient Prefer. Adherence* **2016**, *10*, 1299–1307. [CrossRef] [PubMed]
13. Currie, C.J.; Peyrot, M.; Morgan, C.L.; Poole, C.D.; Jenkins-Jones, S.; Rubin, R.R.; Burton, C.M.; Evans, M. The impact of treatment noncompliance on mortality in people with type 2 diabetes. *Diabetes Care* **2012**, *35*, 1279–1284. [CrossRef] [PubMed]
14. Sherman, L.D.; Grande, S.W. Building better clinical relationships with patients: An argument for digital health solutions with black men. *Health Serv. Insights* **2019**, *12*, 1–4. [CrossRef] [PubMed]
15. Egede, L.E.; Gebregziabher, M.; Echols, C.; Lynch, C.P. Longitudinal effects of medication nonadherence on glycemic control. *Ann. Pharmacother.* **2014**, *48*, 562–570. [CrossRef] [PubMed]
16. DiBonaventura, M.; Wintfeld, N.; Huang, J.; Goren, A. The association between nonadherence and glycated hemoglobin among type 2 diabetes patients using basal insulin analogs. *Patient Prefer. Adherence* **2014**, *8*, 873–882. [CrossRef]
17. Ho, P.M.; Rumsfeld, J.S.; Masoudi, F.A.; McClure, D.L.; Plomondon, M.E.; Steiner, J.F.; Magid, D.J. Effect of medication nonadherence on hospitalization and mortality among patients with diabetes mellitus. *Arch. Intern. Med.* **2006**, *166*, 1836–1841. [CrossRef]
18. Whittemore, R.; Knafl, K. The integrative review: Updated methodology. *J. Adv. Nurs.* **2005**, *52*, 546–553. [CrossRef]
19. Gee, P.M.; Greenwood, D.A.; Paterniti, D.A.; Ward, D.; Miller, L.M. The eHealth Enhanced Chronic Care Model: A theory derivation approach. *J. Med. Internet Res.* **2015**, *17*, e86. [CrossRef]
20. Wagner, E.H. Chronic disease management: What will it take to improve care for chronic illness? *Eff. Clin. Pract.* **1998**, *1*, 2–4.
21. Grover, A.; Joshi, A. An overview of chronic disease models: A systematic literature review. *Glob. J. Health Sci.* **2014**, *7*, 210–227. [CrossRef]
22. Wagner, E.H. Academia, chronic care, and the future of primary care. *J. Gen. Intern. Med.* **2010**, *25*, 636–638. [CrossRef] [PubMed]
23. Wagner, E.H.; Austin, B.T.; Davis, C.; Hindmarsh, M.; Schaefer, J.; Bonomi, A. Improving chronic illness care: Translating evidence into action. *Health Aff. (Proj. Hope)* **2001**, *20*, 64–78. [CrossRef] [PubMed]
24. Bodenheimer, T.; Wagner, E.H.; Grumbach, K. Improving primary care for patients with chronic illness. *JAMA* **2002**, *288*, 1909–1914. [CrossRef] [PubMed]
25. Gugiu, P.C.; Westine, C.D.; Coryn, C.L.; Hobson, K.A. An application of a new evidence grading system to research on the chronic care model. *Eval. Health Prof.* **2013**, *36*, 3–43. [CrossRef] [PubMed]
26. Kleinman, N.J.; Shah, A.; Shah, S.; Phatak, S.; Viswanathan, V. Improved Medication Adherence and Frequency of Blood Glucose Self-Testing Using an m-Health Platform Versus Usual Care in a Multisite Randomized Clinical Trial Among People with Type 2 Diabetes in India. *Telemed. J. E Health* **2017**, *23*, 733–740. [CrossRef]
27. Huang, Z.; Tan, E.; Lum, E.; Sloot, P.; Boehm, B.O.; Car, J. A Smartphone App to Improve Medication Adherence in Patients With Type 2 Diabetes in Asia: Feasibility Randomized Controlled Trial. *JMIR Mhealth Uhealth* **2019**, *7*, e14914. [CrossRef]
28. Xu, R.; Xing, M.; Javaherian, K.; Peters, R.; Ross, W.; Bernal-Mizrachi, C. Improving HbA1c with Glucose Self-Monitoring in Diabetic Patients with EpxDiabetes, a Phone Call and Text Message-Based Telemedicine Platform: A Randomized Controlled Trial. *Telemed. J. E Health* **2020**, *26*, 784–793. [CrossRef] [PubMed]

29. Omar, M.A.; Hasan, S.; Palaian, S.; Mahameed, S. The impact of a self-management educational program coordinated through WhatsApp on diabetes control. *Pharm. Pract.* **2020**, *18*, 1841. [CrossRef]
30. Alamer, A.; Palm, C.; Almulhim, A.S.; Te, C.; Pendergrass, M.L.; Fazel, M.T. Impact of Non-Tailored One-Way Automated Short Messaging Service (OASMS) on Glycemic Control in Type 2 Diabetes: A Retrospective Feasibility Study. *Int. J. Environ. Res. Public Health* **2020**, *17*, 7590. [CrossRef]
31. Shamanna, P.; Saboo, B.; Damodharan, S.; Mohammed, J.; Mohamed, M.; Poon, T.; Kleinman, N.; Thajudeen, M. Reducing HbA1c in Type 2 Diabetes Using Digital Twin Technology-Enabled Precision Nutrition: A Retrospective Analysis. *Diabetes Ther.* **2020**, *11*, 2703–2714. [CrossRef]
32. Katz, L.B.; Aparicio, M.; Cameron, H.; Ceppa, F. Use of a Meter With Color-Range Indicators and a Mobile Diabetes Management App Improved Glycemic Control and Patient Satisfaction in an Underserved Hispanic Population: "Tu Salud"—A Randomized Controlled Partial Cross-Over Clinical Study. *Diabetes Spectr.* **2022**, *35*, 86–94. [CrossRef]
33. Lee, E.Y.; Cha, S.A.; Yun, J.S.; Lim, S.Y.; Lee, J.H.; Ahn, Y.B.; Yoon, K.H.; Hyun, M.K.; Ko, S.H. Efficacy of Personalized Diabetes Self-care Using an Electronic Medical Record-Integrated Mobile App in Patients With Type 2 Diabetes: 6-Month Randomized Controlled Trial. *J. Med. Internet Res.* **2022**, *24*, e37430. [CrossRef]
34. Orozco-Beltrán, D.; Morales, C.; Artola-Menéndez, S.; Brotons, C.; Carrascosa, S.; González, C.; Baro, Ó.; Aliaga, A.; Ferreira de Campos, K.; Villarejo, M.; et al. Effects of a Digital Patient Empowerment and Communication Tool on Metabolic Control in People With Type 2 Diabetes: The DeMpower Multicenter Ambispective Study. *JMIR Diabetes.* **2022**, *7*, e40377. [CrossRef] [PubMed]
35. Al-Mutairi, A.M.; Alshabeeb, M.A.; Abohelaika, S.; Alomar, F.A.; Bidasee, K.R. Impact of telemedicine on glycemic control in type 2 diabetes mellitus during the COVID-19 lockdown period. *Front. Endocrinol.* **2023**, *14*, 1068018. [CrossRef] [PubMed]
36. Heald, A.H.; Roberts, S.; Albeda Gimeno, L.; Gilingham, E.; James, M.; White, A.; Saboo, A.; Beresford, L.; Crofts, A.; Abraham, J. A Randomised Control Trial to Explore the Impact and Efficacy of the Healum Collaborative Care Planning Software and App on Condition Management in the Type 2 Diabetes Mellitus Population in NHS Primary Care. *Diabetes Ther.* **2023**, *14*, 977–988. [CrossRef] [PubMed]
37. Conway, C.M.; Kelechi, T.J. Digital Health for Medication Adherence in Adult Diabetes or Hypertension: An Integrative Review. *JMIR Diabetes* **2017**, *2*, e20. [CrossRef]
38. Zaki, S.; Sharma, S.; Vats, S. Digital Health Technologies for Type 2 diabetes Management: A Systematic Review. In Proceedings of the International Conference on Recent Advances in Electrical, Electronics & Digital Healthcare Technologies (REEDCON), New Delhi, India, 1–3 May 2023; pp. 127–132. [CrossRef]
39. Keidong, H.; Volmer, D. Improved medication adherence with smart applications and medication dispensers—A literature review. *Acta Pol. Pharm. Drug Res.* **2022**, *79*, 451–454. [CrossRef]
40. Piatt, G.A.; Orchard, T.J.; Emerson, S.; Simmons, D.; Songer, T.J.; Brooks, M.M.; Korytkowski, M.; Siminerio, L.M.; Ahmad, U.; Zgibor, J.C. Translating the chronic care model into the community: Results from a randomized controlled trial of a multifaceted diabetes care intervention. *Diabetes Care* **2006**, *29*, 811–817. [CrossRef]
41. Hussein, Z.; Taher, S.W.; Gilcharan Singh, H.K.; Chee Siew Swee, W. Diabetes care in Malaysia: Problems, new models, and solutions. *Ann. Glob. Health* **2015**, *81*, 851–862. [CrossRef]
42. Gabbay, R.A.; Lendel, I.; Saleem, T.M.; Shaeffer, G.; Adelman, A.M.; Mauger, D.T.; Collins, M.; Polomano, R.C. Nurse case management improves blood pressure, emotional distress and diabetes complication screening. *Diabetes Res. Clin. Pract.* **2006**, *71*, 28–35. [CrossRef]
43. Green, B.B.; Cook, A.J.; Ralston, J.D.; Fishman, P.A.; Catz, S.L.; Carlson, J.; Carrell, D.; Tyll, L.; Larson, E.B.; Thompson, R.S. Effectiveness of home blood pressure monitoring, Web communication, and pharmacist care on hypertension control: A randomized controlled trial. *JAMA* **2008**, *299*, 2857–2867. [CrossRef] [PubMed]
44. Shojania, K.G.; Ranji, S.R.; McDonald, K.M.; Grimshaw, J.M.; Sundaram, V.; Rushakoff, R.J.; Owens, D.K. Effects of quality improvement strategies for type 2 diabetes on glycemic control: A meta-regression analysis. *JAMA* **2006**, *296*, 427–440. [CrossRef] [PubMed]
45. Yeoh, E.K.; Wong, M.C.S.; Wong, E.L.Y.; Yam, C.; Poon, C.M.; Chung, R.Y.; Chong, M.; Fang, Y.; Wang, H.H.X.; Liang, M.; et al. Benefits and limitations of implementing Chronic Care Model (CCM) in primary care programs: A systematic review. *Int. J. Cardiol.* **2018**, *258*, 279–288. [CrossRef] [PubMed]

Disclaimer/Publisher's Note: The statements, opinions and data contained in all publications are solely those of the individual author(s) and contributor(s) and not of MDPI and/or the editor(s). MDPI and/or the editor(s) disclaim responsibility for any injury to people or property resulting from any ideas, methods, instructions or products referred to in the content.

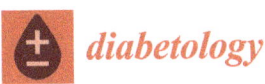

Brief Report

Educating Medical Students on How to Prescribe Anti-Hyperglycaemic Drugs: A Practical Guide

Erik M. Donker [1,2,*,†], Andrej Belančić [3,4,*,†], Joost D. Piët [1,2], Dinko Vitezić [3,4,‡], Jelle Tichelaar [1,2,5,‡] and on behalf of the Clinical Pharmacology and Therapeutics Teach the Teacher (CP4T) Program and the Early Career Pharmacologists of the European Association for Clinical Pharmacology and Therapeutics (EACPT)

[1] Unit Pharmacotherapy, Department of Internal Medicine, Amsterdam UMC, Vrije Universiteit, de Boelelaan 1117, 1081 HV Amsterdam, The Netherlands; j.piet@amsterdamumc.nl (J.D.P.); j.tichelaar@amsterdamumc.nl (J.T.)
[2] Research and Expertise Centre in Pharmacotherapy Education (RECIPE), de Boelelaan 1117, 1081 HV Amsterdam, The Netherlands
[3] Department of Clinical Pharmacology, Clinical Hospital Centre Rijeka, Krešimirova 42, 51000 Rijeka, Croatia; dvitezic@gmail.com
[4] Department of Basic and Clinical Pharmacology with Toxicology, Faculty of Medicine, University of Rijeka, Braće Branchetta 20, 51000 Rijeka, Croatia
[5] Interprofessional Collaboration and Medication Safety at the Faculty of Health, Sports and Social Work, Inholland University of Applied Sciences, de Boelelaan 1109, 1817 MN Amsterdam, The Netherlands
* Correspondence: e.donker@amsterdamumc.nl (E.M.D.); a.belancic93@gmail.com (A.B.)
† These authors contributed equally to this work.
‡ These authors contributed equally to this work.

Abstract: In the light of the rapidly increasing global incidence of, and therapeutic arsenal for, diabetes type 2, this brief report underscores the need for advancements in clinical pharmacology and therapeutics (CPT) education with regard to diabetes type 2. We advocate for the comprehensive training of medical students and junior doctors in line with current guidelines, and emphasize the importance of teaching how to draw up individualized treatment plans based on patients' specific risk factors and conditions, such as cardiovascular risks, weight, and risk of hypoglycaemia. Within the curriculum, traditional teaching approaches should be replaced by innovative methods such as problem-based learning, which has been shown to be more effective in developing prescribing knowledge and skills. The inclusion of real-world experience and interprofessional learning via so-called student-run clinics is also recommended. Subsequently, innovative assessment methods like the European Prescribing Exam and objective structured clinical examinations (OSCE) are highlighted as essential for evaluating knowledge and practical skills. By adopting these educational advances, medical education can better equip future practitioners to adequately manage the complex pharmacological treatment of diabetes.

Keywords: education; clinical pharmacology and therapeutics; undergraduate; postgraduate

1. Introduction

Diabetes mellitus is a disease with a high global health burden [1]. With the alarming surge in people who are overweight and obese (with the latter encompassing 13% or 650 million people globally), more than 500 million individuals are currently diagnosed with diabetes type 2, and it is estimated that more than 1.3 billion people will have the disease by 2050 [1–3]. Diabetes type 2 is accompanied by a spectrum of associated health complications, such as microvascular (e.g., nephropathy, retinopathy, and neuropathy) and macrovascular diseases [4,5]. These complications significantly diminish patients' quality of life and increase the cost of healthcare, which affects high-, middle-, and low-income nations alike [6]. Consequently, there is an urgent need for better preventive strategies, optimal medicinal interventions, and more effective patient education.

Recent years have seen an increase in the number of therapeutic agents available for diabetes management, such as sodium-glucose cotransporter-2 (SGLT2) inhibitors, glucagon-like peptide-1 (GLP-1) receptor agonists, and dual glucose-dependent insulinotropic polypeptide (GIP) and glucagon-like peptide-1 (GLP-1) receptor agonists. This growing therapeutic arsenal makes prescribing challenging, especially for junior doctors who write out most hospital prescriptions, often without direct supervision [7,8]. Worryingly, studies suggest that junior doctors are responsible for the majority of prescribing errors [7–9], which can in part be explained by their limited prescribing competence early in their career [10–14], which do not improve in the year after graduation [11]. This highlights the need for improved teaching and training in prescribing for both medical students and junior doctors.

In this commentary, we focus on salient aspects of education in clinical pharmacology and therapeutics (CPT) with regard to diabetes type 2, one of the diseases considered essential in prescribing education [15]. We make a plea for efficacious pedagogical and assessment strategies, which may in turn help teaching professionals to update medical curricula, especially CPT modules and internal medicine [16].

2. What to Teach

First, although self-evident, it is essential to underscore the importance of a thorough education on diabetes type 2 and its management with anti-hyperglycaemic agents, based on the most recent (inter)national guidelines and evidence-based medicine, such as the guidelines jointly established by the American Diabetes Association (ADA) and the European Association for the Study of Diabetes (EASD) [17]. While we will not discuss these aspects further here, it is essential that students have a comprehensive understanding of the aetiology, pathophysiology, diagnostic criteria, evaluation, and potential complications and comorbidities associated with diabetes. Students need to learn that the initial approach to treating diabetes type 2 hinges on lifestyle recommendations, with an emphasis on factors such as physical activity, a balanced diet, weight management, smoking cessation, and limited alcohol consumption [18].

Students must be familiar with the distinct classes of drugs available for the treatment of diabetes (e.g., biguanides, thiazolidinediones, α-glucosidase inhibitors, sulfonylurea derivatives, glinides, SGLT2 inhibitors, DPP-4 inhibitors, GLP-1 receptor agonists, dual GIP and GLP-1 receptor agonists, and insulin). Table 1 gives the key pharmacodynamic attributes of each drug class, highlighting potential benefits/concerns, prevalent or perilous adverse events, and contraindications. Broadly speaking, when prescribing anti-hyperglycaemic agents, prescribers must be cognizant of differences in drug efficacy/effectiveness (where efficacy is based on randomized controlled trial data and effectiveness on real-word experience), particularly with respect to lowering HbA1c levels, fluctuations in weight, and the risk of hypoglycaemia. For example, weight reduction is associated with better outcomes in terms of metabolic and glycaemic control, disease-modifying effects, cardiometabolic disease, and quality of life determinants [19]. Drug–drug interactions are reported in the Summary of Product Characteristics (SmPC) of all individual drugs. In general, two important interactions are those of drugs associated with a high risk of causing hypoglycaemia given in combination with drugs that can mask the symptoms of hypoglycaemia (e.g., the beta-blocker propranolol) or drugs that can worsen glycaemic control (e.g., corticosteroids) [20,21].

Equipped with the foundational knowledge outlined above, students should be able to understand and implement current (local) guidelines. This proficiency should empower them to write specific prescriptions tailored to the individual patient (i.e., desired drug with correct dosage). A pivotal understanding they must internalize is the difference in treatment strategies for patients with or without a high risk of cardiovascular disease. Notably, SGLT2-inhibitors (i.e., empagliflozin and canagliflozin) and GLP-1 receptor agonists (e.g., semaglutide, liraglutide and dulaglutide) have demonstrated additional efficacy in reducing major adverse cardiovascular events (MACE) in patients at high cardiovascular risk (e.g., those with a stroke or myocardial infarction in their medical history) [17]. Furthermore, students should base their decision-making on a comprehensive risk/benefit assessment, selecting the optimal therapeutic strategy tailored to the circumstances of an individual patient, such as treating professional drivers with drugs that carry a low risk of hypoglycaemia, considering alternatives to insulin for patients with a needle phobia, or opting for gliclazide 80 mg extended-release tablets for patients with irregular eating patterns, instead of 30 mg extended-release tablets. Moreover, when the most appropriate drug therapy is chosen, students have to be knowledgeable about what information should be provided to the patient (with or without a consultation with a pharmacist), and what the correct follow-up management approach is. Although beyond the scope of this paper, students should also be taught about the cardiovascular risk factors associated with diabetes and their treatment, such as hypertension (e.g., preferably renin–angiotensin system inhibitors in patient with diabetes) [22], and hypercholesterolemia (e.g., statins) [23].

Table 1. Overview of anti-hyperglycaemic drug classes with potential benefits and risks.

Anti-Hyperglycaemic Class	Pharmacodynamics	Efficacy *	Safety Profile **	Hypoglycaemic Risk	Weight Change ***	Potential Cardio-Renal Benefits	Contraindications/Special Considerations	Costs
Biguanides	- Inhibition of gluconeogenesis and glycogenolysis - Increase in insulin sensitivity - Delay in the absorption of glucose in the small intestine	++	- GI ADRs - Lactic acidosis	Low	↔	MACE: potential benefit	- Acute metabolic acidosis - eGFR < 30 mL/min - Decompensated heart failure, recent myocardial infarction, shock - Hepatic insufficiency	Low
Thiazolidinediones ****	- PPAR-γ activation	++	- Oedema - Congestive heart failure - Hepatogram alteration	Low	↑	MACE: potential benefit HF: increased risk	- (History of) heart failure - Hepatic insufficiency - Existing or recovered bladder cancer	Low
α-gluconidase inhibitors	- Inhibition of intestinal α-glucosidase	+	- GI ADRs	Low	↔	Neutral	- Inflammatory bowel disease - Colon ulceration - Partial bowel obstruction - Hepatic insufficiency - eGFR <30 mL/min	Low
Sulfonylurea derivates	- β-cytotropic drugs (glucose-independent stimulation)	++	- Hypoglycaemia - GI ADRs - Skin and subcutaneous tissue disorders	High	↑	Neutral	- C-peptide negative DM - Hepatic insufficiency - Severe impairment of renal function (≥G3b); does not apply for gliquidone (dose adjustment per renal function not needed)	Low
Glinides	- β-cytotropic drugs (glucose-independent stimulation)	++	- Hypoglycaemia - GI ADRs	Intermediate	↑	Neutral	- C-peptide-negative DM - Hepatic insufficiency	Low
SGLT2 inhibitors	- Competitive inhibition of SGLT2; renal mechanism	+(+)	- Urinary tract infection - Genital infection - Polyuria, pollakisuria, volume depletion - Euglycaemic ketoacidosis (rare) - Fournier gangrene (extremely rare)	Low	↓	MACE: benefit for canagliflozin and empagliflozin HF: benefit for dapagliflozin and empagliflozin DKD: benefit for canagliflozin, dapagliflozin and empagliflozin	- Recurrent urinary infections Considerations: - Euglycaemic ketoacidosis (rare) - Fournier gangrene (extremely rare)	High

Table 1. Cont.

Anti-hyperglycaemic Class	Pharmacodynamics	Efficacy *	Safety Profile **	Hypoglycaemic Risk	Weight Change ***	Potential Cardio-Renal Benefits	Contraindications/Special Considerations	Costs
DPP-4 inhibitors	- β-cytotropic drugs (glucose-dependent stimulation); - ↑insulin/glucagon ratio	+	- Very good safety profile and tolerability - ADRs are occasional and not typical	No	↔	HF: potential risk of saxaglitptin	- Consider discontinuation in case of acute pancreatitis	High
GLP-1 receptor agonists	- β-cytotropic drugs (glucose-dependent stimulation); - ↑insulin/glucagon ratio	++(+)	- GI ADRs	No	↓(↓)	MACE: benefit for dulaglutide, liraglutide and semaglutide DKD: potential benefit for dulaglutide, liraglutide, and semaglutide (secondary outcomes)	- Gastroparesis - Consider discontinuation in case of acute pancreatitis	High
Insulin (human and analogues)	- Tyrosine kinase receptor activation	++(+)	- Hypoglycaemia - Lipodystrophy - Somogyi effect - Injection site reactions	High	↑	Neutral	- Injection site reactions - Higher risk of hypoglycaemia with human insulin vs. analogues	High

* + Intermediate (HbA1c↓ 0.5–1.0%), ++ High (HbA1c↓ 1.0–1.5%), +++ Super high (HbA1c↓ >1.5%); ** Check the Summary of Product Characteristics for information regarding individual ADR frequency; *** ↓↓ high loss, ↓ loss, ↔ neutral, ↑ gain; **** Benefit in non-alcoholic fatty liver disease and non-alcoholic steatohepatitis. PPAR-γ Peroxisome proliferator-activated receptor gamma; SGLT2 sodium-glucose cotransporter-2; DPP-4 dipeptidyl peptidase 4; GLP-1 glucagon-like peptide-1; GI gastrointestinal; ADR adverse drug reaction; MACE major adverse cardiovascular events; HF Heart failure; DKD diabetic/chronic kidney disease; eGFR estimated glomerular filtration rate; DM Diabetes Mellitus.

The economic dimensions of care, encompassing both the direct costs of medications and the nuances of national or local health insurance reimbursement, are also important within diabetes education, and students should understand this. The general principle is that newer anti-hyperglycaemic drugs are more expensive than older drugs. In the Netherlands, for example, the cost of one tablet of metformin (500 mg) is EUR 0.02 compared with that of EUR 23.84 for one injection of semaglutide (0.25 mg) [24].

Lastly, students need to learn how to interpret new findings and information. They need to become well versed in the principles of evidence-based medicine and understand the distinctions between primary and secondary outcomes (e.g., secondary outcomes often lack sufficient power). In diabetes research, cardiovascular outcomes (MACEs) have often been a secondary concern, despite the recommendations of the Food and Drug Administration and the European Medicines Agency.

In summary, we advocate that students should be able to draw up an individualized therapeutic strategy for patients with diabetes, with a view to achieving the glycaemic target and reducing the risk of cardiovascular disease. The treatment plan should provide clear information about the medication, its route of administration, correct dosage, and any adjustments made on the basis of renal or hepatic function, patient preferences, age, concurrent health conditions, co-administered drugs, frailty, and cost implications.

3. How to Teach

Traditional teaching methods have focused on lectures and self-study, methods that are still common in European universities [25]. However, emerging pedagogical strategies provide innovative alternatives for teaching and training CPT. For instance, problem-based learning has proven more effective than traditional methods in equipping medical students with prescribing knowledge and skills [26–29]. The problem-based approach, in combination with the effective World Health Organisation (WHO)'s six-step model which is currently under revision [30–33], is designed to foster active and collaborative learning by situating learning in real-world contexts or problems [34,35]. For instance, students can learn about anti-hyperglycaemic agents in small group-based discussions of real or hypothetical cases. This approach is particularly effective in the bachelor phase [26]. Supplementary Materials File S1 gives an example case that can be used for such discussions. More cases can be found on the European Open Platform for Prescribing Education (https://www.prescribingeducation.eu/, accessed on 6 November 2023) [36].

The learning context is also important for improving educational outcomes [37]. An enriched learning context, such as one incorporating responsibilities for patient care, significantly improves the prescribing competence of medical students. Competence also improves when students move from studying case-based scenarios to analysing real patient records and preparing for therapeutic consultations [38]. Carrying out real-life consultations helps students to refine their prescription writing abilities. While real-life teaching should be available in the master's degree phase at the latest, it is more effective if it is incorporated during the bachelor's degree phase via, for example, so-called student-run clinics (SRC), which have proven effective in increasing the prescribing competence of medical students [39–44]. In SRCs, students have early exposure to prescribing and taking on authentic patient care responsibilities while assisting physicians in their prescribing tasks [45,46]. SRCs for diabetes management are already available in the United States [46–48], and a SRC for cardiovascular risk management has proven beneficial to patients, students, and general practitioners in the Netherlands [43].

Furthermore, we believe that the interprofessional nature of clinical practice should be mirrored in CPT education. Typically, in diabetes management, the healthcare team comprises different professionals, such as physicians, specialist nurses, and pharmacists. Promoting interprofessional learning in (pre-)clinical stages could help students to understand the role of other health professionals, which might facilitate better interprofessional collaboration in the future. SRCs are a feasible way to incorporate this interprofessional learning [41,44].

Lastly, it is essential to assess students' knowledge and skills regarding the safe and effective prescription of anti-hyperglycaemic drugs. This assessment should not only include theoretical knowledge (e.g., contraindications and interactions) but also practical skills, such as the ability to prescribe or conduct therapeutic consultations. Standardized examinations such as the European Prescribing Exam (https://www.prescribingeducation.eu/, accessed on 6 November 2023) are suitable for assessing both knowledge and the ability to prescribe [49], while objective structured clinical examinations (OSCE) can effectively gauge practical skills [50,51]. Diabetes management is one of the eight main topics of the European Prescribing Exam and is assessed on all levels of Miller's pyramid [49]. OSCEs encourage students' deeper understanding of diabetes management and the reasons why they choose a specific drug.

In summary, CPT education must evolve to incorporate problem-based learning, hands-on experience, and interprofessional collaboration. This will help to prepare medical students better for the demands of their future roles, particularly regarding the prescription of critical therapeutics such as anti-hyperglycaemic drugs.

4. Conclusions and Future Direction

In conclusion, CPT education on diabetes management must evolve to align it with current guidelines, to emphasize the need for a comprehensive understanding of the disease, and to encourage students to make tailored treatment plans. Problem-based learning, real-world experience, and interprofessional learning should shape teaching strategies, preparing students to navigate the complexity of prescribing anti-hyperglycaemic agents in clinical practice. Innovative assessment methods, including the European Prescribing Exam and OSCEs, are crucial to the evaluation of knowledge and practical skills. By embracing these advances, educational institutions can empower (future) healthcare practitioners to effectively manage the pharmacological treatment of diabetes.

Supplementary Materials: The following supporting information can be downloaded at: https://www.mdpi.com/article/10.3390/diabetology4040043/s1, File S1: Example case.

Author Contributions: Conceptualization, E.M.D., A.B. and on behalf of the Clinical Pharmacology and Therapeutics Teach the Teacher (CP4T) Program and the Early Career Pharmacologists of the European Association for Clinical Pharmacology and Therapeutics (EACPT); writing—original draft preparation, E.M.D., A.B. and J.D.P.; writing—review and editing, all authors; visualization, E.M.D. and A.B.; supervision, D.V. and J.T. All authors have read and agreed to the published version of the manuscript.

Funding: This work was supported by Erasmus +, grant number 2022-1-NL01-KA220-HED-000088069.

Institutional Review Board Statement: Not applicable.

Informed Consent Statement: Not applicable.

Data Availability Statement: Not applicable.

Conflicts of Interest: The authors declare no conflict of interest.

References

1. GBD 2021 Diabetes Collaborators. Global, regional, and national burden of diabetes from 1990 to 2021, with projections of prevalence to 2050: A systematic analysis for the Global Burden of Disease Study 2021. *Lancet* **2023**, *402*, 203–234. [CrossRef] [PubMed]
2. Sun, H.; Saeedi, P.; Karuranga, S.; Pinkepank, M.; Ogurtsova, K.; Duncan, B.B.; Stein, C.; Basit, A.; Chan, J.C.N.; Mbanya, J.C.; et al. IDF Diabetes Atlas: Global, regional and country-level diabetes prevalence estimates for 2021 and projections for 2045. *Diabetes Res. Clin. Pract.* **2022**, *183*, 109119. [CrossRef] [PubMed]
3. World Obesity Federation. World Obesity Atlas. 2022. Available online: https://www.worldobesity.org/resources/resource-library/world-obesity-atlas-2022 (accessed on 14 August 2023).
4. Leon, B.M.; Maddox, T.M. Diabetes and cardiovascular disease: Epidemiology, biological mechanisms, treatment recommendations and future research. *World J. Diabetes* **2015**, *6*, 1246–1258. [CrossRef] [PubMed]
5. Bhupathiraju, S.N.; Hu, F.B. Epidemiology of Obesity and Diabetes and Their Cardiovascular Complications. *Circ. Res.* **2016**, *118*, 1723–1735. [CrossRef] [PubMed]
6. Bommer, C.; Heesemann, E.; Sagalova, V.; Manne-Goehler, J.; Atun, R.; Bärnighausen, T.; Vollmer, S. The global economic burden of diabetes in adults aged 20-79 years: A cost-of-illness study. *Lancet Diabetes Endocrinol.* **2017**, *5*, 423–430. [CrossRef] [PubMed]
7. Dornan, T.; Ashcroft, D.; Heathfield, H.; Lewis, P.; Miles, J.; Taylor, D.; Tully, M.; Wass, V. An in Depth Investigation into Causes of Prescribing Errors by Foundation Trainees in Relation to Their Medical Education. EQUIP Study. Available online: http://www.gmc-uk.org/FINAL_Report_prevalence_and_causes_of_prescribing_errors.pdf_28935150.pdf (accessed on 27 December 2009).
8. Ryan, C.; Ross, S.; Davey, P.; Duncan, E.M.; Francis, J.J.; Fielding, S.; Johnston, M.; Ker, J.; Lee, A.J.; MacLeod, M.J.; et al. Prevalence and causes of prescribing errors: The PRescribing Outcomes for Trainee Doctors Engaged in Clinical Training (PROTECT) study. *PLoS ONE* **2014**, *9*, e79802. [CrossRef] [PubMed]
9. Ashcroft, D.M.; Lewis, P.J.; Tully, M.P.; Farragher, T.M.; Taylor, D.; Wass, V.; Williams, S.D.; Dornan, T. Prevalence, Nature, Severity and Risk Factors for Prescribing Errors in Hospital Inpatients: Prospective Study in 20 UK Hospitals. *Drug Saf.* **2015**, *38*, 833–843. [CrossRef]
10. Maxwell, S.R.; Cascorbi, I.; Orme, M.; Webb, D.J. Educating European (junior) doctors for safe prescribing. *Basic Clin. Pharmacol. Toxicol.* **2007**, *101*, 395–400. [CrossRef] [PubMed]
11. Donker, E.M.; Brinkman, D.J.; van Rosse, F.; Janssen, B.; Knol, W.; Dumont, G.; Jorens, P.G.; Dupont, A.; Christiaens, T.; van Smeden, J.; et al. Do we become better prescribers after graduation: A 1-year international follow-up study among junior doctors. *Br. J. Clin. Pharmacol.* **2022**, *88*, 5218–5226. [CrossRef] [PubMed]
12. Lewis, P.J.; Dornan, T.; Taylor, D.; Tully, M.P.; Wass, V.; Ashcroft, D.M. Prevalence, incidence and nature of prescribing errors in hospital inpatients: A systematic review. *Drug Saf.* **2009**, *32*, 379–389. [CrossRef]
13. Tully, M.P.; Ashcroft, D.M.; Dornan, T.; Lewis, P.J.; Taylor, D.; Wass, V. The causes of and factors associated with prescribing errors in hospital inpatients: A systematic review. *Drug Saf.* **2009**, *32*, 819–836. [CrossRef]
14. Farzi, S.; Irajpour, A.; Saghaei, M.; Ravaghi, H. Causes of Medication Errors in Intensive Care Units from the Perspective of Healthcare Professionals. *J. Res. Pharm. Pract.* **2017**, *6*, 158–165. [PubMed]

15. Jansen, B.H.E.; Disselhorst, G.W.; Schutte, T.; Jansen, B.; Rissmann, R.; Richir, M.C.; Keijsers, C.; Vanmolkot, F.H.M.; van den Brink, A.M.; Kramers, C.; et al. Essential diseases in prescribing: A national Delphi study towards a core curriculum in pharmacotherapy education. *Br. J. Clin. Pharmacol.* **2018**, *84*, 2645–2650. [CrossRef] [PubMed]
16. Belančić, A.; Sans-Pola, C.; Jouanjus, E.; Alcubilla, P.; Arellano, A.L.; Žunić, M.; Nogueiras-Álvarez, R.; Roncato, R.; Sáez-Peñataro, J. European association for clinical pharmacology and therapeutics young clinical pharmacologists working group: A cornerstone for the brighter future of clinical pharmacology. *Eur. J. Clin. Pharmacol.* **2022**, *78*, 691–694. [CrossRef] [PubMed]
17. Davies, M.J.; Aroda, V.R.; Collins, B.S.; Gabbay, R.A.; Green, J.; Maruthur, N.M.; Rosas, S.E.; Del Prato, S.; Mathieu, C.; Mingrone, G.; et al. Management of Hyperglycemia in Type 2 Diabetes, 2022. A Consensus Report by the American Diabetes Association (ADA) and the European Association for the Study of Diabetes (EASD). *Diabetes Care* **2022**, *45*, 2753–2786. [CrossRef]
18. Visseren, F.L.J.; Mach, F.; Smulders, Y.M.; Carballo, D.; Koskinas, K.C.; Bäck, M.; Benetos, A.; Biffi, A.; Boavida, J.M.; Capodanno, D.; et al. 2021 ESC Guidelines on cardiovascular disease prevention in clinical practice. *Eur. Heart J.* **2021**, *42*, 3227–3337. [CrossRef] [PubMed]
19. Lingvay, I.; Sumithran, P.; Cohen, R.V.; le Roux, C.W. Obesity management as a primary treatment goal for type 2 diabetes: Time to reframe the conversation. *Lancet* **2022**, *399*, 394–405. [CrossRef] [PubMed]
20. Tamez-Pérez, H.E.; Quintanilla-Flores, D.L.; Rodríguez-Gutiérrez, R.; González-González, J.G.; Tamez-Peña, A.L. Steroid hyperglycemia: Prevalence, early detection and therapeutic recommendations: A narrative review. *World J. Diabetes* **2015**, *6*, 1073–1081. [CrossRef]
21. Dungan, K.; Merrill, J.; Long, C.; Binkley, P. Effect of beta blocker use and type on hypoglycemia risk among hospitalized insulin requiring patients. *Cardiovasc. Diabetol.* **2019**, *18*, 163. [CrossRef]
22. Williams, B.; Mancia, G.; Spiering, W.; Agabiti Rosei, E.; Azizi, M.; Burnier, M.; Clement, D.L.; Coca, A.; De Simone, G.; Dominiczak, A.; et al. 2018 ESC/ESH Guidelines for the management of arterial hypertension: The Task Force for the management of arterial hypertension of the European Society of Cardiology and the European Society of Hypertension: The Task Force for the management of arterial hypertension of the European Society of Cardiology and the European Society of Hypertension. *J. Hypertens.* **2018**, *36*, 1953–2041.
23. Mach, F.; Baigent, C.; Catapano, A.L.; Koskinas, K.C.; Casula, M.; Badimon, L.; Chapman, M.J.; De Backer, G.G.; Delgado, V.; Ference, B.A.; et al. 2019 ESC/EAS Guidelines for the management of dyslipidaemias: Lipid modification to reduce cardiovascular risk. *Eur. Heart J.* **2020**, *41*, 111–188. [CrossRef] [PubMed]
24. Zorginstituut Nederland. GIP Databank. 2020. Available online: https://www.gipdatabank.nl/ (accessed on 6 November 2023).
25. Brinkman, D.J.; Tichelaar, J.; Okorie, M.; Bissell, L.; Christiaens, T.; Likic, R.; Maciulaitis, R.; Costa, J.; Sanz, E.J.; Tamba, B.I.; et al. Pharmacology and Therapeutics Education in the European Union Needs Harmonization and Modernization: A Cross-sectional Survey Among 185 Medical Schools in 27 Countries. *Clin. Pharmacol. Ther.* **2017**, *102*, 815–822. [CrossRef] [PubMed]
26. Brinkman, D.J.; Monteiro, T.; Monteiro, E.C.; Richir, M.C.; van Agtmael, M.A.; Tichelaar, J. Switching from a traditional undergraduate programme in (clinical) pharmacology and therapeutics to a problem-based learning programme. *Eur. J. Clin. Pharmacol.* **2021**, *77*, 421–429. [CrossRef] [PubMed]
27. Brinkman, D.J.; Tichelaar, J.; Schutte, T.; Benemei, S.; Bottiger, Y.; Chamontin, B.; Christiaens, T.; Likic, R.; Ma iulaitis, R.; Marandi, T.; et al. Essential competencies in prescribing: A first european cross-sectional study among 895 final-year medical students. *Clin. Pharmacol. Ther.* **2017**, *101*, 281–289. [CrossRef] [PubMed]
28. De Vries, T.P.G.M.; Henning, R.H.; Hogerzeil, H.V.; Bapna, J.S.; Bero, L.; Kafle, K.K.; Mabadeje, A.F.B.; Santoso, B.; Smith, A.J. Impact of a short course in pharmacotherapy for undergraduate medical students: An international randomised controlled study. *Lancet* **1995**, *346*, 1454–1457. [CrossRef] [PubMed]
29. Smith, A.; Hill, S.; Walkom, E.; Thambiran, M. An evaluation of the World Health Organization problem-based pharmacotherapy teaching courses (based on the "Guide to Good Prescribing"), 1994–2001. *Eur. J. Clin. Pharmacol.* **2005**, *61*, 785–786. [CrossRef] [PubMed]
30. Kamarudin, G.; Penm, J.; Chaar, B.; Moles, R. Educational interventions to improve prescribing competency: A systematic review. *BMJ Open* **2013**, *3*, e003291. [CrossRef] [PubMed]
31. Omer, U.; Danopoulos, E.; Veysey, M.; Crampton, P.; Finn, G. A Rapid Review of Prescribing Education Interventions. *Med. Sci. Educ.* **2021**, *31*, 273–289. [CrossRef]
32. Ross, S.; Loke, Y.K. Do educational interventions improve prescribing by medical students and junior doctors? A systematic review. *Br. J. Clin. Pharmacol.* **2009**, *67*, 662–670. [CrossRef]
33. Tichelaar, J.; Richir, M.C.; Garner, S.; Hogerzeil, H.; de Vries, T.P.G.M. WHO guide to good prescribing is 25 years old: Quo vadis? *Eur. J. Clin. Pharmacol.* **2020**, *76*, 507–513. [CrossRef]
34. Hmelo-Silver, C.E. Problem-Based Learning: What and How Do Students Learn? *Educ. Psychol. Rev.* **2004**, *16*, 235–266. [CrossRef]
35. Dolmans, D.; Michaelsen, L.; van Merriënboer, J.; van der Vleuten, C. Should we choose between problem-based learning and team-based learning? No, combine the best of both worlds! *Med. Teachnol.* **2015**, *37*, 354–359. [CrossRef] [PubMed]
36. Bakkum, M.J.; Richir, M.C.; Papaioannidou, P.; Likic, R.; Sanz, E.J.; Christiaens, T.; Costa, J.N.; Mačiulaitis, R.; Dima, L.; Coleman, J.; et al. EurOP(2)E—The European Open Platform for Prescribing Education, a consensus study among clinical pharmacology and therapeutics teachers. *Eur. J. Clin. Pharmacol.* **2021**, *77*, 1209–1218. [CrossRef] [PubMed]
37. Godden, D.R.; Baddeley, A.D. Context-dependent memory in two natural environments: On land and underwater. *Br. J. Psychol.* **1975**, *66*, 325–331. [CrossRef]

38. Tichelaar, J.; van Kan, C.; van Unen, R.J.; Schneider, A.J.; van Agtmael, M.A.; de Vries, T.P.; Richir, M.C. The effect of different levels of realism of context learning on the prescribing competencies of medical students during the clinical clerkship in internal medicine: An exploratory study. *Eur. J. Clin. Pharmacol.* **2015**, *71*, 237–242. [CrossRef] [PubMed]
39. Dekker, R.S.; Schutte, T.; Tichelaar, J.; Thijs, A.; van Agtmael, M.A.; de Vries, T.P.; Richir, M.C. A novel approach to teaching pharmacotherapeutics--feasibility of the learner-centered student-run clinic. *Eur. J. Clin. Pharmacol.* **2015**, *71*, 1381–1387. [CrossRef] [PubMed]
40. Schutte, T.; Tichelaar, J.; van Agtmael, M. Learning to prescribe in a student-run clinic. *Med. Teachnol.* **2016**, *38*, 425. [CrossRef]
41. Reumerman, M.O.; Richir, M.C.; Sultan, R.; Daelmans, H.E.M.; Springer, H.; Grijmans, E.; Muller, M.; van Agtmael, M.A.; Tichelaar, J. An inter-professional student-run medication review programme. Reducing adverse drug reactions in a memory outpatient clinic: A controlled clinical trial. *Expert Opin. Drug Saf.* **2022**, *21*, 1511–1520. [CrossRef]
42. Reumerman, M.O.; Tichelaar, J.; Richir, M.C.; van Agtmael, M.A. Medical students as junior adverse drug event managers facilitating reporting of ADRs. *Br. J. Clin. Pharmacol.* **2021**, *87*, 4853–4860. [CrossRef]
43. Schutte, T.; Prince, K.; Richir, M.; Donker, E.; van Gastel, L.; Bastiaans, F.; de Vries, H.; Tichelaar, J.; van Agtmael, M. Opportunities for Students to Prescribe: An Evaluation of 185 Consultations in the Student-run Cardiovascular Risk Management Programme. *Basic Clin. Pharmacol.* **2018**, *122*, 299–302. [CrossRef]
44. Sultan, R.; van den Beukel, T.O.; Reumerman, M.O.; Daelmans, H.E.M.; Springer, H.; Grijmans, E.; Muller, M.; Richir, M.C.; van Agtmael, M.A.; Tichelaar, J. An Interprofessional Student-Run Medication Review Program: The Clinical STOPP/START-Based Outcomes of a Controlled Clinical Trial in a Geriatric Outpatient Clinic. *Clin. Pharmacol. Ther.* **2022**, *111*, 931–938. [CrossRef] [PubMed]
45. Cohen, J. Eight steps for starting a student-run clinic. *JAMA* **1995**, *273*, 434–435. [CrossRef] [PubMed]
46. Smith, S.; Thomas, R., 3rd; Cruz, M.; Griggs, R.; Moscato, B.; Ferrara, A. Presence and characteristics of student-run free clinics in medical schools. *JAMA* **2014**, *312*, 2407–2410. [CrossRef] [PubMed]
47. An, M.L.; Laks, K.M.; Long, N.A. Uninsured with Diabetes: How Student-Run Free Medical Clinics Are Filling the Gap. *Clin. Diabetes* **2019**, *37*, 282–283. [CrossRef] [PubMed]
48. Schroeder, M.N.; Hickey, M.O. Patient Satisfaction with Diabetes Care in a Student-Run Free Medical Clinic: A Quality Improvement Study. *J. Pharm. Technol.* **2020**, *36*, 61–67. [CrossRef] [PubMed]
49. Donker, E.M.; Brinkman, D.J.; Richir, M.C.; Papaioannidou, P.; Likic, R.; Sanz, E.J.; Christiaens, T.; Costa, J.N.; De Ponti, F.; Böttiger, Y.; et al. The European Prescribing Exam: Assessing whether European medical students can prescribe rationally and safely. *Eur. J. Clin. Pharmacol.* **2022**, *78*, 1049–1051. [CrossRef] [PubMed]
50. Harden, R.M.; Stevenson, M.; Downie, W.W.; Wilson, G.M. Assessment of clinical competence using objective structured examination. *Br. Med. J.* **1975**, *1*, 447–451. [CrossRef]
51. Khan, K.Z.; Ramachandran, S.; Gaunt, K.; Pushkar, P. The Objective Structured Clinical Examination (OSCE): AMEE Guide No. 81. Part I: An historical and theoretical perspective. *Med. Teachnol.* **2013**, *35*, e1437–e1446. [CrossRef]

Disclaimer/Publisher's Note: The statements, opinions and data contained in all publications are solely those of the individual author(s) and contributor(s) and not of MDPI and/or the editor(s). MDPI and/or the editor(s) disclaim responsibility for any injury to people or property resulting from any ideas, methods, instructions or products referred to in the content.

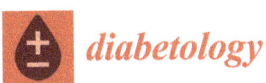

Systematic Review

A Systematic Review of Economic Evaluations of Insulin for the Management of Type 2 Diabetes

Elvira Meni Maria Gkrinia [1,*], Andrea Katrin Faour [2], Andrej Belančić [3,4,*], Jacques Bazile [1], Emma Marland [1] and Dinko Vitezić [3,4]

1. Independent Researcher, 11741 Athens, Greece; jbazile2023@gmail.com (J.B.); emma.s.marland@gmail.com (E.M.)
2. Vancouver Coastal Health, Vancouver, BC V5K 0A1, Canada; andrea.faour@gmail.com
3. Department of Clinical Pharmacology, Clinical Hospital Centre Rijeka, Krešimirova 42, 51000 Rijeka, Croatia; dinko.vitezic@uniri.hr
4. Department of Basic and Clinical Pharmacology with Toxicology, Faculty of Medicine, University of Rijeka, Braće Branchetta 20, 51000 Rijeka, Croatia
* Correspondence: elvira.gkrinia20@alumni.imperial.ac.uk (E.M.M.G.); abelancic93@gmail.com or andrej.belancic@uniri.hr (A.B.)

Abstract: Diabetes is a chronic, metabolic disease characterized by hyperglycemia, which occurs as a result of inadequate production or utilization of insulin. Type 2 diabetes (T2D) is the most common type of diabetes with estimates projecting a prevalence of more than 1 billion people living with T2DM by 2050. Hence, it was decided to conduct a systematic literature review of health economic evaluations of insulin, the most common medication used for the treatment of the disease, to inform policy. Pharmacoeconomic analyses, written in English and published after 2016, were considered for inclusion. PubMed/Medline, Global Health, Embase and Health Management Consortium were searched separately between 5 July 2023 and 17 July 2023. Grey literature articles were searched on ISPOR and the Cost-Effectiveness Analysis Registry during the same period. After the exclusion criteria were applied, 21 studies were included. Using the BMJ checklist, a quality appraisal was performed on all included studies. Data extraction was performed manually. Regarding evidence synthesis, data were heterogenous and are presented based on study type. The results showed a variety of treatment combinations being available for the treatment of diabetes, with insulin degludec/DegLira and semaglutide being cost-effective despite their high cost, due to the effectiveness of managing the disease. Research around the cost-effectiveness or cost-utility of insulin has potential to progress further, to ensure informed policy-making in the future.

Keywords: systematic literature review; cost-effectiveness; cost-utility; diabetes; insulin; pharmacoeconomics

Citation: Gkrinia, E.M.M.; Faour, A.K.; Belančić, A.; Bazile, J.; Marland, E.; Vitezić, D. A Systematic Review of Economic Evaluations of Insulin for the Management of Type 2 Diabetes. *Diabetology* 2023, 4, 440–452. https://doi.org/10.3390/diabetology4040038

Academic Editor: Yoshifumi Saisho

Received: 13 September 2023
Revised: 2 October 2023
Accepted: 9 October 2023
Published: 13 October 2023

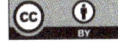

Copyright: © 2023 by the authors. Licensee MDPI, Basel, Switzerland. This article is an open access article distributed under the terms and conditions of the Creative Commons Attribution (CC BY) license (https://creativecommons.org/licenses/by/4.0/).

1. Introduction

Diabetes is a chronic metabolic disorder, caused by defects in insulin secretion and/or insulin action, which results in hyperglycemia; prolonged hyperglycemia can lead to acute complications (e.g., diabetic ketoacidosis), chronic complications (e.g., retinopathy, chronic kidney damage, diabetic foot ulcers) and, consequently, impaired quality of life (QOL) and reduced life-expectancy [1–3]. Over 500 million people were living with diabetes in 2021, with 96% of cases being Type 2 (T2D); T2D is associated with β-cell dysfunction, insulin resistance, and the impairment of incretin signaling, and prevalence is projected to increase to 1.31 billion people worldwide by 2050 [2,4].

Attaining recommended glycaemic targets, a hemoglobin A1c (HbA1c) of around 53 mmol/mol (7%), which is the average blood glucose level over 3 months, results in the substantial reduction in the onset and progression of macrovascular (e.g., coronary heart disease, cerebrovascular disease) and microvascular (e.g., diabetic nephropathy, retinopathy) complications [5–9]. Time-in-range (TIR), i.e., the amount of time (%) that an individual's glucose level remains within the proposed target range, should be more than 70% a day to ensure micro- and macrovascular protection. Other useful clinical targets in terms of preventing/well-managing complications are time below range (TBR) and glycemic variability (GV) [10].

Insulin therapy has been the main treatment option for patients with T2D for over a century and it is ultimately required in the chronic management of T2D, if glycaemic targets are not achieved following dietary intervention, review of physical activity behaviour, and oral anti-hyperglycaemic medication [5,11]. There is often a delay in commencing insulin therapy, due to hesitancy both among patients to take insulin and healthcare providers to prescribe [12]; a survey of 66,000 patients found that average HbA1c was 80 mmol/mol at the start of insulin therapy and over 90% of participants already had associated complications [13]. The American Diabetes Association (ADA) and European Association for the Study of Diabetes (EASD) advocate for early introduction of insulin when glycaemic measurements do not meet targets [5].

Insulin is available in numerous formulations (e.g., rapid-acting, short-acting, intermediate-acting, long-acting) to enable the dose and timing to be matched to an individual's physiological requirements [11]. The global median government procurement price for a standardised 100 U/10 mL vial of human insulin is USD 5, compared to long-lasting 'analogue' insulin at USD 33; the individual pays USD 9 for human insulin at pharmacies and private hospitals [14]. That said, the reimbursement environment and guidelines vary significantly on the national level. In 2022, the global insulin market was valued at approximately USD 20.18 billion; yet, it is estimated that 60% of users lack secure access to affordable insulin [15,16].

There are significant costs associated with diabetes and its complications; in 2021 health expenditures were USD 966 billion globally and are forecast to reach over USD 1054 billion by 2045 [4]. Diabetic peripheral neuropathy alone is estimated to cost USD 10.9 billion per year in the United States, whilst diabetic ulceration and amputation costs the United Kingdom's National Health Service up to GBP 962 million annually [17,18]. By 2030, the global economic burden of diabetes and its complications is estimated to reach USD 2.1 trillion, a 61% rise from 2015, even if countries meet the Sustainable Development Goal of decreasing mortality from diabetes by one third [19].

In addition to the financial burden, the rising prevalence of T2D is a major concern as the condition is associated with a serious deterioration in general QOL [20]; T2D was ranked as the seventh leading cause of DALYs (Disability-Adjusted Life Years) in 2017 [21]. Bearing all this in mind, the aim of this study is to conduct a systematic literature review (SLR) on pharmacoeconomic evaluations of insulin in the management of T2D at a global level.

2. Materials and Methods

The databases, PubMed/Medline, Global Health, Embase and Health Management Consortium, were systematically searched for medical subjects, while manual searching was conducted on ISPOR (The International Society for Pharmacoeconomics and Outcomes Research) and the Cost-Effectiveness Analysis Registry to include grey literature in order to reduce bias [22,23]. Each database and website was searched separately between 5 July 2023 and 17 July 2023. The following key-words were used: (diabetes) AND (insulin) AND (econom* OR economic evaluation). The comprehensive search strategy is included in Appendix A.

The inclusion and exclusion criteria were informed by the PICOS search framework (Table 1). Cost-Effectiveness Analyses (CEA) and Cost-Utility Analyses (CUA) were considered for inclusion, based on the criteria outlined below. Published peer-reviewed SLRs were utilized to confirm that the correct methods were used and the appropriate results were included.

Table 1. The PICOS search framework used to inform the inclusion and exclusion criteria within the study.

Population	Intervention	Comparator	Outcome	Study Design
Patients with T2D *	Insulin	Insulin or other pharmaceutical products	Effectiveness and cost-effectiveness in the management of T2D *	CEA [1] CUA [2]

* T2D—type 2 diabetes; [1] CEA—cost-effectiveness analysis; [2] CUA—cost-utility analysis.

During the process of screening, studies written in English, CEAs and CUAs of insulin in the management of T2D and comparisons of insulin products against other insulin products or pharmaceutical products used for the management of T2D were considered for inclusion. Moreover, studies published between 2016 and July 2023 and using data after 2016 were also deemed appropriate. Including studies that had been published before 2016 may have led to inclusion of out-of-date data, as the reimbursement and health economics environment changes regularly, e.g., in the United Kingdom, drug prices are negotiated every 5 years [24]. The inclusion criteria also included real-world studies, as well as grey literature reports and publications by non-industry organisations, to minimise bias. Studies not written in English, published before 2016 or using data before 2016 and not pertaining to insulin, were excluded. Studies with participants aged <18 years, pertaining to any other disease than T2D (T1D, gestational diabetes, cardiovascular diseases), comparing devices or non-pharmaceutical interventions (e.g., exercise) in the management of diabetes, as well as studies on insulin biosimilars, did not meet the inclusion criteria. Finally, reviews, opinions, SLRs, scoping reviews, cohort studies and case-reports were also excluded.

The search for publications was performed independently by two authors (E.G., A.F.), and all retrieved articles were compared to avoid duplication. Any disagreements were discussed, whilst potential conflicts were then solved by a third reviewer (A.B.). The SLR was performed according to PRISMA (Preferred Reporting Items for Systematic Reviews and Meta-Analyses) guidelines [25]. The titles and abstracts of all studies were screened based on the eligibility criteria by two independent reviewers (E.G., A.F.) and there was 100% agreement between them. Full-text screening was conducted by the two reviewers (E.G., A.F.) for studies that seemed suitable at the abstract and title screening stage or when the title and abstract did not provide enough information. There was 85% agreement between the two reviewers, and a third reviewer (A.B) solved conflicts between them.

For citations published as abstracts that were eligible for inclusion, we attempted to contact the first and/or last author to ask for raw data and/or potential full-text publications. This was applied on 14 ISPOR abstracts, out of which, we identified email addresses for eight authors by searching PubMed/Medline and Google Scholar. However, we did not receive any relevant answers in the 2-week pre-specified deadline. Thus, we believe, the choice to exclude them was justified.

To enhance the reliability and relevance of the review at hand, each study was evaluated for its quality and bias using specific and recognised tools. The health economic evaluations were assessed based on the Consolidated Health Economic Evaluation Reporting Standards (CHEERS) statement and the British Medical Journal (BMJ) checklist for economic evaluations [26,27]. Each analysis was then scored based on the BMJ checklist with a maximum score of 35, while also considering the CHEERS statement. If an analysis had a score of less than 30/35, it was excluded. By scoring each analysis, it was possible to ensure the inclusion of studies with robust results and minimised bias.

Data extraction was performed manually using extraction forms created on Microsoft Excel 360. The following data were extracted from each included study: last name of first author, year of publication, country/ethnicity, sample size/number of patients and controls (where applicable), study inclusion/exclusion criteria, analysis type, type of comparison (insulin vs. insulin or insulin vs. other pharmaceutical products) and additional comments (if applicable). Considering selection heterogeneity across studies, a meta-analysis could not have been conducted. Therefore, the results were grouped based on study type (CEA,

CUA) on the first level and based on comparison (insulin vs. insulin or insulin vs. other pharmaceutical interventions) on the second level.

3. Results

3.1. PRISMA Flowchart

The database search yielded 7745 citations in total, of which, 2301 were duplicates and were excluded. Manual searching identified 23 results, of which 100% were duplicates with the results on the medical databases being consequently excluded, with 2324 duplicates being removed in total. The steps of the study selection, along with the reasons for the exclusion of full texts, are presented in the PRISMA flow diagram (Figure 1).

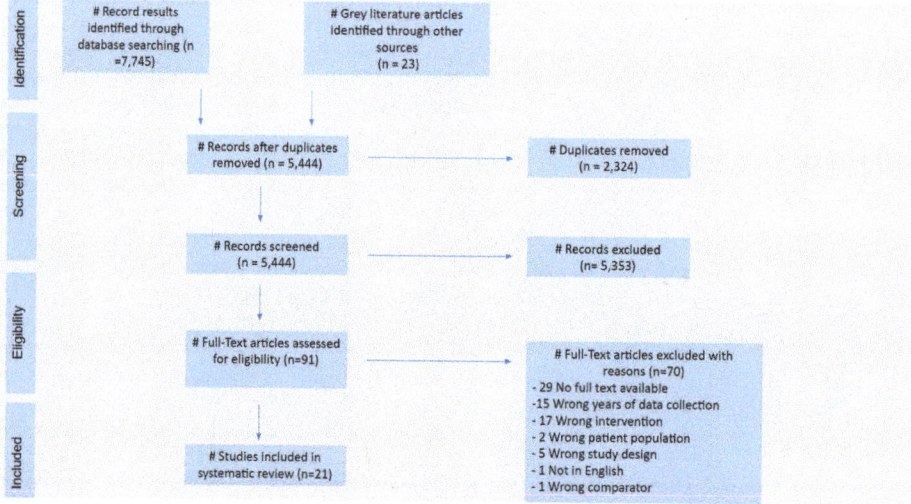

Figure 1. The PRISMA flow diagram of the present systematic review.

3.2. Studies Selected

After the inclusion and exclusion criteria were applied, 21 studies were included in the SLR [28–48]. Overall, 18 CEAs and three CUAs were included. All studies assessed the economic impacts of insulin in the treatment of T2D. Table 2 includes the basic characteristics of each study included.

Table 2. Basic characteristics of each study included in the concept of the present systematic review.

#	First Author	Year of Publication	Setting	Study Type	Comparison
1	Cannon, A.J. [28]	2020	USA	Cost-effectiveness analysis	Insulin degludec/liraglutide versus basal insulin and basal-bolus therapy
2	Cheng, H. [29]	2019	China	Cost-effectiveness analysis	Insulin degludec versus insulin glargine
3	Dempsey, M. [30]	2018	USA	Cost-effectiveness analysis	Insulin degludec/liraglutide versus insulin glargine U100 plus insulin aspart
4	Drummond, R. [31]	2018	UK	Cost-effectiveness analysis	Insulin degludec/liraglutide versus insulin glargine U100 plus insulin aspart
5	Evans, M. [32]	2023	UK	Cost-effectiveness analysis	Insulin aspart versus once-weekly semaglutide

Table 2. Cont.

#	First Author	Year of Publication	Setting	Study Type	Comparison
6	Gu, S. [33]	2020	China	Cost-effectiveness analysis	Insulin vs. other agents (10 pharmacologic combination strategies overall)
7	Han, G. [34]	2022	China	Cost–utility analysis	Insulin degludec/liraglutide versus its single components—degludec or liraglutide
8	Hunt, B. [35]	2017	USA	Cost-effectiveness analysis	Insulin degludec/liraglutide versus insulin glargine U100
9	Jiang, Y. [36]	2023	China	Cost-effectiveness analysis	Insulin glargine U100/lixisenatide versus insulin degludec/insulin aspart
10	Kvapil, M. [37]	2017	Czech Republic	Cost-effectiveness analysis	Insulin degludec/liraglutide versus basal insulin intensification strategies
11	Langer, J. [38]	2019	Japan	Cost-effectiveness analysis	Insulin degludec vs. other basal insulins
12	Lau, E. [39]	2019	Hong Kong	Cost-effectiveness analysis	Insulin glargine U100 versus NPH * insulin
13	Luo, Q. [40]	2022	China	Cost-effectiveness analysis	Insulin degludec/insulin aspart versus biphasic insulin aspart 30
14	McCrimmon, R.J. (iGlarLixi vs. basal insulin plus metformin) [41]	2021	UK	Cost-effectiveness analysis	Insulin glargine U100/lixisenatide versus insulin degludec/liraglutide and the free-combination comparators insulin glargine plus dulaglutide and basal insulin plus liraglutide
15	McCrimmon, R.J. (iGlarLixi Versus iDegLira) [42]	2021	UK	Cost-effectiveness analysis	Insulin glargine U100/lixisenatide versus insulin degludec/liraglutide
16	Pöhlmann, J. (ClinicoEcon Outcomes) [43]	2019	Italy	Cost-effectiveness analysis	Insulin degludec/liraglutide versus insulin glargine U100/lixisenatide
17	Pöhlmann, J. (Diabetes Ther.) [44]	2019	Czech Republic	Cost-effectiveness analysis	Insulin degludec/liraglutide versus insulin glargine U100/lixisenatide
18	Pollock, R.F. [45]	2019	Canada	Cost-utility analysis	Insulin glargine versus dulaglutide
19	Pollock, R.F. [46]	2018	UK	Cost-utility analysis	Insulin degludec versus insulin glargine U100
20	Pollock, R.F. (Applied Health Economics and Health Policy) [47]	2019	UK	Cost-effectiveness analysis	Insulin degludec versus insulin glargine U100
21	Raya, P.M. [48]	2019	Spain	Cost-effectiveness	Insulin degludec/liraglutide versus comparator regimens

UK—United Kingdom; USA—United States of America; * NPH—Neutral Protamine Hagedorn.

3.3. Methodology of Selected Studies

Most selected studies included data from clinical trials or pooled analyses and literature reviews to populate the models. Studies #1, #3, #4, #5, #7, #8, #9, #10, #13, #14, #15, #16, #17, #18, #19 and #20 included data from clinical trials and reviews, with some studies including data from local cohort studies. Study #7 used real-world-data (RWD) in addition to clinical trial data. The authors of studies #2, #6, #11, #12 and #21 used RWD. The original authors of all studies used publicly available data and monetary information to construct the economic variables of the models.

3.4. Quality Appraisal

All studies that were selected met the inclusion/exclusion criteria and the BMJ score threshold. Comprehensive quality appraisal results are presented in Table 3 below.

Table 3. Overview of quality appraisal of individual studies based on BMJ health economics checklist and associated scoring.

#	First Author	Score on BMJ * Checklist
1	Cannon, A.J. [28]	34/35
2	Cheng, H. [29]	35/35
3	Dempsey, M. [30]	35/35
4	Drummond, R. [31]	34/35
5	Evans, M. [32]	35/35
6	Gu, S. [33]	34/35
7	Han, G. [34]	35/35
8	Hunt, B. [35]	35/35
9	Jiang, Y. [36]	32/35
10	Kvapil, M. [37]	33/35
11	Langer, J. [38]	35/35
12	Lau, E. [39]	34/35
13	Luo, Q. [40]	35/35
14	McCrimmon, R.J. (iGlarLixi vs. basal insulin plus metformin) [41]	34/35
15	McCrimmon, R.J. (iGlarLixi Versus iDegLira) [42]	34/35
16	Pöhlmann, J. (ClinicoEcon Outcomes) [43]	35/35
17	Pöhlmann, J. (Diabetes Ther.) [44]	34/35
18	Pollock, R.F. (2019) [45]	35/35
19	Pollock, R.F. (2018) [46]	35/35
20	Pollock, R.F. (Applied Health Economics and Health Policy) [47]	35/35
21	Raya, P.M. [48]	34/35

* BMJ—British Medical Journal.

3.5. Evidence Synthesis

3.5.1. CEA Studies

Cheng et al. found that treatment with insulin degludec (IDeg), when compared to insulin glargine (iGlar), was associated with improved Quality-Adjusted Life years (QALYs) (+0.0053) and life expectancy (0.0082 years) in insulin-naive patients with T2D living in China, with an additional total mean lifetime cost of USD 3278 and an Incremental Cost-Effectiveness Ratio (ICER) of USD 613,443 per QALY gained [29]. The authors assert that reduced cumulative incidence of myocardial infarction, stroke and congestive heart failure in the IDeg arm might have been potential reasons for their findings.

Moreover, Langer et al. state improved effectiveness in terms of QALYs (+0.0354), slightly higher annual treatment costs (JPY 9510) and a better value-for-money assessment (JPY 268,811 per QALY gained) for Japanese patients switching from basal insulin to IDeg [38].

Pollock et al., based on evidence from DEVOTE 16, found that treatment with IDeg in UK-based patients was associated with superior cost-effectiveness in contrast to IGlar U100 (ICER GBP 14,956/QALY) [47]. Treatment with IDeg had also slightly superior results pertaining to life expectancy (6.8980 years vs. 6.7825 years) at mean costs of GBP 47,311 (versus GBP 45,582) per patient.

Cannon et al. conducted a short-term CEA in the US, comparing insulin degludec/liraglutide (IDegLira) with basal insulin and basal-bolus therapy, using DUAL V and DUAL VII clinical study data [28]. The rates of reaching double or triple composite outcomes (HbA1c $\leq$ 7.5%, $\leq$8.0%, and $\leq$9.0%) were significantly higher for IDegLira versus IGlar U100 or other basal-bolus regimens for all targets, both in DUAL V and DUAL VII. For each USD 1 spent on IDegLira, the equivalent annual costs per patient to achieve the aforementioned HbA1c targets without hypoglycemia and without weight gain were USD 2.43, USD 2.10 and USD 2.05 for IGlar U100, and USD 6.33, USD 5.80 and USD 6.06, respectively for basal-bolus therapy. A long-term US CEA by Dempsey et al. outlined that IDegLira usage (in comparison to iGlar U100 + insulin aspart) was associated with an increase in discounted life expectancy and discounted quality-adjusted life expectancy (QALE) by 0.02 years and 0.22 QALYs, respectively [30]. The authors argued that these increases were driven primarily by a small reduction in the cumulative incidence of diabetes-related complications and delayed time to their onset. Regarding direct mean medical costs over a patient lifetime, treatment with IDegLira resulted in a USD 3571 cost saving; mostly due to lower acquisition costs as well as lower rates of hypoglycaemia and cardiovascular complications in the IDegLira arm.

Drummond et al. suggested an annual improvement of 0.0512 QALYs for IDegLira; however direct costs were somewhat higher (GBP 303) because of higher acquisition costs in the UK market (GBP 828) [31]. When combining clinical and cost outcomes, an ICER of GBP 5924 per QALY was reported for IDegLira in the treatment of patients with TD2 not reaching glycaemic targets on basal insulin therapy. Hunt et al. also observed IDegLira superiority over iGlar U100 up-titration in terms of annual costs among HbA1c $\leq$ 6.5 without hypoglycaemia (USD 10,608), weight gain (USD 29,215) and their combination (USD 57,351) in US-based patients [35]. Furthermore, in a CEA study in the Czech Republic, treatment with IDegLira was associated with a gain in QALE of 0.31 QALYs, with an additional cost of CZK 107,829 (Czech Koruna) over a patient's lifetime (compared to insulin intensification regimens), which corresponds to an ICER of CZK 345,052 per QALY gained [37]. The authors theorised that the latter was mostly driven by a reduction in the incidence of diabetes-related complications and in the prolongation of symptom onset.

Pöhlmann et al. (ClinicoEcon Outcomes) associated treatment with IDegLira with superior outcomes, when compared to insulin glargine/lixisenatide (iGlarLixi) (gained 0.09 LY and 0.13 QALYs) in Italian patients, as a result of lower cumulative incidence of diabetes-related complications and their delayed onset [43]. Treatment with IDegLira (versus iGlarLixi) yielded an ICER of EUR 7368 per QALY, which fell below the Willingness-To-Pay (WTP) threshold and confirmed its cost-effectiveness. In addition, Pöhlmann et al. (Diabetes Ther.) mentioned an association of IDegLira treatment with superior cost-effectiveness over iGlarLixi in Czech patients [44], a gain in life expectancy of 0.11 years, QALE of 0.14 QALYs (mainly driven by the same diabetes complication reasons) and an ICER of CZK 695,998 (versus iGlarLixi pens containing 33 lg/mL of lixisenatide) and CZK 348,223 (versus 50 lg/mL) per QALY gained, which was below the pre-specified WTP threshold.

Treatment with IDegLira was associated with improved clinical outcomes, i.e., decreased diabetes-related complications and increased QALE, and reduced costs compared with other injectable regimens in a CEA conducted in Spain [48]. When compared to multiple daily insulin injections and basal insulin, ICERs of EUR 3013/QALY and EUR 6890/QALY were reported.

Jiang et al. found that treatment with iGlarLixi (net increase of 0.08 QALYs and 0.07 LE over a patient's lifetime) was dominant over insulin degludec/insulin aspart (IDegAsp) with the projection of an annual medication cost of USD 590.41 to USD 865.03 in Chinese patients [36]. McCrimmon et al. conducted a CEA on a population of UK citizens with TD2, who were suboptimally controlled on basal insulin plus metformin, and demonstrated lower estimated costs with iGlarLixi (GBP 31,295) compared with iGlar plus dulaglutide (Dula) (GBP 38,790), iDegLira (GBP 40,179), and BI plus liraglutide (Lira) (GBP 42,467) [41]. Total QALYs gained were 8.438 with iGlarLixi and iDegLira, 8.439 with iGlar plus Dula, and 8.466 with BI plus Lira; and the net monetary benefit was positive when compared to all other comparators. In another study by the same leading author, conducted on a population of UK citizens with TD2 inadequately controlled by GLP-1 receptor agonists (GLP-1RA) and oral antihyperglycemic therapy, iGlarLixi was reported to be less costly (owing to acquisition costs) compared to iDegLira (GBP 30,011 versus GBP 40,742), whilst at the same time being associated with similar QALYs: 8.437 and 8.422, respectively [42]. The net monetary benefit of iGlarLixi was GBP 11,030.

Luo et al. compared biphasic insulin aspart (BIAsp) 30 and IDegAsp strategy and found an incremental benefit of 0.0001 LYs (12.439 for BIAsp 30 versus 12.438 for IDegAsp), a 0.280 QALYs gain (9.522 versus 9.242) over a 30-year period, and an ICER of Chinese Yuan (CNY) 13.886/QALY for the IDegAsp strategy [40].

Evans et al. conducted a study evaluating the long-term cost-effectiveness of once-weekly semaglutide 1 mg versus insulin aspart in the UK [32]. Despite higher treatment costs (GBP 800) in the semaglutide arm, it was associated with superior cost-effectiveness due to an improvement in QALE of 0.18 QALYs, as a result of a decreased incidence in diabetes complications and delay in disease progress, while also having an ICER of GBP 4457/QALY.

In a comparison between iGlar U100 and Neutral Protamine Hagedorn (NPH) insulin, the former was associated with an incremental gain of 0.217 QALYs and a cost of Hong Kong Dollar (HKD) 21,360, which coincided with an ICER of HKD 98,663/QALY [39].

Gu et al. showed that metformin + insulin (following a second-line treatment with metformin + glinide) had superior cost-effectiveness results in Chinese patients, gaining 14.085 QALYs, among the ten treatment strategies assessed by the authors (extensively described within Gu et al.) [33]. Scenario analyses showed that patients who report adherence on pharmacologic treatments increased their QALYs (0.456~0.653) at an acceptable range of cost increase (ICERs, USD 1450/QALY~USD 12,360/QALY) and in some cases, at decreased costs compared with those not receiving treatment.

3.5.2. CUA Studies

A combination therapy of IDegLira did not demonstrate 'financial superiority' over its monotherapy components (IDeg and Lira) in the treatment of T2D in a CUA conducted in China [34]. No gains were observed in QALYs (11.79, 11.62, and 11.73, respectively), medications costs (USD 20,281.61, USD 3726.76 and USD 11,941.26, respectively), complication costs (USD 25,274.22, USD 25,016.67 and USD 25,204.84, respectively), total costs (USD 45,555.83, USD 28,743.43 and USD 36,660.18, respectively), incremental cost–utility ratio values (USD 99,464.12/QALYs and USD 143,348.26/QALYs, respectively; both surpassed the WTP threshold) nor net monetary benefits (−10,447.67 and −6200.68, respectively).

Both CUA studies positioning iGlar U100 as a 'financial protagonist' were published by Pollock et al. and conducted in Canada and the UK, respectively. Treatment with iGlar U100 was inferior to GLP-1RA agent dulaglutide (when used as a third-line therapy in Canada) in terms of QALE (12.52 vs. 12.90 QALYs) and ICER (CAD 52,580 per QALY gained) [45]. In the second study, treatment with IDeg was superior to iGlar U100 (when compared with basal-bolus regimens in the treatment of patients with T2D in the UK), reporting cost savings of GBP 28.78 per patient (particularly among a population at high risk of the development of heart disease) and a 0.0064 increase in QALYs (1.4778 versus 1.4715, mostly due to lower hypoglycemia risk) [46].

4. Discussion

There are many blood-glucose-lowering treatments with varied clinical outcomes and costs available worldwide. Insulin and GLP-1RA therapies have been continuously developed and approved in order to help patients better manage glycemic control. Generally, newer products such as insulin degludec/DegLira and semaglutide with more positive clinical outcomes were associated with higher acquisition costs but lower healthcare costs due to mitigated hypoglycemia or other T2D complications during short and long-term CEAs. Specifically, IDeg and DegLira were always found to be more cost-effective therapies than basal-bolus or insulin glargine therapies when hypoglycemic events were considered. The studies where they were not found to be suitable cost-effective alternatives included a UK study where a lower cost generic biosimilar of iGlarLixi was used to calculate the iGlarLixi acquisition cost, which was then compared to branded iDegLira and a study conducted in China where hypoglycemic events were not considered a potential risk factor for subsequent cardiovascular outcomes [36,42]. The latter of these is significant, as all of the studies reporting IDeg and similar insulin mixes to be more effective than insulin glargine variants considered hypoglycemic events, which were key in determining IDeg variants to be more cost-effective. Additionally, a CUA in China found treatment with combination therapy iDegLira to be significantly less cost-effective than either degludec or liraglutide monotherapy despite achieving the highest QALY, due to its high cost in the Chinese market [34].

Cost-effectiveness assessments are important due to the high absolute costs of insulin therapy. Though markets for insulin across the nine countries covered in this review vary in both size and most commonly prescribed insulin analogue, significant healthcare resources are dedicated to procuring insulin for T2D patients.. The average standard unit of insulin (100 units of insulin/mL of fluid) in each of the countries covered in this review cost USD 98.7 in the USA, USD 14.4 in Japan, USD 12 in Canada, USD 10.03 in Italy, USD 9.04 in Spain, USD 8.18 in the Czech Republic and USD 7.52 in the UK. The wide range of insulin prices is due to both reimbursement practices and the types of insulin analogues most commonly prescribed.

New therapies, whether novel compounds or combination therapies, are often associated with high prices that can negatively impact their cost-effectiveness despite clear clinical benefits. In wealthier countries where payer systems have a higher capacity to absorb increased upfront acquisition costs, these products can be attractive, cost-effective alternative treatments compared to established lower-cost alternatives when downstream associated health costs are substantially decreased. The characteristics of countries' health payer systems and their approaches to optimising health can impact criteria used to determine whether interventions are cost effective. Beyond using different criteria to assess the cost-effectiveness of therapeutics, systems may approach allocating scarce resources differently, perhaps opting to prioritise acquisition costs over potential downstream savings. Other factors impacting CEAs and CUAs in different markets are the variance in availability and acquisition costs of therapeutic products and reimbursement for care. Combined, all these factors have the collective effect of creating country-specific scenarios that are not necessarily directly comparable or generalizable. Despite this heterogeneity, assessing the global cost-effectiveness of insulin therapies in the management of T2D allows for the care landscape to be better understood, hopefully leading to better outcomes for all patients with T2D.

The primary strengths of this SLR include the robustness of the study selection process and inclusion of studies across low-, medium- and high-income levels, with a variety of payer systems. Both reviewers assessing all 5444 abstracts sourced from the databases listed in the Methods section allowed for early consensus building and the mitigation of selection bias. Among the 21 studies that met the inclusion/exclusion criteria, 6 were UK-focused, 5 China-focused, 3 USA-focused, 2 Czech Republic-focused, 1 Spain-focused, 1 Japan-focused, 1 Italy-focused, 1 Canada-focused and 1 Hong Kong-focused.

Limitations to this review include the inability to directly compare studies due to different data sources, variables or heterogeneous results, and the majority of the reviewed studies having received industry funding from an organisation manufacturing at least one of the assessed products. Studies used different clinical outcomes, assumptions and models even when using similar methodologies to conduct CEAs or CUAs. The studies focussing on China differed from the rest of the studies reviewed as they did not consider hypoglycemic events caused by insulin when assessing cost-effectiveness; however besides this, there were not significant regional differences in health economic evaluations of insulin. Lastly, though seven diverse regions were assessed in this SLR, the findings may not be generalizable to other regions due to differences in therapeutic availability, pricing and reimbursement. This review could still be used as a foundation for more directly applicable research in regions not directly addressed. Despite these weaknesses, we are confident that the comprehensive search and selection process, following PRISMA guidelines and using quality assessment tools for each included study, has allowed for a strong review of the literature focused on pharmacoeconomic evaluations of insulin in the management of T2D.

To the best of our knowledge, no SLR including CUAs and CEAs published after 2016 on the use of insulin in the management of T2D has been published recently. In 2015, Zhong et al. published an SLR including CUAs in the management of both types of diabetes, while Saunders et al. conducted an SLR on the cost-effectiveness of intermediate-acting, long-acting, ultralong-acting, and biosimilar insulins in the treatment of T1D [49,50]. In addition, Shafie et al. and Suh et al. performed SLRs on the cost-effectiveness of insulin in the management of both types of diabetes [51,52]. The authors of the latter concluded that insulin detemir is more cost-effective than NPH and as cost-effective as iGlar. Saunders et al., writing about T1D, reported superior cost-effectiveness of long-acting insulin over intermediate-acting insulin. Shafie et al. called for more research to be conducted on the cost-effectiveness of insulin analogues in the treatment of T2D and Zhong et al. asserted that practice needs to be optimised with the use of value-for-money interventions. Hence, we are positive that our work provides an updated insight in the research around insulin and T2D management.

Novel, increasingly expensive therapies based on innovative science are being continuously developed to combat T2D, and as such, it is important for healthcare providers and payers to be able to identify optimal therapies and treatment algorithms for their healthcare settings. Growing understanding of and ability to affect mechanisms of T2D yield new treatment options with new therapeutic outcomes and risks. However, newer therapies are not always necessarily better for patients and health systems, whether looking at therapeutic outcomes, cost, or a combination of both. Novel therapies associated with increased therapeutic benefit are often expensive during their exclusivity period, which can negatively impact their cost-effectiveness. This relationship is not static however, as generic and biosimilar therapies can often offer similar or identical benefits at a lower price point, positively improving the cost-effectiveness of a given therapy. These lower-cost options are not ubiquitous in their availability, meaning that different settings may still generate heterogenous assessments of the most cost-effective T2D interventions. Regardless of setting, healthcare needs are far vaster than the available finite resources, marking the importance of cost–benefit analyses spanning the therapeutic landscape. Reviews such as this can be helpful tools for collating work conducted in a variety of settings to help build understanding of the therapeutic landscape. More research exploring etiologies of T2D and associated therapeutic outcomes linked to existing and novel interventions will help bolster the foundation of knowledge that can better help payers, providers, and patients make more optimal care decisions. Developing more consistent models with these acquired data will allow for more effective cross-market comparisons of cost effectiveness, helping all patients with T2D receive more cost-effective care while mitigating the burden on healthcare systems.

Author Contributions: Project administration, E.M.M.G. and A.B.; Methodology, E.M.M.G.; Investigation, E.M.M.G., A.K.F. and A.B.; Writing—Original Draft, E.M.M.G., A.B., E.M. and J.B.; Conceptualization, E.M.M.G. and A.B.; Supervision, D.V. All authors have read and agreed to the published version of the manuscript.

Funding: This research received no external funding.

Institutional Review Board Statement: Not applicable.

Data Availability Statement: Data sharing is not applicable to this article as no new data were created or analysed in this study.

Conflicts of Interest: The authors declare no conflict of interest.

Appendix A

Table A1. The comprehensive search strategy that was used on Pubmed/Medline, Embase, and Global Health.

	Search Strategy
PubMed	(diabetes) AND (insulin) AND (econom* OR economic evaluation). af
Embase	(diabetes) AND (insulin) AND (econom OR economic evaluation). af
Global Health	(diabetes) AND (insulin) AND (econom* OR economic evaluation). af
Medline	(diabetes) AND (insulin) AND (econom* OR economic evaluation). af
	Limitations
PubMed	2016–2023 The results of the search were filtered only for English papers
Embase	English Language 2016–Current
Global Health	English Language 2016–Current
Medline	2016–Current The results of the search were filtered only for English papers

af—All fields.

References

1. World Health Organisation: Diabetes. Available online: https://www.who.int/news-room/fact-sheets/detail/diabetes (accessed on 12 September 2023).
2. Alshammary, A.F.; Alshammari, A.M.; Alsobaie, S.F.; Alageel, A.A.; Ali Khan, I. Evidence from genetic studies among rs2107538 variant in the CCL5 gene and Saudi patients diagnosed with type 2 diabetes mellitus. *Saudi J. Biol. Sci.* **2023**, *30*, 103658. [CrossRef]
3. Farmaki, P.; Damaskos, C.; Garmpis, N.; Garmpi, A.; Savvanis, S.; Diamantis, E. Complications of the Type 2 Diabetes Mellitus. *Curr. Cardiol. Rev.* **2020**, *16*, 249–251. [CrossRef]
4. Ong, K.L.; Stafford, L.K.; McLaughlin, S.A.; Boyko, E.J.; Vollset, S.E.; Smith, A.E.; Dalton, B.E.; Duprey, J.; Cruz, J.A.; Hagins, H.; et al. Global, regional, and national burden of diabetes from 1990 to 2021, with projections of prevalence to 2050: A systematic analysis for the Global Burden of Disease Study 2021. *Lancet* **2023**, *402*, 203–234. [CrossRef]
5. Davies, M.J.; Aroda, V.R.; Collins, B.S.; Gabbay, R.A.; Green, J.; Maruthur, N.M.; Rosas, S.E.; Del Prato, S.; Mathieu, C.; Mingrone, G.; et al. Management of Hyperglycemia in Type 2 Diabetes, 2022: A Consensus Report by the American Diabetes Association (ADA) and the European Association for the Study of Diabetes (EASD). *Diabetes Care* **2022**, *45*, 2753–2786. [CrossRef] [PubMed]
6. Draznin, B.; Aroda, V.R.; Bakris, G.; Benson, G.; Brown, F.M.; Freeman, R.; Green, J.; Huang, E.; Isaacs, D.; Kahan, S.; et al. Glycemic Targets: Standards of Medical Care in Diabetes-2022. *Diabetes Care* **2022**, *45*, S83–S96. [CrossRef]
7. Viigimaa, M.; Sachinidis, A.; Toumpourleka, M.; Koutsampasopoulos, K.; Alliksoo, S.; Titma, T. Macrovascular Complications of Type 2 Diabetes Mellitus. *Curr. Vasc. Pharmacol.* **2020**, *18*, 110–116. [CrossRef] [PubMed]
8. Faselis, C.; Katsimardou, A.; Imprialos, K.; Deligkaris, P.; Kallistratos, M.; Dimitriadis, K. Microvascular Complications of Type 2 Diabetes Mellitus. *Curr. Vasc. Pharmacol.* **2020**, *18*, 117–124. [CrossRef] [PubMed]
9. Saboo, B.; Kesavadev, J.; Shankar, A.; Krishna, M.B.; Sheth, S.; Patel, V.; Krishnan, G. Time-in-range as a target in type 2 diabetes: An urgent need. *Heliyon* **2021**, *7*, e05967. [CrossRef]
10. Poretsky, L. *Principles of Diabetes Mellitus*, 2nd ed.; Springer: New York, NY, USA, 2009; pp. 645–658.
11. Coetzee, A. An introduction to insulin use in type 2 diabetes mellitus. *S. Afr. Fam. Pract.* **2004**, *65*, e1–e5. [CrossRef]
12. Peyrot, M.; Rubin, R.R.; Lauritzen, T.; Skovlund, S.E.; Snoek, F.J.; Matthews, D.R.; Landgraf, R.; Kleinebreil, L. Resistance to insulin therapy among patients and providers: Results of the cross-national Diabetes Attitudes, Wishes, and Needs (DAWN) study. *Diabetes Care* **2005**, *28*, 2673–2679. [CrossRef]

13. Home, P.; Naggar, N.E.; Khamesh, M.; Gonzalez-Galvez, G.; Shen, C.; Chakkarwar, P.; Wenying, Y. An observational non-interventional study of people with diabetes beginning or changed to insulin analogue therapy in non-Western countries: The A1chieve study. *Diabetes Res. Clin. Pract.* **2022**, *94*, 352–363. [CrossRef]
14. Grand Review Research: Insulin Market Size & Share Trends Analysis by Product Type (Rapid-Acting Insulin, Long-Acting Insulin, Combination Insulin, Biosimilar), by Application, by Type (Type 1, Type 2), by Distribution Channel, by Region, and Segment Forecasts, 2022–2030. Available online: https://www.grandviewresearch.com/industry-analysis/insulin-market-report (accessed on 12 September 2023).
15. Beran, D.; Lazo-Porras, M.; Mba, C.M.; Mbanya, J.C. A global perspective on the issue of access to insulin. *Diabetologia* **2021**, *64*, 954–962. [CrossRef] [PubMed]
16. Basu, S.; Yudkin, J.S.; Kehlenbrink, S.; Davies, J.I.; Wild, S.H.; Lipska, K.J.; Sussman, J.B.; Beran, D. Estimation of global insulin use for type 2 diabetes, 2018–2030: A microsimulation analysis. *Lancet Diabetes Endocrinol.* **2019**, *7*, 25–33. [CrossRef] [PubMed]
17. Hicks, C.W.; Selvin, E. Epidemiology of Peripheral Neuropathy and Lower Extremity Disease in Diabetes. *Curr. Diab. Rep.* **2019**, *19*, 86. [CrossRef] [PubMed]
18. Kerr, M.; Barron, E.; Chadwick, P.; Evan, T.; Kong, W.M.; Rayman, G.; Sutton-Smith, M.; Todd, G.; Young, B.; Jeffcoate, W.J. The cost of diabetic foot ulcers and amputations to the National Health Service in England. *Diabet. Med.* **2019**, *36*, 995–1002. [CrossRef]
19. Bommer, C.; Sagalova, V.; Heesemann, E.; Manne-Goehler, J.; Atun, R.; Bärnighausen, T.; Davies, J.; Vollmer, S. Global Economic Burden of Diabetes in Adults: Projections from 2015 to 2030. *Diabetes Care* **2018**, *41*, 963–970. [CrossRef]
20. Trikkalinou, A.; Papazafiropoulou, A.K.; Melidonis, A. Type 2 diabetes and quality of life. *World J. Diabetes* **2017**, *8*, 120–129. [CrossRef]
21. Khan, M.A.B.; Hashim, M.J.; King, J.K.; Govender, R.D.; Mustafa, H.; Al Kaabi, J. Epidemiology of Type 2 Diabetes—Global Burden of Disease and Forecasted Trends. *J. Epidemiol. Glob. Health* **2020**, *10*, 107–111. [CrossRef]
22. ISPOR Presentations Database. Available online: https://www.ispor.org/heor-resources/presentations-database/search (accessed on 12 September 2023).
23. Tufts Medical Centre: CEA Registry. Available online: https://cear.tuftsmedicalcenter.org/ (accessed on 12 September 2023).
24. Houses of Parliament, Parliamentary Office of Science & Technology: Drug Pricing. Available online: https://www.parliament.uk/globalassets/documents/post/postpn_364_Drug_Pricing.pdf (accessed on 12 September 2023).
25. PRISMA Transparent Reporting of Systematic Reviews and Meta-Analyses. Available online: http://www.prisma-statement.org/?AspxAutoDetectCookieSupport=1 (accessed on 12 September 2023).
26. The BMJ Health Economics Checklist. Available online: https://www.bmj.com/content/suppl/2004/05/06/328.7448.1102.DC1 (accessed on 12 September 2023).
27. Equator Network, Consolidated Health Economic Evaluation Reporting Standards 2022 (CHEERS 2022) Statement: Updated Reporting Guidance for Health Economic Evaluations. Available online: https://www.equator-network.org/reporting-guidelines/cheers/ (accessed on 12 September 2023).
28. Cannon, A.J.; Bargiota, A.; Billings, L.; Hunt, B.; Leiter, L.A.; Malkin, S.; Mocarski, M.; Ranthe, M.F.; Schiffman, A.; Doshi, A. Evaluation of the Short-Term Cost-Effectiveness of IDegLira versus Basal Insulin and Basal-Bolus Therapy in Patients with Type 2 Diabetes Based on Attainment of Clinically Relevant Treatment Targets. *J. Manag. Care Spec. Pharm.* **2020**, *26*, 143–153. [CrossRef] [PubMed]
29. Cheng, H.; Wan, X.; Ma, J.; Wu, B. Cost-effectiveness of Insulin Degludec versus Insulin Glargine in Insulin-naive Chinese Patients with Type 2 Diabetes. *Clin. Ther.* **2019**, *41*, 445–455.e4. [CrossRef]
30. Dempsey, M.; Mocarski, M.; Langer, J.; Hunt, B. Long-term cost-effectiveness analysis shows that IDegLira is associated with improved outcomes and lower costs compared with insulin glargine U100 plus insulin aspart in the US. *J. Med. Econ.* **2018**, *21*, 1110–1118. [CrossRef]
31. Drummond, R.; Malkin, S.; Du Preez, M.; Lee, X.Y.; Hunt, B. The management of type 2 diabetes with fixed-ratio combination insulin degludec/liraglutide (IDegLira) versus basal-bolus therapy (insulin glargine U100 plus insulin aspart): A short-term cost-effectiveness analysis in the UK setting. *Diabetes Obes. Metab.* **2018**, *20*, 2371–2378. [CrossRef] [PubMed]
32. Evans, M.; Chubb, B.; Malkin, S.J.P.; Berry, S.; Lawson, J.; Hunt, B. Once-weekly semaglutide versus insulin aspart for the treatment of type 2 diabetes in the UK: A long-term cost-effectiveness analysis based on SUSTAIN 11. *Diabetes Obes. Metab.* **2023**, *25*, 491–500. [CrossRef] [PubMed]
33. Gu, S.; Shi, L.; Shao, H.; Wang, X.; Hu, X.; Gu, Y.; Dong, H. Choice across 10 pharmacologic combination strategies for type 2 diabetes: A cost-effectiveness analysis. *BMC Med.* **2020**, *18*, 378. [CrossRef] [PubMed]
34. Han, G.; Hu, S.; Zhang, X.; Qiu, Z.; Huang, Z. Insulin degludec/liraglutide versus its monotherapy on T2D patients: A lifetime cost-utility analysis in China. *Front. Pharmacol.* **2022**, *13*, 1011624. [CrossRef]
35. Hunt, B.; Mocarski, M.; Valentine, W.J.; Langer, J. Evaluation of the Short-Term Cost-Effectiveness of IDegLira Versus Continued Up-Titration of Insulin Glargine U100 in Patients with Type 2 Diabetes in the USA. *Adv. Ther.* **2017**, *34*, 954–965. [CrossRef]
36. Jiang, Y.; Liu, R.; Xuan, J.; Lin, S.; Zheng, Q.; Pang, J. A Cost-effectiveness Analysis of iGlarLixi Versus IDegAsp and Appropriate Price Exploration of iGlarLixi for Type 2 Diabetes Mellitus Patients in China. *Clin. Drug Investig.* **2023**, *43*, 251–263. [CrossRef]
37. Kvapil, M.; Prázný, M.; Holik, P.; Rychna, K.; Hunt, B. Cost-Effectiveness of IDegLira Versus Insulin Intensification Regimens for the Treatment of Adults with Type 2 Diabetes in the Czech Republic. *Diabetes Ther.* **2017**, *8*, 1331–1347. [CrossRef]

38. Langer, J.; Wolden, M.L.; Shimoda, S.; Sato, M.; Araki, E. Short-Term Cost-Effectiveness of Switching to Insulin Degludec in Japanese Patients with Type 2 Diabetes Receiving Basal-Bolus Therapy. *Diabetes Ther.* **2019**, *10*, 1347–1356. [CrossRef]
39. Lau, E.; Salem, A.; Chan, J.C.N.; So, W.Y.; Kong, A.; Lamotte, M.; Luk, A. Insulin glargine compared to Neutral Protamine Hagedorn (NPH) insulin in patients with type-2 diabetes uncontrolled with oral anti-diabetic agents alone in Hong Kong: A cost-effectiveness analysis. *Cost Eff. Resour. Alloc.* **2019**, *17*, 13. [CrossRef]
40. Luo, Q.; Zhou, L.; Zhou, N.; Hu, M. Cost-effectiveness of insulin degludec/insulin aspart versus biphasic insulin aspart in Chinese population with type 2 diabetes. *Front. Public Health* **2022**, *10*, 1016907. [CrossRef]
41. McCrimmon, R.J.; Falla, E.; Sha, J.Z.; Alsaleh, A.J.O.; Lew, E.; Hudson, R.; Baxter, M.; Palmer, K. Cost-Effectiveness of iGlarLixi in People with Type 2 Diabetes Mellitus Suboptimally Controlled on Basal Insulin Plus Metformin in the UK. *Diabetes Ther.* **2021**, *12*, 3217–3230. [CrossRef] [PubMed]
42. McCrimmon, R.J.; Lamotte, M.; Ramos, M.; Alsaleh, A.J.O.; Souhami, E.; Lew, E. Cost-Effectiveness of iGlarLixi Versus iDegLira in Type 2 Diabetes Mellitus Inadequately Controlled by GLP-1 Receptor Agonists and Oral Antihyperglycemic Therapy. *Diabetes Ther.* **2021**, *12*, 3231–3241. [CrossRef] [PubMed]
43. Pöhlmann, J.; Montagnoli, R.; Lastoria, G.; Parekh, W.; Markert, M.; Hunt, B. Value For Money In The Treatment Of Patients With Type 2 Diabetes Mellitus: Assessing The Long-Term Cost-Effectiveness of IDegLira Versus iGlarLixi In Italy. *Clin. Outcomes Res.* **2019**, *11*, 605–614. [CrossRef]
44. Pöhlmann, J.; Russel-Szymczyk, M.; Holík, P.; Rychna, K.; Hunt, B. Treating Patients with Type 2 Diabetes Mellitus Uncontrolled on Basal Insulin in the Czech Republic: Cost-Effectiveness of IDegLira Versus iGlarLixi. *Diabetes Ther.* **2019**, *10*, 493–508. [CrossRef] [PubMed]
45. Pollock, R.F.; Norrbacka, K.; Cameron, C.; Mancillas-Adame, L.; Jeddi, M. A cost-utility analysis of dulaglutide versus insulin glargine as third-line therapy for Type 2 diabetes in Canada. *J. Comp. Eff. Res.* **2019**, *8*, 229–240. [CrossRef]
46. Pollock, R.F.; Valentine, W.J.; Marso, S.P.; Gundgaard, J.; Hallén, N.; Hansen, L.L.; Tutkunkardas, D.; Buse, J.B. DEVOTE 5: Evaluating the Short-Term Cost-Utility of Insulin Degludec versus Insulin Glargine U100 in Basal-Bolus Regimens for Type 2 Diabetes in the UK. *Diabetes Ther.* **2018**, *9*, 1217–1232. [CrossRef] [PubMed]
47. Pollock, R.F.; Valentine, W.J.; Marso, S.P.; Andersen, A.; Gundgaard, J.; Hallén, N.; Tutkunkardas, D.; Magnuson, E.A.; Buse, J.B. Long-term Cost-effectiveness of Insulin Degludec Versus Insulin Glargine U100 in the UK: Evidence from the Basal-bolus Subgroup of the DEVOTE Trial (DEVOTE 16). *Appl. Health Econ. Health Policy* **2019**, *17*, 615–627. [CrossRef]
48. Raya, P.M.; Blasco, F.J.A.; Hunt, B.; Martin, V.; Thorsted, B.L.; Basse, A.; Price, H. Evaluating the long-term cost-effectiveness of fixed-ratio combination insulin degludec/liraglutide (IDegLira) for type 2 diabetes in Spain based on real-world clinical evidence. *Diabetes Obes. Metab.* **2019**, *21*, 1349–1356. [CrossRef] [PubMed]
49. Zhong, Y.; Lin, P.J.; Cohen, J.T.; Winn, A.N.; Neumann, P.J. Cost-utility analyses in diabetes: A systematic review and implications from real-world evidence. *Value Health* **2015**, *18*, 308–314. [CrossRef]
50. Saunders, H.; Pham, B.; Loong, D.; Mishra, S.; Ashoor, H.M.; Antony, J.; Darvesh, N.; Bains, S.K.; Jamieson, M.; Plett, D.; et al. The Cost-Effectiveness of Intermediate-Acting, Long-Acting, Ultralong-Acting, and Biosimilar Insulins for Type 1 Diabetes Mellitus: A Systematic Review. *Value Health* **2022**, *25*, 1235–1252. [CrossRef] [PubMed]
51. Shafie, A.A.; Ng, C.H.; Tan, Y.P.; Chaiyakunapruk, N. Systematic Review of the Cost Effectiveness of Insulin Analogues in Type 1 and Type 2 Diabetes Mellitus. *Pharmacoeconomics* **2017**, *35*, 141–162. [CrossRef] [PubMed]
52. Suh, D.C.; Aagren, M. Cost-effectiveness of insulin detemir: A systematic review. *Expert Rev. Pharmacoeconomics Outcomes Res.* **2011**, *11*, 641–655. [CrossRef] [PubMed]

Disclaimer/Publisher's Note: The statements, opinions and data contained in all publications are solely those of the individual author(s) and contributor(s) and not of MDPI and/or the editor(s). MDPI and/or the editor(s) disclaim responsibility for any injury to people or property resulting from any ideas, methods, instructions or products referred to in the content.

MDPI
St. Alban-Anlage 66
4052 Basel
Switzerland
www.mdpi.com

Diabetology Editorial Office
E-mail: diabetology@mdpi.com
www.mdpi.com/journal/diabetology

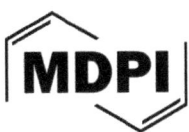

Disclaimer/Publisher's Note: The statements, opinions and data contained in all publications are solely those of the individual author(s) and contributor(s) and not of MDPI and/or the editor(s). MDPI and/or the editor(s) disclaim responsibility for any injury to people or property resulting from any ideas, methods, instructions or products referred to in the content.